Earn CME Credits while you learn!

Up to 75 *AMA PRA Category 1 Credits*™ available with the
MedStudy 2009 Internal Medicine Board-Style Questions & Answers

Release Date: April 1, 2009   **Expiration Date: April 1, 2012**

This CME credit is provided by MedStudy. To apply for CME credit, you must complete the *Verification of Credit* form and Product *Evaluation* found on the following pages. Then submit this completed form and evaluation, along with the $40 CME processing fee, to MedStudy. All necessary contact information is included on the Verification of Credit form.

Please note: CME credit is available only to the original purchaser of this product – issuance of CME credit is subject to verification of product ownership.

The Release Date for the 2009 Internal Medicine Board-Style Questions & Answers is April 1, 2009. To be eligible for CME credit, you must study the content in the books and submit your Verification of Credit form and Evaluation no later than April 1, 2012.

Accreditation / Designation Statements
MedStudy is accredited by the Accreditation Council for Continuing Medical Education (ACCME) to provide continuing medical education for physicians. MedStudy designates this educational activity for a maximum of 75 AMA PRA Category 1 Credits™. Physicians should claim credit only commensurate with the extent of their participation in the activity (one hour = one credit).

Learning Objectives

As a result of participation in this activity, learners should be able to:

- Integrate and demonstrate increased overall knowledge of Internal Medicine

- Identify and remedy areas of weakness (gaps) in knowledge and clinical competencies

- Describe the clinical manifestations and treatments of diseases encountered in Internal Medicine and effectively narrow the differential diagnosis list by utilizing the most appropriate medical studies

- Apply the competence and confidence gained through participation in this activity to both a successful Board exam-taking experience and daily practice

Target Audience / Method of Participation
Participants in this educational activity are those physicians interested in expanding their knowledge in General Internal Medicine, focusing one's learning on subjects that are directly relevant to clinical scenarios and associated questions that will be encountered on the ABIM Board certifying and recertifying (MoC) exam. Use the question-answer content as a self-study, self-testing exercise, attempting to answer questions as though they are part of an actual Board exam. Compare your selected answers against the answers given as "correct" in the Answer Book to assess your level of knowledge and recall of pertinent medical facts and clinical decision-making. Review your results to see your relative strengths and weaknesses by topic areas. Repeat the self-testing process as often as necessary to improve your knowledge and proficiency and ultimately to ensure your mastery of the material.

Author / Reviewer Disclosure Summary

MedStudy adheres to the AMA PRA system requirements and the ACCME's Policies, Essential Areas and Accreditation Criteria, including the Standards for Commercial Support regarding industry support of continuing medical education. Disclosures of authors/reviewers and commercial relationships have been documented below, and any perceived conflicts of interest have been resolved by MedStudy's CME Physicians Oversight Council prior to publication. This pertains to any entity producing, marketing, re-selling, or distributing health care goods or services consumed by, or used on, patients.

I. The following authors/reviewers have openly indicated any affiliation with organizations that may have interests related to the content of their contributions: None

II. The following authors/reviewers have documented that they have nothing to disclose:
J. Thomas Cross, Jr., MD, MPH, FACP   Robert A. Hannaman, MD

III. The following authors/reviewers have received requests but have not provided disclosure information: None

IV. Good Practices Agreement: Authors/reviewers have signed a Good Practices Agreement affirming that their contributions are based upon currently available, scientifically rigorous data; that the content is free from commercial bias; and that clinical practice and patient care recommendations presented in the content are based on the best available evidence for these specialties and subspecialties.

MedStudy presents this activity for educational purposes only. Material is prepared based on multiple sources of information, but content is not intended to be exhaustive of the subject matter. Participants are expected to utilize their own expertise and judgment while engaged in the practice of medicine.

Provider Disclosure Statement

In accordance with the requirements of the AMA PRA system and the ACCME's Policies, Essential Areas, and Accreditation Criteria, which include the Standards for Commercial Support regarding industry support of continuing medical education, MedStudy Corporation documents the following with regard to the 2009 Internal Medicine Board-Style Questions & Answers:

MedStudy Corporation, including all of its employees, *does not* have a financial interest, arrangement or affiliation with any commercial organization that may have a direct or indirect interest in the content of this product. This includes any entity producing, marketing, re-selling, or distributing health care goods or services consumed by, or used on, patients. Furthermore, MedStudy complies with the AMA Council on Ethical and Judicial Affairs (CEJA) opinions that address the ethical obligations that underpin physician participation in CME: 8.061, "Gifts to physicians from industry," and 9.011, "Ethical issues in CME."

Author / Reviewer Disclosure Summary

J. Thomas Cross, Jr., MD, MPH, FACP (Author)
Vice President, Education
Author / Editor
Member, MedStudy CME Physicians Oversight Council
MedStudy Corporation
Colorado Springs, CO

Robert A. Hannaman, MD (Reviewer)
President/CEO
Author/Editor
Member, MedStudy CME Physicians Oversight Council
MedStudy Corporation
Colorado Springs, CO

MedStudy®

Internal Medicine Board-Style Questions & Answers 2009

Questions

Edited by J. Thomas Cross, Jr., MD, MPH, FACP and Robert A. Hannaman, MD

TABLE OF CONTENTS

Note: Many of the images you see throughout this Questions book can be viewed in color in the image atlas at the back of the book.

IMPORTANT: These Q&A books are meant to be used as an adjunct to the MedStudy Internal Medicine Review Core Curriculum. The ABIM exams cover a vast realm of diagnostic and treatment knowledge. Board-simulation exercise such as these self-testing Q&As are valuable tools, but these alone are not adequate preparation for a Board exam. Be sure you use a comprehensive IM review resource in addition to these Q&As for adequate exam preparation.

GOOD STUDYING!

MEDSTUDY
P.O. Box 38148
Colorado Springs, CO 80937-8148
(800) 841-0547

GASTROENTEROLOGY

1.

A 50-year-old man had an inferior myocardial infarction one week ago. He was discharged 5 days after admission in stable condition. He has a follow-up appointment scheduled for one week after discharge. His wife (an attorney) calls and says that he woke up throwing up about a ¼ cup of blood. You meet him at the Emergency Room and discover that he is now well appearing. His vital signs via the ER are normal and he feels quite well at the moment.

PAST MEDICAL HISTORY: Besides the recent MI, hypertension for 20 years treated with various calcium-channel blockers

CURRENT MEDICATIONS: Propranolol 25 mg q day
Enteric-coated ASA 80 mg q day

SOCIAL HISTORY: Smoking: hasn't smoked since his MI; before that, 1 pack/day x 30 years
Alcohol: drinks 2 beers a day until recent MI; now abstinent
Illicit drugs: never used

FAMILY HISTORY: Father died of MI at age 50
Mother died of MI at age 70
Brother with MI at age 60

REVIEW OF SYSTEMS: Mild epigastric pain
No fever, chills, weight loss, or night sweats

PHYSICAL EXAM: BP 120/60, P 64, RR 18, Temp 99° F
    HEENT: PERRLA, EOMI, sclera nonicteric
    Neck: Supple; no bruits
    Heart: RRR without murmurs, rubs, or gallops
    Lungs: Clear to auscultation
    Abdomen: Mild epigastric tenderness to deep palpation
    Extremities: No cyanosis, clubbing, or edema
    GU: Mild heme-positive stool; no melena

Laboratory values are normal except for his platelet count, which is 100,000.

An esophagogastroduodenoscopy (EGD) is contraindicated for which of the following reasons:

    A. He is on enteric-coated ASA, and he might bleed during the procedure.
    B. His platelet count is too low.
  ✓C. He had a recent MI.
    D. He is stable, and EGD is not indicated at this point.
    E. His wife is an attorney.

2.

A 60-year-old Native American woman with a history of hypertension and hyperlipidemia presents with right upper quadrant pain and fever. She has been ill for several days and reports that she has been vomiting on occasion during the last day or so. She denies recent travel.

PAST MEDICAL HISTORY:	Hypertension for 20 years, currently treated with fosinopril 20 mg q day Hyperlipidemia diagnosed 5 years ago, currently on pravastatin 20 mg q hs
SOCIAL HISTORY:	Smokes ½ pack a day for 45 years Alcohol: occasional glass of wine on weekends
FAMILY HISTORY:	Mother died from acute MI at age 75 Father died from "old age" at 99 Sister with gallstones and HTN Brother with HTN
REVIEW OF SYSTEMS:	Decreased appetite, recent fatty food intolerance; fever for 2 days, chills

PHYSICAL EXAMINATION:

General:	Moderately ill-appearing woman
VS:	Temp 102.2° F, BP 110/70, Pulse 105, RR 25
HEENT:	Scleral icterus, PERRLA, EOMI Throat: clear
Heart:	RRR with no murmurs, rubs, or gallops; tachycardic
Lungs:	CTA
Abdomen:	Diminished bowel sounds, right upper quadrant tenderness to palpation; she has rebound tenderness also
GU:	Normal female genitalia, no tenderness on bimanual palpation
Extremities:	No cyanosis, clubbing, or edema

LABORATORY:

White Blood Count (WBC): 18,500 with 70% neutrophils, 15% band forms, 10% monocytes

Hematocrit: 37.2%

Platelet count: 522,000/µL

Serum chemistries: Sodium 140 mg/dL, chloride 110 mg/dL, potassium 4.2 mg/dL

Total bilirubin 6 mg/dL with a direct bilirubin of 4 mg/dL

Serum aminotransferases: AST 90 IU/L, ALT 75 IU/L; alkaline phosphatase 300 IU/L

Computed tomography of the abdomen shows a dilated common bile duct and no other abnormalities.

The next appropriate diagnostic study is which of the following?

A. Endoscopic retrograde cholangiopancreatography (ERCP) with laparoscopic cholecystectomy
B. Ultrasonography
C. Liver biopsy
D. Magnetic resonance imaging of the biliary system
E. Exploratory laparotomy

3.

A 60-year-old Asian woman presents with a chief complaint of difficulty in swallowing solid foods for the past 2 weeks. She noted this while attending her friend's wedding reception. At the wedding, she noted that she could not swallow the fried shrimp very easily. Since then, she has noted that the only things she can swallow easily are soft foods like gelatin and bananas. She does not seem to have difficulty with liquids.

PAST MEDICAL HISTORY:	Healthy, no problems Normal GYN exams
SOCIAL HISTORY:	Lives with her husband in Alabama Smokes 3 packs/day of cigarettes Drinks beer on occasion, but only with fried shrimp
FAMILY HISTORY:	Mother healthy, HTN Father died 2 years ago at age 75 of CVA Sister in good health 6 brothers, all in relatively good health except her youngest brother, who has severe coronary artery disease
REVIEW OF SYSTEMS:	Essentially unremarkable; except for 15-lb weight loss

Which of the following is the next diagnostic test you should order?

A. Esophagogastroduodenoscopy (EGD)
B. Barium swallow
C. MRI of chest
D. Tensilon test
E. Motility studies

4.

A 50-year-old man with negative past medical history presents with progressive dysphagia for both liquids and solids. Recently he has started to regurgitate food, especially while bending over. He reports that this has occurred gradually over the past year and he now has had a 10-lb weight loss, which was unintentional. He denies any other symptoms and has been healthy except for a viral illness 6 months ago.

PAST MEDICAL HISTORY: Negative for anything of significance

SOCIAL HISTORY:
      Never smoked
      Doesn't drink alcohol except at "special occasions"
      Works as a writer for a medical publishing company—reports being very highly stressed at all times by deadlines
      No travel history; specifically not to South America

FAMILY HISTORY: Noncontributory

REVIEW OF SYSTEMS:
      No fever
      No chest pain or discomfort
      No rash
      Denies tinnitus

PHYSICAL EXAMINATION: Generally well-appearing man
      VSS, afebrile

HEENT:	PERRLA, EOMI,
	Tympanic membranes clear
	Throat clear
Neck:	Supple, no bruits
Heart:	RRR without murmurs, rubs, or gallops
Lungs:	CTA
Abdomen:	Benign, no tenderness, no hepatosplenomegaly
Extremities:	No cyanosis, clubbing, or edema
GU:	Deferred
Neurological:	Reflexes equal and symmetrical throughout; no sensory or motor deficits noted

LABORATORY:
   CBC: Normal
   Electrolytes: Normal
   CXR: Widened mediastinum with an air-fluid level and no gastric air bubble

Barium Swallow:

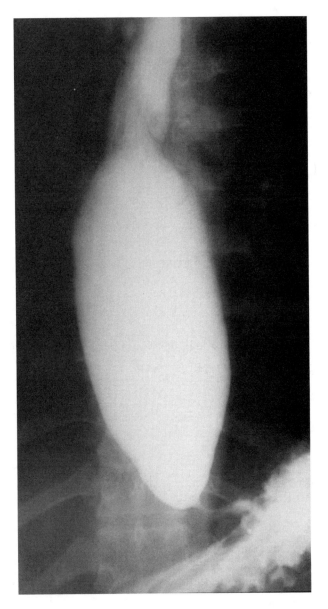

Based on your findings, which of the following is the most likely diagnosis for this patient?

A. Gastroesophageal reflux
B. Esophageal ulcer
C. Chagas disease
D. Achalasia
E. Plummer-Vinson syndrome (Patterson-Kelly syndrome)

5.

A 55-year-old woman presents as a new patient for a routine checkup. On questioning, you determine that she has been relatively healthy and has not required any hospitalizations since the delivery of her last child over 20 years ago. She notes that she recently has had swelling of her hands and occasionally of her feet. She relates this to "eating too much salt." Her only other complaint is that she has frequent heartburn, and occasionally notes "food sticks when it goes down." She does not report any other problems.

PAST MEDICAL HISTORY: As above, noncontributory

SOCIAL HISTORY:
Works as a 4th grade elementary teacher
Quit smoking 30 years ago
Alcohol: Drinks on occasion with her church group
Married, husband is a forester

FAMILY HISTORY:
Mother: Still living; has hypertension, had CVA 3 years ago
Father: Died 2 years ago from emphysema
Sister: Diagnosed with lupus 10 years ago

REVIEW OF SYSTEMS:
Skin: On questioning, she notes that when she is outside in the winter her hands turn white and occasionally even have a bluish color to them
GI: Recurrent reflux on a regular basis
"Food sticking" as described above
Occasional diarrhea
Eyes: She notes dryness of her eyes on occasion
No visual changes have been noted
General: Mild weight gain in the last year
GU: Vaginal dryness noted in the last year
Has noted dyspareunia in the last few months

PHYSICAL EXAMINATION:
General: Well-developed, well-nourished woman in no distress
Vitals: BP 120/70, P56, RR 18, Temp 96.7° F
HEENT: Noted that she has difficulty opening her mouth fully—says she can't open very wide
PERRLA, EOMI, Discs sharp
Tympanic membranes intact
Teeth normal in appearance
Throat clear; tonsils present
Neck: Supple, No bruits
Heart: Slight bradycardia, RRR with no murmurs, rubs, or gallops
Lungs: CTA
Abdomen: Bowel sounds present in all 4 quadrants, no tenderness to palpation; no hepatosplenomegaly
Extremities: Skin over fingers is shiny
Skin creases and hair follicles are not present
No cyanosis, clubbing noted
No noticeable joint abnormalities
GU: Dry vaginal mucosa noted; otherwise nothing abnormal

LABORATORY:

    CBC: WBC 8,700 $10^3/\mu L$ with normal differential

    Electrolytes: WNL

    ESR: 48 mm/hour

    ANA present in nucleolar pattern at 1:640

Which of the following can be predicted with regard to her esophageal disease?

    A. She will gradually improve over time without medical therapy.

    B. It is unlikely that her esophageal disease is related to her skin findings.

    C. Progression is likely to occur and stricture formation with nearly complete loss of peristalsis will be seen in later forms of this disease.

    D. Treatment with H-2 blockers will provide complete recovery from the esophageal disease.

    E. The gastrointestinal findings with her illness will be usually confined to the esophagus.

6.

A 16-year-old male with a history of acne is brought in by his mother because of acute onset of difficulty swallowing since breakfast. He notes nothing unusual before this and had a good night's sleep. He says school is going very well, and he really enjoys being in the band. He did not notice a problem until he tried to eat his breakfast, which consisted of a chocolate pop tart and tortilla chips.

PAST MEDICAL HISTORY: Acne for about 2 years treated with topical agents initially and now on doxycycline 100 mg PO bid for the past 3 months. He has been adherent to his medication regimen and took the medication this morning.

SOCIAL HISTORY: In 10th grade at Holy Redeemer High School
                            Denies smoking or alcohol use
                            Makes mostly A's except a C in PE

FAMILY HISTORY: Father: 45 and healthy
                             Mother: 48 suffers from chronic depression
                             Sister: 17 y/o and pregnant

ROS: No fever, chills, night sweats
                             Has difficulty swallowing only solids, not liquids
                             No nausea or vomiting
                             No diarrhea
                             No skin changes

PHYSICAL EXAMINATION: Well-developed, obese WM in no apparent distress

    VS: BP 130/70, P 90, RR 16, Temp 98.5° F, Height 5'10, Weight 250 lbs

    HEENT: PERRLA, EOMI
                     No oral thrush
                     No abnormalities seen

    Neck: Supple, non-tender examination

    Heart: RRR with 2/6 systolic flow murmur (not new, heard in the past)

    Lungs: CTA

    Abdomen: Bowel sounds heard in all quadrants; no hepatosplenomegaly

    Extremities: No cyanosis, clubbing, or edema

    Skin: Acne is very mild compared to 3 months ago; no back lesions are present

Which of the following is the likely etiology of his swallowing complaint?

    A. Gastroesophageal reflux
    B. Scleroderma
    C. Cocaine abuse
    D. Pill-induced esophagitis
    E. Bulimia

7.

A 45-year-old woman with history of hypertension and diet-controlled diabetes presents with complaints of "heartburn" for several days. She has been taking over-the-counter agents for heartburn without much relief. Today she is feeling better but is still worried about the possibility of something more serious.

PAST MEDICAL HISTORY: Negative except for hospitalizations for childbirth

MEDICATIONS: None except over-the-counter calcium carbonate for heartburn

SOCIAL HISTORY:
Smokes 1 pack/day of cigarettes
Drinks a 6-pack of beer on weekends
Works as a waitress at a cocktail bar

FAMILY HISTORY:
Mother with peptic ulcer disease diagnosed at age 42
Father with hypertension
Son with lymphoma 10 years ago

REVIEW OF SYSTEMS: Deferred; see question below

PHYSICAL EXAMINATION: Well-appearing woman in no distress
VSS Afebrile

HEENT:	PERRLA, EOMI
	Throat normal
	Normal dentition
Neck:	Supple, no thyromegaly
Heart:	RRR without murmurs, rubs, or gallops
Lungs:	CTA
Abdomen:	Mild epigastric discomfort with palpation; no rebound
Extremities:	No cyanosis, clubbing, or edema
GU:	Normal female genitalia
	Heme-positive rectal exam
Psych:	Oriented x 3
	No outward signs of depression

LABORATORY:
Routine CBC, electrolytes ordered

All choices are indications for endoscopy <u>except</u> which of the following?

   A. Weight loss
   B. Heme-positive stool
   C. Rapid onset of dysphagia
   D. Anemia
   E. Improvement with therapeutic trial of anti-GERD medication

---

8.

A 30-year-old man with recent history of gastroesophageal reflux disease (GERD) returns for follow-up. He has a lengthy history with you as follows:

You first saw him a little over 9 months ago and recommended that he sleep with the head of his bed elevated by 6 to 9 inches, lose 10-15 pounds of weight, eat small meals, and eat dinner 3 hours before bedtime. You additionally strongly recommended that he stop smoking. At that time you started him on ranitidine 150 mg twice daily.

He returned 1 month later saying that he had done everything that you recommended, but his GERD was still quite severe. You started him on omeprazole 20 mg daily and discontinued the ranitidine.

He returned a month after that and said his symptoms were markedly improved and that he could sleep flat without discomfort. He continued to lose weight and also quit smoking. You recommended he complete a 3-month course of therapy with omeprazole.

He returned 4 months later (now, off of omeprazole) and told you that his symptoms had all returned and actually seemed worse. You restarted his omeprazole for another 3-month course. His symptoms resolved and he was doing well.

He now returns again today, 2 weeks off therapy, reporting that his symptoms have returned again.

PAST MEDICAL HISTORY: Nothing significant except for motor vehicle accident when he was 18

SOCIAL HISTORY: Quit smoking as you recommended about 8 months ago
                        Alcohol: glass of wine on the weekend
                        Employment: Works at a donut shop, making donuts
                        Started exercising 6 months ago, now runs 3 miles every other day

FAMILY HISTORY: Mother, 65, healthy
                        Father, 66, known coronary artery disease, diabetes
                        Brother, 32, GERD

ROS: Non-contributory

PHYSICAL EXAMINATION: Unremarkable, very healthy 30-year-old man

LABORATORY: EGD done 11 months ago showed grade 3 esophagitis (circumferential erosions and exudative lesions)

He tells you today that he is tired of taking these medications and realizes that he may need to take them chronically. He asks you what would be his best option for treatment of his GERD, based on his age and current health status.

Which of the following should be your response?

A. Because he is young, it may be best to begin metoclopramide for long-term therapy.
B. He has severe disease that will likely require long-term medical therapy, so the best option is chronic proton-pump inhibitor therapy.
C. Because he is young, the best therapy is over-the-counter medications such as calcium-containing antacids, because they are much safer than the proton-pump inhibitors.
D. Omeprazole cannot be used for long-term maintenance therapy.
E. Even though he currently has frequent recurrences, it is likely as he gets older that these episodes will become less frequent; therefore, medical management with omeprazole is the most prudent choice to see if his GERD will resolve over time.

9.

A 48-year-old Caucasian male with a history of Barrett esophagus presents for follow-up. He has been doing fairly well on omeprazole 20 mg daily, which seems to reduce his GERD symptoms to a minimum. Additionally, he stopped smoking several years ago and has lost about 20 pounds in the last 4 years. Today, he is returning for the pathology report from his last endoscopy, performed last week. Clinically, he has been doing well.

LABORATORY: Pathology report: High-grade dysplasia confirmed by two pathologists.

Now that he has confirmed high-grade dysplasia, which of the following is one of the currently recommended treatment options?

A. Increase dose of omeprazole to 40 mg and repeat EGD in 1 month; if no change, then recommend surgery or ablation.
B. Increase endoscopy frequency to every 6 months and intervene in 1 year if changes still exist.
C. Perform EGD monthly and watch for changes.
D. Refer for surgery.
E. Apply low-grade beam radiation to the affected area.

10.

A 35-year-old personal trainer with a negative past medical history presents for a routine check-up. She is concerned because she says that at a supermarket health fair last week, she took a "home breath test" for "ulcer bacteria," which came up positive. She denies any symptoms of heartburn or excessive belching. She came in only out of concern from this testing.

PAST MEDICAL HISTORY: Negative; no hospitalizations

MEDICATIONS: Takes multi-vitamin daily

SOCIAL HISTORY: Works as a personal trainer; denies use of supplements
Never smoked
Drinks glass of wine rarely on special occasion
Single, sexually active

FAMILY HISTORY: Father age 62 in good health
                                     Mother died age 55 of breast cancer
                                     Sister age 28 in good health

ROS: No dyspepsia
                                     No diarrhea
                                     No chest discomfort
                                     No use of antacids
                                     No use of NSAIDs or iron products

PHYSICAL EXAMINATION:
    Vitals: BP 110/50; P 55; RR 18; Temp 97.8º F; Weight 110 lbs.; Height 5'6"
                              Healthy energetic woman in no distress
    HEENT: PERRLA, EOMI
                              TMs clear
                              Throat clear
    Neck: Supple
                              No thyromegaly
    Heart: RRR with S_4 gallop
    Lungs: CTA
    Abdomen: Bowel sounds present in all quadrants; no hepatosplenomegaly; no tenderness to
                              palpation
    Extremities: No cyanosis, clubbing, or edema
    Breast: No masses or abnormalities noted
    GU: Normal external genitalia; pelvic examination normal; nontender; no discharge
    Rectal: Normal; heme negative

LABORATORY: Pap smear sent

Which of the following can you tell her about her positive test for "ulcer bacteria"?

  A. Since she has known *Helicobacter pylori,* it is prudent to treat her with appropriate antimicrobial therapy.
  B. Because she is asymptomatic, further investigation is not indicated or necessary; treatment is also not required.
  C. Because the test she received in the supermarket is likely a false positive, it is best to repeat the test in the office with a more specific test for *Helicobacter pylori* to determine if therapy is indicated.
  D. She should undergo endoscopy.
  E. She should undergo barium swallow.

11.

A 25-year-old male presents with a history of deep burning epigastric pain for the past week. The pain is worse 1 to 3 hours after eating and is relieved by ingestion of antacids or food. The pain has also awakened him from sleep at night on occasion. He has no anorexia, dysphagia, vomiting, or weight loss. He smokes a pack of cigarettes daily. He denies use of NSAIDs.

PAST MEDICAL HISTORY: Gonorrhea at age 18
                                  Syphilis at age 19

SOCIAL HISTORY:
Waiter at local Mexican restaurant
Smoking history as above; started smoking at age 15
No illicit drug use since age 19 (cocaine and marijuana); no IV drug history
Alcohol: Abstinent since age 19; attends regular AA meetings
Sex: Uses condoms every time; no sexual encounters in 6 months

FAMILY HISTORY:
Father 55 with diabetes
Mother 60 with hypertension, mild CVA last year
Sister 23 with no health problems

REVIEW OF SYSTEMS:
No fever or chills
No tachycardia
Frequent dyspepsia
Frequent burping
No heartburn while lying flat
No regurgitation
No other pain besides the deep epigastric pain
No nausea or vomiting
No GU symptoms

PHYSICAL EXAMINATION:

Vital signs: BP 130/80, P 75, RR 14, Temp 99° F, Ht 6'1", Wt 220
HEENT: PERRLA, EOMI
TMs clear
Throat clear
Neck: Supple; no thyromegaly
Heart: RRR with murmurs, rubs, or gallops
Lungs: CTA
Abdomen Bowel sounds present in all 4 quadrants, slightly hyperactive; no hepatomegaly; spleen tip non-palpable; mid-epigastric tenderness to deep palpation; no rebound
Extremities: No cyanosis, clubbing, or edema
Skin: No rash, except mild acne
Rectal: External hemorrhoids, heme negative
GU: No lesions noted; normal male genitalia

LABORATORY:

CBC: WBC 8,500 with 60% polys, 40% lymphocytes;
hemoglobin 15.5 mg/dL, hematocrit is 55%
MCV 90
Electrolytes: Normal

Based on your history, physical, and laboratory tests, which of the following is the next step in evaluation of this patient?

A. Non-invasive testing for *Helicobacter pylori*.
B. Barium swallow.
C. Esophagogastroduodenoscopy (EGD).
D. Treat empirically with H-2 blockers; if no improvement in 2 weeks, then test for *Helicobacter pylori*.
E. Esophagogastroduodenoscopy (EGD) with biopsy, because this is the only definitive method to determine if *Helicobacter pylori* is the etiology of his symptoms.

12.

A 50-year-old man presents for follow-up of a gastric ulcer diagnosed 8 weeks ago. It was a relatively large, non-bleeding ulcer located in the duodenum. *Helicobacter pylori* was found in the biopsy specimen, as well as with a rapid urease test on the clinical specimen taken at biopsy. He took 14 days of a prepackaged triple-therapy agent (Prevpac®—consists of 30 mg lansoprazole, 1 g amoxicillin, and 500 mg clarithromycin). He was adherent with his medication regimen and reports no problem taking the medication correctly. He returns for follow-up 6 weeks after the completion of therapy.

PAST MEDICAL HISTORY: No prior episodes of ulcer disease
                                      HTN for 20 years; currently on propranolol 20 mg q day

SOCIAL HISTORY: Quit smoking 6 weeks ago; before then, 1 pack/day for 30 years
                                        No alcohol in last 6 months
                                        Works in a staple factory; packages staples

FAMILY HISTORY: Non-contributory

ROS: All symptoms now resolved
                                          No dyspepsia
                                          No chest discomfort
                                          No epigastric pain
                                          No difficulty with nocturnal pain
                                          No difficulty with pain after eating

PHYSICAL EXAMINATION:
                                  VSS stable and documented correctly for Medicaid rules

    HEENT: No problems noted; non-icteric
    Heart: RRR without murmurs, rubs or gallops
    Lungs: CTA
    Abdomen: Bowel sounds present in all 4 quadrants, no hepatosplenomegaly, no tenderness elicited
                        on deep palpation of epigastric area
    Extremities: No cyanosis, clubbing, or edema
    Rectal: Heme negative

Which of the following tests should he be scheduled for now as follow-up?

  A. None; patients who are treated with triple therapy for *H. pylori* do not require follow-up assessment for cure because known cure rates with current regimens are nearly 95%.
  B. Repeat endoscopy is indicated because the other non-invasive tests are likely to still be false positive this early after therapy is completed.
  C. Convalescent serology for *H. pylori* to look for 4-fold fall in titers.
  D. A urea breath test is indicated at this point to determine cure.
  E. It is too early to test for cure; you must wait until 3 months after therapy is complete.

13.

A 45-year-old man presents with recently diagnosed peptic ulcer disease. His ulcer was found on esophagoduodenostomy (EGD) and was in the 2nd portion of the duodenum. Also on EGD, he was noted to have fairly significant esophagitis. He had presented with an upper gastrointestinal bleed yesterday. On further questioning, he relates that he has been doing well except for dyspepsia on occasion after eating "spicy" foods and has noted increasing episodes of diarrhea for the last few months.

PAST MEDICAL HISTORY: Non-contributory

FAMILY HISTORY:
Mother with peptic ulcer disease in her mid-40s, died at age 50 of severe upper GI bleed
Brother: Hx of peptic ulcer disease

SOCIAL HISTORY:
Works as a carpenter
Smokes 1 ppd x 30 years
Alcohol: 6 pack of beer on weekends

REVIEW OF SYSTEMS:
Negative for fever, chills
Denies night sweats
No tachycardia
No vomiting
No burning on urination
No hair loss or changes in hair character

PHYSICAL EXAM:
Vital signs: BP 140/50, P 88, RR 15, Temp 98.7° F, Ht 5'5, Wt 170 lbs.
HEENT: PERRLA, EOMI
TMs clear
Throat clear
Neck: Supple, no thyromegaly
Heart: RRR with murmurs, rubs, or gallops
Lungs: CTA
Abdomen: Bowel sounds present in all 4 quadrants, slightly hyperactive; no hepatomegaly, spleen tip non-palpable, mid-epigastric tenderness to deep palpation; no rebound
Extremities: No cyanosis, clubbing, or edema
Skin: No rash
Rectal: Heme positive
GU: No lesions noted; normal male genitalia

LABORATORY: A rapid urease test was done on the biopsy specimen and was positive for *H. pylori*.

Based on his history and findings at EGD, which of the following tests or diagnostic studies should you order now?

    A. Computed tomography of the abdomen to rule out malignancy.
    B. Repeat EGD in 5 days.
    C. Barium swallow.
    D. Fasting serum gastrin level.
    E. Follow-up *H. pylori* serology in 1 month to look for cure.

14.

A 60-year-old Asian male who immigrated to the United States in 1950 was recently diagnosed with gastric carcinoma that is distal in character. He has started adjuvant combination chemotherapy. His oldest son comes in with his father today and asks what things he, the son, can do to prevent "from getting this type of cancer."

All of the following are risk factors for gastric carcinoma <u>except</u>:

A. Pernicious anemia
B. *H. pylori* infection independent of known ulcer disease
C. Blood type A
D. Alcohol consumption
E. Diet low in fruits and vegetables

15.

A 25-year-old woman presents with a history of recurrent diarrhea. Recently, she has become concerned because the diarrhea has occurred while she is sleeping. Additionally, she notes that she has had abdominal pain on occasion. The pain is relieved by defecation. Usually the pain is located in the right lower quadrant. She describes it as a chronic nagging type pain ("colicky"). On further questioning, she relates a 10-lb weight loss over the past 5 months. Her husband has noted that she sweats "a lot" during the night, and occasionally she has had to change her bedclothes. Also, she reports that on occasion she is "feverish" but has not taken her temperature. She has not traveled anywhere outside of Colorado where she lives, but she and her husband did go camping during the past summer at Pike's Peak. Their last camping trip was 3 months ago. They boiled water for drinking while camping and did not go swimming. Her husband has not been ill.

PAST MEDICAL HISTORY: History of frequent episodes of diarrhea intermittently over the past 5 years
                                  On oral contraceptives; no change in medication in 6 years
                                  Allergies: none

FAMILY HISTORY: Mother with episodes of diarrhea on occasion
                           Father with coronary artery disease, hypertension
                           Sister healthy, no problems
                           Brother healthy, no problems

SOCIAL HISTORY: Works for a telecommunication company in Colorado Springs, CO; does phone-messaging services
                           Lives with husband and 2 dogs in the city limits
                           Dogs are healthy, no problems
                           Never has smoked
                           Drinks a margarita on weekends

ROS: Most reviewed above
      No blood noted in stool
      Stools of normal caliber when she is not having diarrhea

PHYSICAL EXAMINATION: Well-appearing woman in no distress
                      BP 110/65, P 68, RR 16, Temp 99.2° F

HEENT:	PERRLA, EOMI
	Throat normal
	Normal dentition
Neck:	Supple, no thyromegaly
Heart:	RRR without murmurs, rubs, or gallops
Lungs:	CTA
Abdomen:	Bowel sounds hyperactive, present in all 4 quadrants equally
	Mild epigastric discomfort with deep palpation; no rebound
	No hepatosplenomegaly
Extremities:	No cyanosis, clubbing, or edema
GU:	Normal female genitalia
	Heme-positive rectal exam

LABORATORY:

CBC:	WBC 12,500 with 60% polys, 20% lymphocytes, 15% monocytes
	Hemoglobin 10.5 g/dL
	Platelets: 450,000
Stool Studies:	Marked number of fecal leukocytes seen on direct smear
	Negative for enteric pathogens, ova and parasites, *Giardia*-specific antigen, and
	Clostridium difficile toxin
Electrolytes:	Normal
Liver transaminases: Normal for age	
ESR: 50	

Based on your history and physical examination, which of the following studies is most likely to confirm your diagnosis?

- A. MRI of the abdomen and pelvis
- B. Endoscopic laparotomy
- C. Repeat ova and parasite studies x 3
- D. Rectal biopsy
- E. Colonoscopy with upper endoscopy

16.

A 30-year-old Hispanic male with history of Crohn disease presents for usual routine checkup. He has been doing very well on his current regimen, which includes sulfasalazine and metronidazole. Initially during the office visit he has no complaints. However, during the end of your examination he jokes that he and his wife have been trying to get pregnant during the last year without any luck. He says that they have been reading suggestions in books and on the Internet without any luck. His wife is healthy—they have had 2 children, now ages 8 and 7. His Crohn's was diagnosed 6 years ago, and he essentially has been in remission for 5 years on his current therapy. He asks if his Crohn's could be related to the inability to conceive.

PAST MEDICAL HISTORY: As above; before diagnosis of Crohn's had intermittent diarrhea for 5–6 years

MEDICATIONS: Sulfasalazine 1 gram PO bid
                        Metronidazole 500 mg PO bid

SOCIAL HISTORY: Works as photographer
        Lives with wife and 2 children in El Paso, TX

FAMILY HISTORY: Non-contributory

REVIEW OF SYSTEMS: Sexual libido has been normal
        No problems with erections
        He wears "briefs"
        No change in ejaculate
        No rash
        No urinary complaints

PHYSICAL EXAMINATION: Muscular athletic male in no distress
    BP 125/62, P 56, RR 12, Temp 98.3° F

HEENT:	PERRLA, EOMI,
	Tympanic membranes clear
	Throat clear
Neck:	Supple, no masses
Heart:	RRR without murmurs, rubs, or gallops
Lungs:	CTA
Abdomen:	Bowel sounds present in all 4 quadrants, no tenderness, no hepatosplenomegaly
Extremities:	No cyanosis, clubbing, or edema
GU:	Normal male genitalia, Tanner V staging
	No testicular masses
Rectal:	Heme negative, tone normal
Neurological:	Reflexes equal and symmetrical throughout; no sensory or motor deficits noted

LABORATORY:

CBC:	Normal
Electrolytes:	Normal

Liver function tests: Normal
Semen analysis: Volume 4 mL; pH 7.5; sperm count 10 million/mL with 85% motile
(Normal values volume 2–5 mL; pH 7.2–8.0; sperm count 70–150 million/mL; sperm activity > 80% is normal)

Based on your history, physical examination, and laboratory studies, which of the following would be the next best course of action?

  A. Formal urological evaluation.
  B. Fertility testing of his wife.
  C. Stop sulfasalazine and use another agent for control of his disease.
  D. Check serum testosterone.
  E. Have him wear boxers instead of briefs.

17.

A 35-year-old man with ulcerative colitis (UC) presents for follow-up. He has been doing well, except recently he had an exacerbation with severe bleeding and anemia. He has a history of pancolitis, and on his recent colonoscopy, the biopsy showed high-grade dysplasias in flat mucosa. He did not have a mass lesion to biopsy. Previous colonoscopies have shown mild dysplasia with inflammation. Since his recent exacerbation, he has been doing well without any further episodes of bleeding. Of significance is that his last exacerbation prior to this was over 10 years ago.

PAST MEDICAL HISTORY: Besides UC, stable

SOCIAL HISTORY:
Smokes ½ ppd x 10 years
Abstains from alcohol
Married for 10 years
Works as a carpet layer

FAMILY HISTORY:
Mother, healthy, age 65
Father, healthy, age 70
No family history of colon cancer or other malignancies

ROS:
Negative for weight loss
Negative for fever, chills
Negative for rash
Negative for joint complaints

PHYSICAL EXAMINATION: Generally well-appearing man
VSS Afebrile

HEENT: PERRLA, EOMI,
                Tympanic membranes clear
                Throat clear
Neck: Supple, no bruits
Heart: RRR without murmurs, rubs, or gallops
Lungs: CTA
Abdomen: Benign, no tenderness, no hepatosplenomegaly
Extremities: No cyanosis, clubbing, or edema
GU: Normal male genitalia
                No testicular masses
Rectal: Heme negative, brown stool
Neuro: Reflexes equal and symmetrical throughout; no sensory or motor deficits noted

LABORATORY:
CBC: WBC 8,500 with 50% polys, 50% lymphs
                Hemoglobin 13 mg/dL (after transfusion last week)
                Platelets: 275,000
Electrolytes: Normal
Liver function tests: ALT 40 U/L; AST 23 U/L; alkaline phosphatase 180 mU/mL;
                Albumin 3.6 mg/dL; total bilirubin 0.5 mg/dL

Based on the findings, which of the following is the next step in management?

A. Re-institute maintenance therapy and repeat colonoscopy in 6 months to see if the "dysplasia" is just a side effect of his exacerbation.
B. Re-institute maintenance therapy, assuming that he will continue to do well long-term based on his relapse rate of every 10 years.
C. Continue routine colonoscopy on a yearly basis unless another exacerbation occurs; then repeat colonoscopy at that time.
D. Recommend referral to surgery.
E. Repeat colonoscopy in 2 weeks.

18.

An 18-year-old hip-hop singer presents with diarrhea for the past 2 weeks. She says that she noted the diarrhea began while she was performing in Mexico. You are the physician for the cruise line on which she is performing now. You really like her song, "OOPS, here I go again." But we digress from the topic at hand....

Anyway, she tells you that she has had a low-grade temperature since returning from Mexico. She did not eat any fresh vegetables (unless you call French fries a fresh vegetable). She likes to eat beef jerky and prefers the "extra salty" version. She drank only bottled water and a soft drink for which she is a national spokesperson. She did drink these drinks poured over ice, but she thought that the "frozen stuff would kill the cooties."

She has not noted any blood in her stool. She has lost about 2 pounds in the last week.

PAST MEDICAL HISTORY: Syphilis at the age of 15
Depression since age 16; on no medications at the moment

SOCIAL HISTORY: Sexually active with multiple partners
Smokes 1 pack/day for the past 3 years
Denies illicit drug use
Denies use of alcohol

FAMILY HISTORY: Mother with alcoholism; they are estranged at the moment
Father left when she was 2 years of age
Sister healthy 20-year-old nun

REVIEW OF SYSTEMS: Diarrhea is intermittent and she has crampy abdominal pain on occasion
No rash
No burning on urination
No chills
Diminished appetite

PHYSICAL EXAMINATION:
General: Pink hair with numerous piercings
VS: Temp 100° F, BP 110/70, Pulse 95, RR 16

HEENT: PERRLA, EOMI
Throat clear
Heart: RRR with no murmurs, rubs, or gallops
Lungs: CTA
Abdomen: Hyperactive bowel sounds, nontender examination; no hepatosplenomegaly
GU: Normal female genitalia, no tenderness on bi-manual palpation; no discharge noted
Extremities: No cyanosis, clubbing, or edema
Rectal: Heme positive (slight)

LABORATORY:
Check for stool leukocytes: positive
Giardia specific antigen: negative
Stool culture: *Salmonella enteritidis* β-lactamase producing

Based on this information, which of the following is the best treatment?

A. Ciprofloxacin 500 mg bid for 10 days
B. Erythromycin 500 mg bid for 5 days
C. Tetracycline 500 mg qid for 10 days
D. Amoxicillin 500 mg tid for 10 days
E. No antibiotic therapy

19.

A 19-year-old lifeguard at the local water park in your area presents for his final routine hepatitis B vaccine before going to college. Recently, there has been an outbreak of diarrhea at the water park confirmed as *E. coli* O157:H7. He is concerned about the diarrhea at the park and asks what he can do to limit his exposure. You explain that the outbreak has been linked to hamburgers at the park that were undercooked. He is concerned because he eats hamburgers twice daily. You explain that it is unlikely that he will become ill but to call you at the first sign of diarrhea.

The next morning, you receive a call from him saying that he has diarrhea. It is bloody in character. You tell him to come in right away.

He arrives and is ill appearing. He says the diarrhea started early this morning, and he has gone about 5 times since. He noted large amounts of blood in the initial stool, but it has since tapered off to a few streaks. He says he is lightheaded and dizzy.

PAST MEDICAL HISTORY: Healthy

SOCIAL HISTORY: As above
                         Doesn't smoke
                         Doesn't drink alcohol
                         Not sexually active

FAMILY HISTORY: Non-contributory

ROS: Fever, chills noted early this morning
        Weight loss of approximately 5 pounds since yesterday, he thinks
        Dizzy when standing
        No vomiting

PHYSICAL EXAMINATION:
        Lying down: BP 120/80, Pulse 80
        Sitting up: BP 100/65, Pulse 110
        Temperature: 99.5° F, RR 18

HEENT: PERRLA, EOMI
            Tympanic membranes clear
            Throat clear; mucous membranes dry
Neck: Supple, no bruits
Heart: RRR without murmurs, rubs, or gallops
Lungs: CTA
Abdomen: Benign, no tenderness, no hepatosplenomegaly
Extremities: No cyanosis, clubbing, or edema

GU: Deferred
Neurological: Reflexes equal and symmetrical throughout; no sensory or motor deficits noted

LABORATORY: All pending

Assuming that this also is going to be invasive diarrhea with *E. coli* O157:H7 and after starting supportive fluid therapy, which of the following antibiotics is the best treatment choice for his infection?

A. Penicillin 3 million units IV q 4 hours
B. Ceftriaxone 1 gm IV q day
C. Await sensitivities before starting therapy
D. Ciprofloxacin 400 mg IV bid
E. None of the choices is correct

20.

A 45-year-old man presents with new onset of a debilitating neurological syndrome. He has been healthy until about a month ago when he had gastroenteritis. He says the gastroenteritis lasted about a week and then resolved without any specific therapy. Most of the disease was a diarrheal illness. He has a puppy that also had diarrhea just before he became ill. His diarrhea was bloody in character, and he had crampy abdominal pain. (As opposed to the puppy's diarrhea.) The diarrhea lasted about 5 days. The dog's disease also lasted about that long.

He noted painless onset of mild weakness in the lower extremities, often accompanied by tingling paresthesias in his toes and fingers. He became aware of this first with difficulty walking up stairs. Over a period of days, the weakness progressed rapidly and ascended from the lower extremities to the upper extremities and finally to the face.

PAST MEDICAL HISTORY: Noncontributory

SOCIAL HISTORY: Works as a harmonica player for a popular jazz band
                Smokes 3 packs of cigarettes a day
                Drinks only on weekends; about a 6-pack of beer
                No travel history

FAMILY HISTORY: Non-contributory

REVIEW OF SYSTEM: No fevers, no chills
                No weight loss
                No recent diarrhea
                No vomiting
                No rashes
                No headache
                No vision changes

PHYSICAL EXAMINATION:

    BP 110/70, P100, RR 18, Temp 98.5° F

    HEENT: PERRLA, EOMI,
            Tympanic membranes clear
            Throat clear

Neck:	Supple, no bruits
Heart:	RRR without murmurs, rubs, or gallops
Lungs:	CTA
Abdomen:	Benign, no tenderness, no hepatosplenomegaly
Extremities:	No cyanosis, clubbing, or edema
Neuro:	Deep tendon reflexes are not present
	He has lost proprioceptive perception in his arms and legs
	He has symmetrical motor weakness of both proximal and distal muscles of all the extremities
	He has bilateral VII nerve palsies
	Currently swallowing and breathing are intact

Which of the following organisms is the likely antecedent to this constellation of findings?

    A. *Campylobacter jejuni*
    B. *Shigella dysenteriae*
    C. *Salmonella enteritidis*
    D. *E. coli* O157:H7
    E. Rotavirus infection

21.

A 20-year-old woman presents with a history of chronic diarrhea for over a year. She has complained of diarrhea on many visits to your office. Listed below is the laboratory work that has been done to date, including a few tests done today. The diarrhea is intermittent in character, lasts 3–5 days, and then her stools gradually return to normal. She has not noticed any blood in the stool. She has no nausea or vomiting. She has no other health problems. No one that she lives with (her boyfriend and 1-year-old) have problems with diarrhea. She has not had significant weight loss. The stools are not foul smelling and are usually fairly watery in character.

PAST MEDICAL HISTORY:	History of depression at age 16 requiring hospitalization; since then doing well on Prozac 20 mg q day
SOCIAL HISTORY:	Beauty College student Smokes ½ pack day for 3 years Alcohol—doesn't drink
FAMILY HISTORY:	Mother, healthy, no health problems Father, healthy, no health problems Sister, anorexia Brother, bulimia
REVIEW OF SYSTEMS:	No fever, chills No sore throats No increased nervousness No chest discomfort No wheezing No stomach pain No rashes No travel

PHYSICAL EXAMINATION: Well-appearing WF, with excessive amounts of makeup

BP 120/60, P 64, RR 18, Temp 98.3° F

HEENT:	PERRLA, EOMI, sclera non-icteric
Neck:	Supple; no masses
Heart:	RRR without murmurs, rubs or gallops
Lungs:	Clear to auscultation
Abdomen:	Mild epigastric tenderness to deep palpation
Extremities:	No cyanosis, clubbing, or edema
GU:	Heme-negative stool; scant amount of stool in vault

LABORATORY:
 CBC x 2 normal
 Electrolytes normal x 3
 Liver transaminases normal x 2
 Stool ova and parasites and fecal leukocytes x 3—all negative
 C. difficile toxin negative
 Chem 20—all within normal limits
 TSH normal
 T4 normal
 Gastrin level: normal
 Giardia-specific antigen negative
 Sigmoidoscopy negative
 Sodium hydroxide added to stool: turns red

Which of the following do the history, physical, and laboratory findings suggest?

 A. Bisacodyl abuse
 B. Irritable bowel syndrome
 C. Phenolphthalein abuse
 D. Carcinoid
 E. Need to proceed with colonoscopy

22.

A 40-year-old Irish-American man with a history of celiac disease presents with complaint of increasing fatigue for the past 3 months. He reports he has been compliant with his diet. He was not diagnosed until several years ago. His celiac disease resulted in growth retardation as a child. He currently plays a leprechaun in a revival of "Finnegan's Rainbow." He occasionally suffers from dermatitis herpetiformis. He has a pale pallor to his skin and he looks "run down" to you.

PAST MEDICAL HISTORY: As above

MEDICATIONS: None

SOCIAL HISTORY:	Married, with 2 children
	Works, as above, as a leprechaun
	Has never smoked
	Drinks an occasional pint of beer

| FAMILY HISTORY: | Sister has celiac sprue also; found to have HLA-B8 |
| | Mother and father healthy |

ROS:	Severe fatigue
	Dyspnea on exertion with walking 1 block
	No chest pain
	No swelling in his legs
	No constipation

PHYSICAL EXAMINATION: BP 120/60, P100, RR 18, Temp 99.0° F

HEENT:	PERRLA, EOMI, sclera non-icteric, very pale conjunctiva
Neck:	Supple; no bruits; no masses
Heart:	RRR with new II/VI systolic flow murmur
Lungs:	Clear to auscultation
Abdomen:	Mild epigastric tenderness to deep palpation
Extremities:	No cyanosis, clubbing, or edema
GU:	Heme-negative stool

LABORATORY:

CBC:	WBC 8,500 with 60% polys, 30% lymphs
	Hemoglobin 8.5 mg/dL (previous hemoglobin 14 mg/dL)
	Rest of CBC pending…the machine just broke

Based on your extensive knowledge of celiac disease and putting together the physical exam findings with the laboratory (what limited things they give you), which of the following is the most likely diagnosis?

A. B_{12} deficiency anemia
B. Toxicity from wearing green leprechaun paint
C. Celiac sprue exacerbation
D. Iron deficiency anemia
E. Primary intestinal lymphoma

23.

A 45-year-old man presents with a wasting type illness for the past 6 months. He describes arthralgias and frank arthritis of the larger joints that seem to come and go. He has fever associated with these episodes up to 102° F on occasion. He has had marked episodes of diarrhea over the past 6 months and has lost 20 pounds. Additionally, he describes "swollen glands" for the past few months.

| PAST MEDICAL HISTORY: | Nothing at all; a very healthy man; athletic |

SOCIAL HISTORY:	Lives in Philadelphia, PA
	Works as a guard at the Liberty Bell
	Married with 3 children, ages 14, 12, 10

| FAMILY HISTORY: | Mother 70 with hypertension |
| | Father 75 with diabetes, hypertension |

REVIEW OF SYSTEMS: Difficulty seeing at night—he noticed this in the past month
         Swelling of the joints noted on occasion
         Noted increased bleeding of his gums

PHYSICAL EXAMINATION:

 BP 120/60, P64, RR 18, Temp 99.0° F

HEENT:	PERRLA, EOMI, sclera non-icteric
Teeth:	Gingivitis present
Mouth:	Glossitis present
Neck:	Supple; no bruits
Heart:	RRR without murmurs, rubs or gallops
Lungs:	Clear to auscultation
Abdomen:	Hyperactive bowel sounds; distended abdomen; no hepatosplenomegaly
Extremities:	No cyanosis, clubbing, or edema; joint swelling noted of the right knee; no frank deforming arthritis noted
GU/Rectal:	Mild heme-positive stool; no melena
Skin:	Diffuse hyperpigmentation, particularly around the orbital and malar face areas

LABORATORY: Significant tests for you to consider:
 Sudan stain of stool shows malabsorption
 Serum carotene level 5 mg/dL (normal 40–180 mg/dL)
 Serum albumin 2.4 mg/dL
 Prothrombin time prolonged at 16 secs

Further workup is done and a biopsy is taken of the small intestine that shows the lamina propria contains macrophages containing periodic acid-Schiff (PAS) material.

Based on these findings, which of the following is your diagnosis?

 A. Celiac sprue
 B. AIDS-related complex
 C. Infection with *Tropheryma whippelii*
 D. *Mycobacterium avium intracellulare* infection
 E. Abdominal angina

24.

A 45-year-old African-American woman presents for her routine job screening physical examination. She is applying to be a security guard at her local airport. She is very healthy and works out at her local gym on a regular basis.

PAST MEDICAL HISTORY:
       Negative except for hospitalizations for her 2 children, which required C-section
       On no medications

SOCIAL HISTORY: Lives with her husband and 2 sons, ages 15 and 13
       Never has smoked
       Drinks Mai Tais on a regular basis; one q day

FAMILY HISTORY: Father diagnosed at age 48 with colon cancer; died 2 years later
                    Mother healthy, age 70
                    Brother 42, obese

REVIEW OF SYSTEMS: No headaches
                        No sore throat
                        No eye changes
                        No muscle aches or pains
                        No chest pain
                        No cough
                        No diarrhea
                        No constipation
                        No rashes
                        Poor dentition—has been to dentist multiple times in last few months for cavities

PHYSICAL EXAMINATION: Well-developed, well-nourished woman in no distress
        BP 110/70, P 65, RR 14, Temp 98.6° F

    HEENT: PERRLA, EOMI
                    TMs clear
                    Throat clear; poor dentition noted
    Neck: Supple, no masses
    Heart: RRR with murmurs, rubs, or gallops
    Lungs: CTA
    Abdomen: Auscultation normal; no hepatosplenomegaly
    Extremities: No cyanosis, clubbing, or edema
    GU: Normal female external genitalia; pelvic examination: Normal findings; non-tender exam
    Rectal: Done—no results because you have to answer the question without knowing the answer

Which of the following would be the most appropriate colorectal cancer screening for her?

   A. Begin annual fecal occult blood testing and flexible sigmoidoscopy every 5 years starting at age 50.
   B. Begin annual fecal occult blood testing and flexible sigmoidoscopy every 5 years starting at age 60.
   C. Colonoscopy every 5 years beginning now.
   D. Colonoscopy every 5 years beginning at age 50.
   E. Colonoscopy every 10 years beginning now.

25.

A 49-year-old man presents after undergoing a screening colonoscopy last week. It was normal except for the finding of a 0.5 cm polyp. He is healthy otherwise and has no risk factors for colorectal carcinoma except for his age. He reports that he exercises regularly and eats plenty of fruits and vegetables.

PAST MEDICAL HISTORY: Normal treadmill stress test done 3 years ago; otherwise no problems
                         HTN, benign

MEDICATIONS: ECASA q daily
                         Propranolol 20 mg PO q daily

FAMILY HISTORY: Negative for any type of GI malignancy

SOCIAL HISTORY: Works as a tailor
                         Lives with his mother

REVIEW OF SYSTEMS: Non-contributory

PHYSICAL EXAMINATION:
    BP 130/50, P 88, R 14, Temp 98.5° F

    HEENT: PERRLA, EOMI
                 Throat clear
    Heart: RRR without murmurs, rubs, or gallops
    Lungs: CTA
    Abdomen: Bowel sounds present; no hepatosplenomegaly
    Extremities: No cyanosis, clubbing, or edema

LABORATORY: Path report from biopsy: hyperplastic polyp

Based on these findings, which of the following do you recommend?

   A. Repeat colonoscopy in 3–6 months to be sure the polyp was completely resected.
   B. Repeat colonoscopy in 1 year.
   C. Order CEA level.
   D. Repeat colonoscopy in 3 years.
   E. Repeat colonoscopy in 10 years.

26.

You are seeing a 48-year-old Puerto Rican man with a history of colonoscopic excision of a 3 cm sessile polyp earlier today. He is otherwise healthy and has not had any health issues come up in the past 3 years that you have been following him. He has a history of mild hypertension controlled with diet but otherwise has not been into the office except for an occasional upper respiratory infection.

PAST MEDICAL HISTORY: As above

SOCIAL HISTORY: Works as an attorney
Smokes 2 packs/day of cigarettes
Drinks 3–4 beers nightly

FAMILY HISTORY: Father, healthy
Mother, 75, lives in Puerto Rico, healthy
No siblings

REVIEW OF SYSTEMS: No headache
No sore throat
No fevers
No night sweats
No chest discomfort
Chronic smoker-type cough; worse in the morning on awakening
No weight loss

PHYSICAL EXAMINATION: Had complete physical 2 months ago; nothing has changed since that visit

LABORATORY: Pathology shows resection of a large 3 cm sessile polyp with villous tissue. The pathologist reports that she is reasonably sure the polyp was completely removed—the edges are distinct; no malignancy was found in the biopsy taken.

Based on these findings, which of the following should be your recommendation?

    A. Schedule for routine colonoscopy in 5 years.
    B. Schedule for routine colonoscopy in 10 years.
    C. Repeat colonoscopy in 1 year.
    D. Repeat colonoscopy in 3–6 months to be sure that resection was complete.
    E. Refer to surgeon for surgical resection of affected area.

27.

A 52-year-old man presents for routine colonoscopy.

PAST MEDICAL HISTORY: Insulin-dependent diabetes for 4 years
Hypertension for 3 years
Hyperlipidemia for 2 years

SOCIAL HISTORY: Works as a waiter
Smokes 2 packs/day of cigarettes
Drinks 3–4 beers nightly

FAMILY HISTORY: Father 80 y/o, a minister with diabetes
Mother 75 y/o lives in Florida, osteoporosis
Sister 55 y/o with SLE

REVIEW OF SYSTEMS: No headache
No sore throat
No fevers
No night sweats
No chest discomfort
Chronic "smoker" type cough; worse in the morning on awakening
No weight loss

PHYSICAL EXAMINATION:
BP 130/60, P 90, RR 18, Temp 99.0° F

HEENT:	PERRLA, EOMI, sclera non-icteric
Neck:	Supple; no bruits; no masses
Heart:	RRR with new II/VI systolic flow murmur (old)
Lungs:	Clear to auscultation
Abdomen:	Mild epigastric tenderness to deep palpation; positive bowel sounds in all 4 quadrants, no hepatosplenomegaly
Extremities:	No cyanosis, clubbing, or edema
Genitourinary:	Normal male; no masses
Rectal:	Deferred because about to have colonoscopy

PROCEDURES:
Colonoscopy: 1 suspicious polyp was found in the right colon near the sigmoid junction; completely resected.

He returns in 1 week for his pathology report. These findings show:
The polyp was completely excised and submitted *in toto* for pathological examination. The polyp was fixed and sectioned so that it was possible to accurately determine the depth of invasion, grade of differentiation, and completeness of the excision of the polyp. Carcinoma unfortunately is found in the tissue. The cancer is well differentiated. There is **no** vascular or lymphatic involvement. The margin of the excision is not involved.

Repeat colonoscopy in 3 months shows no residual abnormal tissue at the polypectomy site.

Based on your findings, which of the following should be your recommendation?

- A. Repeat colonoscopy in 3 months.
- B. Repeat colonoscopy in 6 months.
- C. Determine CEA levels.
- D. Refer for surgical intervention and chemotherapy.
- E. Because the incidence of recurrent cancer is small, no other laboratory or imaging studies are indicated for this patient; follow-up should proceed as with benign adenomas.

28.

A 55-year-old woman has been diagnosed with colon cancer. She was diagnosed by colonoscopy and had a left hemicolectomy performed 3 days ago. You are seeing her in the hospital to discuss the results of her pathology specimens from surgery. Other than this new diagnosis, she has been very healthy. The cancer was found on a routine screen, and she had not been having any symptoms.

Pathology report: Cancer was present in the left portion of the colon just proximal to the sigmoid colon and has spread to the regional lymph nodes. Only 2 nodes are positive.

CT Scan: No evidence of distant metastases; liver is normal in appearance. No lung, bone, or rectal mets.

Which of the following treatment options would you recommend?

- A. Her left hemicolectomy alone is adequate therapy.
- B. Besides the hemicolectomy, institute local radiation therapy.
- C. Start adjuvant chemotherapy and initiate local radiation therapy.
- D. Start adjuvant chemotherapy without radiation therapy.
- E. She will need to return to surgery for a complete colectomy with local radiation therapy.

29.

An 85-year-old African-American woman presents to your office with complaints of lower abdominal pain. Her pain is crampy and bilateral but worse on the right side. The pain started approximately 24 hours ago. The location has not changed, but the intensity of the pain increased overnight. The pain is accompanied by nausea. She vomited two or three times the preceding day. She also reports diarrhea and chills during the past 24 hours.

PAST MEDICAL HISTORY:
        Coronary artery disease, for which she had angioplasty three years ago; no angina symptoms since
        Diverticulosis without history of diverticulitis since 1989
        She has well-controlled hypertension, gout, and chronic low back pain
        Past surgical history: hysterectomy/bilateral salpingo-oophorectomy in 1976

MEDICATIONS: Atenolol 50 mg q day
                    Allopurinol
                    Tramadol prn
                    ECASA 81mg q day

SOCIAL HISTORY: No alcohol consumption
                    No cigarette smoking; but does chew tobacco
                    She has no history of drug abuse

FAMILY HISTORY: No living relatives; doesn't know her parents or siblings

PHYSICAL EXAMINATION: Temperature of 101.3° F, pulse 128 bpm, BP 127/50 mmHg, RR 18 breaths/min, oxygen saturation of 98% on room air; she is 5 feet tall and weighs 163 pounds; she appears to be in mild distress secondary to pain; she is alert and fully oriented

HEENT:	Her oral mucosa appears dry; PERRLA, EOMI
Neck:	No masses, no bruits
Heart:	RRR with tachycardia
Lungs:	Clear to auscultation
Abdomen:	Relatively diffuse tenderness over the lower abdomen, more severe over the right lower quadrant; the abdomen was soft without hepatomegaly or splenomegaly; there was no rebound or guarding; bowel sounds were hypoactive
Rectal:	Heme-negative stool

Neurological examination was intact.

LABORATORY:

Leukocyte count was 10.0×10^9/L with 84% neutrophils; hemoglobin concentration was 12.1 g/dL; platelet count was 181,000

Chemistries: sodium 143 mEq/L, serum potassium 4.6 mEq/L, serum chloride 108 mEq/L, serum bicarbonate 21 mEq/L, blood urea nitrogen 44 mg/dL, serum creatinine 1.5 mg/dL, glucose 169 mg/dL

Amylase 113 U/L, lipase 50 U/L, aspartate aminotransferase 44 U/L (14–36), alanine aminotransferase 59 U/L (9–52), alkaline phosphatase 68 U/L, and low-density lipoprotein 784 U/L (313–618)

Urinalysis showed 1–2 white blood cells, +1 leukocyte esterase, +1 bacteria, and nitrite negative

Electrocardiogram showed sinus tachycardia with a rate of 103 without ST segment or T wave changes

Chest x-ray showed minimal bibasilar atelectasis

Flat and upright abdomen x-ray was negative

Ultrasonography of the right upper quadrant showed no signs of cholecystitis

Computed tomography of the abdomen without intravenous contrast showed mild circumferential mural thickening of the terminal ileum, mild inflammation of mesenteric fat, the appendix not visualized, and no free or localized fluid

Which of the following is the most likely diagnosis based on these findings?

A. Diverticulitis
B. Appendicitis
C. Crohn disease
D. Colon carcinoma
E. Viral gastroenteritis

30.

A 55-year-old Caucasian woman presents with history of abdominal complaints off and on "for years." She presents with acute onset of severe pain in her left abdomen. She has fever to 101° F at home and appears ill. She has had some associated diarrhea with the pain.

PAST MEDICAL HISTORY: History of GI disease. See attached figure from endoscopy in 2000:

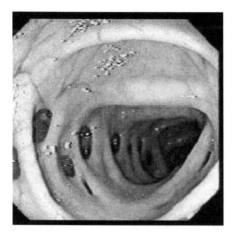

SOCIAL HISTORY:	Housewife, volunteers at her church quite often
	Lives at home with her husband, a retired stripper

FAMILY HISTORY:	Mother died at age 78; renal failure
	Father died at age 25; industrial accident

REVIEW OF SYSTEMS:
No headache
No sore throat
No runny nose; congestion
Occasional dry cough
No tachycardia
No chest pain
No constipation
Diarrhea frequently, usually with emotional upset
No burning on urination

PHYSICAL EXAMINATION:
BP 130/88, P 100, RR 18, Temp 101.5° F

Ill-appearing woman in mild distress

HEENT:	PERRLA, EOMI
	TMs clear
	Throat clear
Neck:	Supple; no masses
Heart:	RRR without murmurs, rubs or gallops
Lungs:	Clear to auscultation

Abdomen:	Hyperactive bowel sounds; tender and palpable mass in left lower quadrant; rebound tenderness noted and involuntary abdominal rigidity noted
Rectal:	Heme positive
Extremities:	No rashes, cyanosis or edema

LABORATORY: pending

Based on her physical findings, which of the following is the most appropriate next step?

A. Emergent colonoscopy
B. Emergent barium enema
C. Bowel rest only is adequate at this point
D. Bleeding scan
E. Abdominal CT scan

31.

All of the following are indications for colonoscopy <u>except</u>:

A. Bright red blood on toilet paper in a 25-year-old man
B. Gross lower gastrointestinal bleeding in a 60-year-old man
C. *Streptococcus bovis* bacteremia
D. Hemoccult-positive screen in a 50-year-old woman
E. Iron deficiency anemia in a 40-year-old man

32.

A 55-year-old man complains of abdominal pain after eating meals and has noted a 25-lb weight loss. The pain is "gnawing" and lasts from 1–3 hours after eating. The weight loss, he says, is because he cannot eat very much without having the pain. It is really bothering him because he has to go to banquets all the time, and he just doesn't enjoy food anymore because of the pain associated with eating.

PAST MEDICAL HISTORY: Hypertension for 20 years; on lisinopril
Obesity

SOCIAL HISTORY: Married
Smokes 3 cigars a day
Doesn't drink anymore; stopped 6 months ago

Pertinent positives from review of systems: Known history of peripheral vascular disease—can walk only 3–4 blocks and then has severe leg pains. Otherwise negative.

PHYSICAL EXAMINATION:
BP 130/70, P90, RR 18, Temp 99.0° F
HEENT: PERRLA, EOMI, sclera non-icteric
Teeth: Mostly capped
Mouth: No lesions noted
Neck: Supple; no bruits
Heart: RRR without murmurs, rubs or gallops
Lungs: Clear to auscultation

Abdomen:	Hyperactive bowel sounds; abdominal bruit heard
Extremities:	Mild clubbing, 2+ peripheral edema
GU/Rectal:	Mild heme-positive stool; no melena
Skin:	Numerous chronic breakdown areas on his lower legs, particularly his shins
Neuro:	Diminished sensation to touch and palpation of lower extremities in stocking distribution
	Reflexes equal and symmetrical; loss of hair over lower extremities

LABORATORY: Pending

Based on your findings so far, which of the following is the most appropriate next step?

A. Colonoscopy
B. Barium swallow with enteroclysis
C. Ultrasound of abdomen
D. Arteriogram
E. Trial of omeprazole

33.

A 24-year-old man with history of chronic alcohol abuse presents with complaint of severe abdominal pain for the past 8 hours. He tried to relieve the pain by drinking beer. He eventually drank 12 beers without relief of the pain. He then started to vomit and noted that his abdominal pain was even worse. He has vomited about 5 times in the past 3 hours.

| PAST MEDICAL HISTORY: | Has never been hospitalized in the past |
| | No medications |

SOCIAL HISTORY:	Works as an air traffic controller in Chicago
	Drinks 6–12 beers usually after work
	Smokes 2 packs/day of cigarettes
	Lives with his girlfriend; she is a country western singer

| FAMILY HISTORY: | Father 50; alcoholic |
| | Mother 50; alcoholic |

REVIEW OF SYSTEMS:	No fever, no chills
	Occasional headache in the mornings after drinking
	Vomiting about once a week
	Diarrhea on occasion

PHYSICAL EXAMINATION:
BP 120/50, RR 22, P 110, Temp 99.9° F

HEENT:	Poor dentition; severe halitosis; alcohol on breath
	PERRLA, EOMI
Neck:	No meningismus
Heart:	RRR without murmurs, rubs, or gallops
Lungs:	CTA
Abdomen:	+BS in all 4 quadrants; severe epigastric tenderness; won't let sheet stay on his belly; writhing in the bed; liver is 3 cm below the right costal margin; no spleen palpated

Rectal: Heme negative
Extremities: No cyanosis or edema; no rash

LABORATORY: Amylase 400 U/L
               Lipase 500 U/L
               WBC 15,000 x 10^9/L with 80% polynuclear forms
               Hemoglobin 15.0 mg/dL
               Platelets: 450,000
               Calcium 9.5 mg/dL
               Albumin 3.5 mg/dL
               Creatinine 0.5 mg/dL

Initial CT scan is shown in this figure:

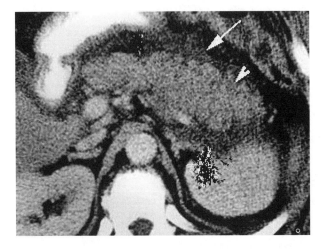

You start appropriate therapy. In a few hours after initiating therapy, you note on physical examination that he now has a faint blue discoloration around the umbilicus.

This finding indicates that he may have developed which of the following?

A. Tissue catabolism of hemoglobin
B. A milder form of pancreatitis
C. Fluid overload and you need to back down on fluid resuscitation
D. Hemoperitoneum
E. A pseudocyst

34.

A 22-year-old man with a negative past medical history presents with a chief complaint of "turning yellow." He noticed that he was becoming yellow in the eyes yesterday. Today he said he noted that his skin was also yellow. He has no nausea, vomiting, or other complaints.

PAST MEDICAL HISTORY: Negative

SOCIAL HISTORY:

Works at Taco Ringer as a cook
Lives with his girlfriend of 3 months
Became sexually active and had multiple sexual partners starting one year ago
Has been monogamous for 3 months and 1 day
Smokes marijuana on weekends
Drink on weeknights

ROS:

Essentially non-contributory

PHYSICAL EXAMINATION:

Only pertinent findings:

Scleral icterus
Liver down about 5 cm and has a span of 17 cm; slightly tender
Spleen tip palpable
No spider angiomas

LABORATORY:

Anti HAV IgM Negative
Anti HAV IgG Positive
Anti-HBc IgM Positive
HBsAg negative
Anti-HBc IgG negative

Which of the following is the best interpretation of the laboratory data?

A. He has acute hepatitis A and past infection with hepatitis B.
B. He has chronic hepatitis A and acute hepatitis B.
C. He has chronic hepatitis A and chronic hepatitis B.
D. He has acute hepatitis B and past infection with A.
E. He has neither hepatitis A or hepatitis B; he is just antibody positive.

35.

A 17-year-old Caucasian male comes in as a referral from his pediatrician. Mark has been having difficulty in the last few months. Initially, he started having bizarre behaviors and was admitted for inpatient psychiatric therapy for a strange psychoneurosis: He kept thinking that if he didn't pass an important test that the world would implode. (Hmm...are *you* feeling this way?). His pediatrician has also been following him for chronic active hepatitis, with all serologies for hepatitis A, B, and C being negative. EBV studies are also negative, as well as CMV.

His physical exam is remarkable for this finding when you look in his eyes (see Figure):

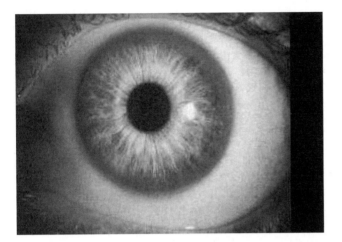

Additionally, on physical exam he has hepatomegaly with a span of about 13 cm. Besides his psychosis (which appears now to be under control), he has a slight tremor to his left upper extremity.

Laboratory from his pediatrician:
His AST and ALT are 3–5 times normal and fluctuate. He has no sign of biliary obstruction. Additionally he has a Coombs-negative hemolytic anemia.

Based on your findings, which of the following is the most likely diagnosis?

    A. Alcohol-induced cirrhosis
    B. Unexplained hepatitis
    C. Drug abuse
    D. Wilson disease
    E. Cross-Hannaman syndrome

36.

A 75-year-old patient presents to the hospital with his second cerebrovascular accident. Although he was functional after his first episode, after 3 days in the hospital he is still unable to speak, and attempts at swallowing liquids have led to coughing.

Which of the following is true?

    A. Percutaneous endoscopic gastrostomy (PEG) is appropriate intervention to allow hydration and nutrition.
    B. Antibiotics are not required before a PEG since this is a sterile procedure.
    C. Most patients with a PEG placement have severe reflux afterwards; therefore, one should consider a surgical jejunostomy instead.
    D. Upper endoscopy should be done to evaluate the cause of dysphagia prior to any decision on long-term management.
    E. None of the choices is true.

37.

A 50-year-old male presents to the office with 10 years of typical heartburn symptoms. The symptoms typically occur after large meals or when he lies down at night. He has treated these with OTC dosing of famotidine, as well as frequent use of antacids. The symptoms are non-progressive but present 4 days out of each week. He recently read a newspaper article about the increased risk of esophageal cancer in patients with reflux and is upset and wants to get "checked out."

Past medical history is significant for hypertension treated with amlodipine. He is overweight by about 20 pounds.

ROS: He denies any dysphagia, hoarseness, or sore throat; he has never had any asthma or wheezing

SOCIAL HISTORY: Significant for the patient being a non-smoker who drinks 1–2 glasses of alcohol per day

PHYSICAL EXAMINATION: Unremarkable except for a mildly overweight, middle-aged man

You schedule an upper endoscopy that reveals a small hiatal hernia and several erosions in the distal esophagus consistent with Grade II reflux esophagitis. No Barrett esophagus changes are identified. The rest of the exam is normal.

Your recommendation to the patient for the most complete relief of his symptoms would be which of the following?

   A. Omeprazole 20 mg PO, before breakfast
   B. Omeprazole 20 mg PO q hs
   C. Ranitidine 150 mg bid, before breakfast and hs
   D. Ranitidine 150 mg bid and sucralfate 1 gm PO qid – before meals and hs

38.

A 30-year-old male with a long history of asthma is admitted to the Intensive Care Unit with severe respiratory failure. He requires intubation, ventilatory support, bronchodilators, and IV corticosteroids. He has no other medical problems. After 3 days of therapy, the critical care physicians are able to extubate the patient. However, once there is initiation of oral feedings, the patient complains of severe pain while swallowing. Upper endoscopy is performed and reveals multiple small, shallow ulcers in the distal esophagus. Biopsies are pending at this time.

Which of the following is the least likely diagnosis?

   A. Herpes esophagitis
   B. *Candida* esophagitis
   C. Pill-induced esophagitis
   D. Reflux esophagitis
   E. Mechanical injury related to nasogastric tube

39.

A 25-year-old male presents to the office complaining of intermittent chest pain for the past year. This is a brief pain that lasts only 1–2 minutes in duration. It is unpredictable and not related to meals. It never wakes him. He says that it can radiate into the left chest, and he describes it as a sharp stabbing pain. There are no other factors in his past medical history. He does have a family history of premature coronary artery disease. In his social history, he admits to significant stress in his job as an IRS auditor. In review of systems, he denies any dysphagia or any typical reflux symptoms. Physical examination is normal.

Stress echo: normal
EGD: normal
Esophageal motility: This demonstrated mostly normal peristalsis, but there were intermittent simultaneous contractions seen. Lower esophageal sphincter pressure was 40, but with complete relaxation. The amplitude in the esophageal body was 140 (normal 40–180).

Which of the following is true?

    A. Nitrates are effective therapy and well tolerated for this condition.
    B. Empiric dilatation may help this pain.
    C. 24-hour ambulatory pH probe may reveal abnormal reflux even without typical reflux symptoms.
    D. Additional cardiac tests are needed (e.g., cardiac catheterization).
    E. You should get a CT of the chest.

40.

Which of the following is the <u>least</u> common GI location for carcinoid tumor?

    A. Rectum
    B. Ileum
    C. Stomach
    D. Appendix
    E. Colon

41.

A 25-year-old patient with ulcerative colitis, who has been in clinical remission for the past year on mesalamine, develops diarrhea and abdominal pain. She denies rectal bleeding. This is similar to past flares of the colitis except for the lack of bleeding.

PAST MEDICAL HISTORY: Ulcerative colitis for 5 years; on mesalamine 2.4 gm per day

ROS: Recent abscessed tooth that required 5 days of clindamycin; complains of occasional joint pain

PHYSICAL EXAMINATION: Temperature 99° F, no apparent distress; abdomen is soft and nontender, although slightly distended

LABORATORY TESTS: Hgb 12.0, WBC 15,500

You recommend which of the following?

A. Check the stool for *Clostridium difficile* toxin before initiating therapy.
B. Admit to the hospital for IV corticosteroids and careful monitoring for possible toxic megacolon.
C. Check for fecal leukocytes and if positive, treat with metronidazole.
D. Perform an unprepped flexible sigmoidoscopy to assess for pseudomembranes.
E. Send a stool culture for *Clostridium difficile*.

42.

A 45-year-old woman presents with abdominal discomfort, distention, and diarrhea. These symptoms have been present about 6 months. She describes 5–6 bowel movements a day that are loose and foul smelling. Her past medical history is significant in that she has been told by one of her physicians in the past that she may have scleroderma. Review of systems is significant for a 5-lb. weight loss.

PHYSICAL EXAMINATION: The skin over the face and hands is tight, consistent with scleroderma. There is slight distention of the abdomen with tympany. There is no focal tenderness or any palpable masses.

Upper GI/small bowel series: This demonstrated decreased gastric motility and numerous diverticula present coming off the jejunum.

Which of the following pharmacologic interventions is most appropriate?

A. Metoclopramide 10 mg PO qid
B. Amoxicillin-clavulanate 875 mg PO bid plus metronidazole
C. Erythromycin 250 mg PO tid
D. Octreotide 200 mcg SubQ bid
E. Azithromycin 500 mg PO q day x 5 days

43.

Which of the following is true regarding the treatment of chronic hepatitis C?

A. By attaching a polyethylene glycol moiety to interferon alpha, there is an increased response rate.
B. Interferon alpha given alone 6 million units three times a week is more efficacious than when used with ribavirin.
C. Infectious complications related to neutropenia frequently require cessation of antiviral therapy.
D. Patients rarely respond to therapy.
E. HCV genotype I is more responsive to therapy.

44.

A 45-year-old patient with known cirrhosis secondary to alcoholic liver disease presents with hematemesis and melena. He has no prior history of gastrointestinal bleeding. He was stabilized in the ER and transferred to the Intensive Care Unit. Upper endoscopy reveals bleeding esophageal varices that are successfully treated with band ligation. Over the next several days, he shows no signs of further bleeding. He is improving overall and tolerating oral feedings. On the third day, he develops a fever to 102° F and is noted to have a decrease in his mental status.

Physical exam reveals a jaundiced male. He has prominent ascites in the abdomen. The abdomen does not have any focal tenderness. There is enlargement of the spleen and the liver edge is 3 cm below the right costal margin.

LABORATORY TESTS: WBC 18,500; Hgb 9; Bili 4.0; AST 70; ALT 45

Which of the following is true?

A. This is unlikely to be spontaneous bacterial peritonitis, since he has no abdominal pain or tenderness.
B. Paracentesis is the appropriate diagnostic test at this time.
C. Antibiotics have not been shown to be beneficial when given prophylactically to cirrhotics with upper GI hemorrhage.
D. If the paracentesis yields acidic fluid with a PMN count greater than 250, this confirms SBP and treatment should be initiated with gentamicin.
E. If the paracentesis yields acidic fluid with a PMN count greater than 100, this confirms SBP and treatment should be initiated with gentamicin.

45.

A 40-year-old man presents to the office with a chief complaint of fatigue. He has been very distressed and upset since his older brother recently required a liver transplantation for hemochromatosis. He has been told that this disease can be hereditary and that he needs to be "checked out." He is an otherwise healthy man who has never had any significant medical problems. He has 1 drink of alcohol per night. He takes no other medications. On review of systems, he complains of occasional knee pain after tennis.

PHYSICAL EXAMINATION: The skin is normal pigmentation. The sclera is anicteric, and there is no sign of jaundice. There is no hepatomegaly or enlargement of the spleen. No ascites felt on exam.

Lab tests included a normal CBC, AST 28, ALT 24, alk phos 72.
You consider further testing.

Which of the following is true?

A. A serum ferritin of greater than 500 is diagnostic for hereditary hemochromatosis.
B. Laboratory tests for iron are notoriously unreliable and therefore not needed. This patient should have a liver biopsy looking for hepatic iron concentration.
C. Transferrin saturation greater than 50% should prompt further evaluation, including HFE gene determination.
D. No further testing is necessary with normal laboratories and no hepatomegaly or abnormal skin color.
E. A serum ferritin of greater than 700 is diagnostic for hereditary hemochromatosis.

46.

Which of the following is the most common cause of acute fulminant liver failure in the United States?

    A. Wilson disease
    B. Hepatitis B virus
    C. Ingestion of amanita species mushrooms
    D. Drug hepatotoxicity
    E. Hepatitis C virus

47.

A 55-year-old male is referred for evaluation of microcytic anemia. He was recently in the hospital after presenting to the Emergency Room with a Hgb of 7, and an MCV of 65. He had noticed gradual weakness for 3 months prior to this but thought it was due to a viral syndrome. He denied any specific complaints and, in fact, denied any overt rectal bleeding or change in bowel movements. While he was in the hospital, he had an upper endoscopy, which was normal. Colonoscopy was also performed with good visualization of the colon to the cecum, again without any abnormalities. He received 2 units of packed RBCs and was discharged on oral iron.

PAST MEDICAL HISTORY: Otherwise unremarkable; he is on no medications; he does not take aspirin or NSAIDs

FAMILY HISTORY: Negative for any specific diseases of the GI tract

SOCIAL HISTORY: Otherwise negative

REVIEW OF SYSTEMS: Significant for fatigue and dyspnea on exertion; otherwise negative

PHYSICAL EXAMINATION: Healthy 55-year-old; although he was pale at the time of admission, his color has now returned after the blood transfusion

At this point, you recommend which of the following?

    A. Upper GI small bowel series
    B. Trial of estrogen empirically for presumed AV malformation bleeding
    C. CT scan of the abdomen and pelvis
    D. Tagged RBC bleeding scan
    E. Ultrasound of the liver

48.

A 70-year-old male patient has absolutely no complaints. He is in for his routine checkup. At this time, he is found to have a Hgb of 10.7 with an MCV of 72. He denies any weakness or fatigue.

PAST MEDICAL HISTORY:	Significant for hypertension; his only medication is lisinopril
SOCIAL HISTORY:	Non-contributory with no alcohol or tobacco history; he is active and walks every day
FAMILY HISTORY:	Negative for gastrointestinal disease
REVIEW OF SYSTEMS:	Denies any abdominal pain, reflux, or change in bowel movements; he has never had any overt bleeding
PHYSICAL EXAMINATION:	Healthy 70-year-old patient
HEENT:	Normal
Chest:	Clear and has a normal cardiac exam
Abdomen:	Soft and nontender without organomegaly; his stool is brown and heme negative

You schedule a colonoscopy, which reveals moderate diverticulosis in the sigmoid colon. There is a single 5-mm AVM found in the cecum. There is also a 5-mm sessile rectal polyp, which was removed.

At this point, which of the following would you recommend?

    A. Endoscopic ablation of the AV malformation, because this was the likely cause of anemia.
    B. Elective sigmoid resection, because diverticulosis was the most likely cause of bleeding.
    C. Place patient on estrogen therapy to stop the bleeding from the AV malformation.
    D. Start patient on iron and monitor the Hgb every 2 months.
    E. Administer an H-2 blocker initially.

49.

A 45-year-old male presents to the Emergency Room with hematemesis that occurred 8 hours before presentation. Just prior to presentation, he noted a black tarry stool. He does not remember vomiting prior to the episode, but admits to heavy drinking and poor recollection of some events.

PAST MEDICAL HISTORY:	Significant for no medical problems
SOCIAL HISTORY:	Significant in that he says he drinks a 6-pack of beer every night and smokes 1 pack of cigarettes per day
REVIEW OF SYSTEMS:	Significant for his denial of abdominal pain, reflux symptoms, chest pain, dyspnea, or syncope

PHYSICAL EXAMINATION:

HR 120, BP 90/60; after 1 liter of IV fluid, the HR is 100 and BP is 120/80

HEENT:	Sclera anicteric
Chest:	Clear to auscultation
Cardiac:	Normal
Abdomen:	Soft and non-tender without hepatosplenomegaly; stool black and heme positive

LABORATORY: Significant for Hgb 11.6

Endoscopy: Reveals a 2-cm linear tear in the distal esophagus without active bleeding or visible vessel. The rest of the stomach is normal. There is no blood present in the stomach, and the duodenum is clear as well.

Which of the following is true?

A. Endoscopic treatment should be performed using a heater probe applied to the length of the tear.
B. Mallory-Weiss tears rarely bleed sufficiently to require blood transfusions.
C. This patient will likely not have recurrent bleeding after admission, though his HCT will likely fall with hydration.
D. The linear erosion is probably due to reflux rather than Mallory-Weiss tear, since there is no report of prior retching.

50.

A 60-year-old female comes in the office with the complaint that 7 days ago she had a dark tarry stool. For several days after that, she didn't have any bowel movements. Yesterday she had her normal brown stool. She initially thought the dark stool was due to something that she might have eaten, but her daughter convinced her to come and get checked out. She denies any weakness or lightheadedness. At no time has she had any abdominal pain recently.

PAST MEDICAL HISTORY:	Unremarkable; she has no medical problems; she does take an aspirin everyday for general purposes
SOCIAL HISTORY:	Significant for no alcohol or tobacco use
FAMILY HISTORY:	Negative
REVIEW OF SYSTEMS:	She denies any chest pain, syncope, reflux symptoms or SOB
LABS:	Hgb 12, MCV 88; other labs are normal

Urgent EGD done in an outpatient facility reveals a 1-cm duodenal ulcer with a clean base. CLO test is done from an antral biopsy, and the preliminary result is negative.

Which of the following should you recommend?

A. Discharge home on lansoprazole 30 mg qd with caution to return to the ER in case of another black stool.
B. Endoscopic treatment with a heater probe to the entire base of the ulcer, and then admit to the ICU for careful observation overnight.
C. Admit to General Medicine ward, and obtain a surgery consult in case of rebleeding.
D. Admission to an observation unit with HCT every 4 hours and discharge the next day if stable.

51.

A 50-year-old woman of Irish descent is referred to your office after another internist noted microcytic anemia on a routine test. She has no specific complaints. She describes 2 soft and slightly loose bowel movements every day, but this has been her normal pattern for many years. It has not progressed in any way. She denies any abdominal pain, although admits to some non-specific bloating, again present for many years.

PAST MEDICAL HISTORY: She is on thyroid replacement for hypothyroidism; she is status-post hysterectomy and is on replacement estrogen as well

FAMILY HISTORY: Negative for any gastrointestinal disease

SOCIAL HISTORY: Negative

REVIEW OF SYSTEMS: She denies fever, chills, weight loss, chest pain, or dyspnea

PHYSICAL EXAMINATION:
Unremarkable except for slight paleness to the skin

HEENT:	Sclera anicteric
Chest and Cardiac exam:	Normal
Abdomen:	Soft and nontender without organomegaly; stool brown and heme negative

LABS: Hgb 9.0, MCV 70, serum iron 8, TIBC 400
You order stools for occult blood and these are negative x 3.

Which of the following should you recommend?

    A. Flat plate x-ray of the abdomen and a trial of pancreatic enzymes if calcifications are found.
    B. IgG antigliadin and antiendomysial antibodies; if positive, treat with steroids and gluten-free diet.
    C. Colonoscopy and endoscopy. If the latter is grossly normal, obtain oriented biopsies of the duodenum.
    D. Order upper GI small bowel series.

52.

A 40-year-old patient has had ulcerative colitis since age 20. In the past 5 years, he has been completely asymptomatic and in remission since the initiation of therapy with azathioprine. His bowel movements are normal, and he never notices rectal bleeding. He further denies any abdominal pain.

PAST MEDICAL HISTORY: Significant only for ulcerative colitis; his medications include sulfasalazine 2 gm a day and azathioprine 100 mg a day

FAMILY HISTORY: Positive for 1 cousin with Crohn disease

REVIEW OF SYSTEMS: Denies any jaundice, itching, or abdominal pain

LABS: Alk phos 410, AST 50, ALT 68, bili 2.2, d. bili 1.8, Hgb 12, WBC 5,000

Ultrasound reveals a normal size liver and no enlargement of the bile ducts

Which of the following studies should you recommend as the next best step?

    A. Liver biopsy
    B. ERCP
    C. Laparoscopic cholecystectomy
    D. Abdominal CT scan

53.

A 52-year-old female originally presented to the ER with severe acute abdominal pain. This pain was unlike any pain she had ever experienced in the past. It radiated to the back and was associated with nausea and vomiting. The pain started 8 hours earlier and had been constant since that time.

PAST MEDICAL HISTORY: Significant for hyperlipidemia; the only medicine is atorvastatin

FAMILY HISTORY: Positive for CAD

SOCIAL HISTORY: Denies any alcohol use; does not smoke cigarettes

REVIEW OF SYSTEMS: She denies any change in her bowel habits, chest pain, or SOB

PHYSICAL EXAMINATION: She is in moderate distress; HR 110, BP 110/60
    Skin: Turgor is normal
    HEENT: Unremarkable
    Chest: Clear to auscultation
    Cardiovascular: Normal, except for the tachycardia
    Abdominal exam: Tender in the epigastrium to mild palpation; there is no rebound or guarding; there is no referred pain on exam; stool is heme negative
    Extremities: Normal

LABS: Amylase 1242, lipase 865, bili 1.9, AST 86, ALT 92, alk phos 245, Hgb 15, WBC 13,000

An ultrasound was done on admission, which revealed a gallbladder with multiple filling defects consistent with stones. The pancreas is edematous. The common bile duct was identified and was of normal diameter.

On the 2nd day of admission, the amylase increased to 1450, and the bilirubin climbed to 3.5. However, at the time, the patient felt much better. She was receiving IV meperidine, but felt she didn't need this anymore.

It is now the 5th day and her amylase has been rechecked and found to be completely normal. Her abdomen is soft and nontender. She is not jaundiced and is now tolerating a liquid diet.

Which of the following studies would you recommend?

    A. ERCP now, since there is a high likelihood of stones present in the CBD
    B. Discharge from the hospital now and then elective cholecystectomy in 2 weeks
    C. Open cholecystectomy with common bile duct exploration now before discharge from the hospital
    D. Percutaneous transhepatic cholangiogram

54.

A 70-year-old female complains of vague abdominal discomfort. She has never had any severe pain. This discomfort has been present for several months. It is located in the middle-to-upper abdomen.

PAST MEDICAL HISTORY: Unremarkable; she is healthy and does not take medications except for a multi-vitamin

SOCIAL HISTORY: She is a very healthy woman who enters 10k races on a regular basis

FAMILY HISTORY: Positive for brother with colon cancer

ROS: She denies any jaundice, weight loss, or change in bowel habits; she has not had any back pain or itching

LABS: CBC and LFTs are all within normal limits

You order an abdominal CT scan, which demonstrates a 7-cm cyst in the tail of the pancreas.

Which of the following should you recommend?

A. Check CA19-9 level; if normal, reassure the patient and recommend no further workup.
B. CT-directed needle aspiration. If the fluid is negative for cytology, then you can reassure the patient.
C. Consult surgery for elective resection of the tail of the pancreas with removal of the cyst.
D. Start pancreatic enzymes, because this is likely a pseudocyst from occult chronic pancreatitis. If the cyst is persistent 3 months later, then recommend percutaneous drainage by the radiologist.

55.

Four people present to the Emergency Room—all within 30 minutes of each other—with similar symptoms. They all describe the sudden onset of nausea and severe vomiting. Shortly thereafter, all of them developed profuse diarrhea, and now all complain of severe weakness. All 4 people had been together that afternoon—they all work for a company in Colorado Springs that provides study material for doctors taking Board exams. The company was celebrating the summer with a picnic. There were a variety of different foods that were brought by different people, including deviled eggs, ham sandwiches, jambalaya, sashimi, barbecued chicken, and hamburgers on the grill, as well as raspberries and melon balls. None of the people involved remember eating any other items. All had been swimming in a creek, and 2 admit to possibly ingesting some of the creek water. The nausea started almost exactly 4 hours after the picnic.

On presentation to the ER, the person complaining of the most profound weakness has a blood pressure of 80/40 with a heart rate of 140 and decreased skin turgor. Temperature is 97° F. Abdomen is soft and nontender. IV fluids have been started.

Which of the following is true?

A. This is probable *Salmonella* related to undercooking of poultry.
B. This is likely a *Staphylococcus aureus* food poisoning.
C. This is likely giardiasis from drinking the creek water in Colorado, which is commonly infested with *Giardia*.
D. This is likely *E. coli* O157 related to the undercooked hamburger.

PULMONARY MEDICINE

56.

Three dishwashers started working at 8:30 a.m. By 1:00 p.m., 11 workers were involved in washing the dishes since there was a huge banquet the previous night, leaving lots of dirty dishes.
The dishwashing procedures consisted of:

1. Pre-rinsing the dirty dishes by hand in a water tank.
2. Washing the pre-rinsed dishes in the automatic dishwasher.
3. Draining the washed dishes and placing them in cupboards.

Starting around 2:00 p.m., workers began complaining of such symptoms as headaches and dizziness. By 2:30 p.m., all workers showed the same symptoms. Two seriously affected workers were taken to a local hospital by ambulance; the other nine workers were also eventually taken to the hospital for treatment.

One of the workers arriving in the ER is a 54-year-old woman whose last memory was washing asparagus off a plate. The next thing she remembers was riding in the ambulance.

PAST MEDICAL HISTORY:	Peptic ulcer disease, fibromyalgia
MEDICATIONS:	Unknown anxiolytic, estrogen
FAMILY HISTORY:	Unknown
SOCIAL HISTORY:	Divorced; lives with her boyfriend in a trailer park; smokes 3 packs/cigarettes/day; drinks a 6-pack of beer daily
ROS:	Positives: Headache Dizziness Weakness Nausea Difficulty concentrating Dyspnea Visual changes

PHYSICAL EXAMINATION:
BP 126/91, HR 86, RR 30, T 98.8° F

MS:	Oriented to name only; speech without dysarthria; 2/3 recall at 5 minutes
General:	Erythema to face and trunk
HEENT:	PERRLA, EOMI, Throat clear
Neck:	No masses
Heart:	RRR without murmurs
Lungs:	CTA
Abdomen:	+BS, soft, nontender
Neuro:	CN grossly intact; reflexes equal and symmetrical
Motor:	Full strength throughout with normal muscle tone and bulk
Sensory:	Unremarkable

ABG: 7.41/30/370 with O_2 Sat 98% on 100% FiO_2; carboxyhemoglobin level is 26%

Which of the following is the most likely diagnosis based on the epidemiology of multiple people being ill and this woman's ABG results?

   A. Allergic reaction to dishwasher detergent
   B. Carbon monoxide poisoning
   C. Influenza A outbreak
   D. Meningococcemia
   E. Asthma

57.

A 45-year-old man presents with a history of stable asthma on the following regimen of medications for 20 years: Cromolyn sodium, theophylline, and inhaled steroids.

He is doing well; however, last weekend he developed a sore throat and a cough. He went to a local "doc in the box" and was prescribed an unknown antibiotic, which he has continued to take. You are appalled that he was put on an antibiotic for a viral infection. Meanwhile, the patient throws up on your shoe and says he has been really nauseated for 2 days and hasn't been able to keep anything down.

Physical exam findings are within normal limits except that his mucous membranes are a little dry. His vital signs are normal and he does not have any signs of dehydration at this point.

Which of the following antibiotics could be causing his troubles (and the need for you to get new shoes)?

   A. Amoxicillin
   B. Sulfamethoxazole
   C. Cefixime
   D. Ciprofloxacin

58.

A 38-year-old man presents with an acute asthma attack. He has been feeling bad for a few days. This morning he awakened and could not breathe. When you see him in the ER, he is anxious and cannot talk because of his discomfort. You realize that you have to act quickly and note in his chart that he has had to be ventilated 3 times in the past for severe asthma exacerbations.

PAST MEDICAL HISTORY:	As above Most recent hospitalization was 1 year ago at another hospital Has been on an inhaled medium-dose steroid, an inhaled long-acting beta$_2$-agonist, and zafirlukast
SOCIAL HISTORY:	Works as a puppet maker Lives with his friend Poppito
FAMILY HISTORY:	Mother with severe asthma Father with coronary artery disease
REVIEW OF SYSTEMS:	Deferred for the moment—he is about to CRASH!

PHYSICAL EXAMINATION:
BP 150/95, RR 40 with shallow breaths and marked accessory muscle use, P 120

HEENT:	Cyanotic around his lips
Heart:	RRR without murmurs, rubs, or gallops
Lungs:	Faint squeaks is all you hear
Abdomen:	Benign

LABORATORY:

ABG: pH 7.06
PCO_2 90
PaO_2 55
Oxygen Saturation 84%
On 100% FiO_2

You realize that you are not going to be able to ventilate him effectively without putting him on mechanical ventilation.

Which of the following ventilator settings are appropriate for a severely ill asthmatic patient?

A. High rate, small tidal volume, high flows
B. Low rate, high tidal volume, high flows
C. Low rate, high tidal volume, low flows
D. Low rate, small tidal volume, high flows
E. High rate, high tidal volume, low flows

59.

You are seeing a 70-year-old man with severe COPD for follow-up. He quit smoking about 5 years ago, but his health has continued to deteriorate. He is at the point now where he cannot ambulate in his home without getting severely short of breath. He wants to know if there is anything else that he can do to improve his health status. You explain to him that supplemental oxygen may be beneficial to him, but you will have to do some laboratory studies to demonstrate to Medicare that they should pay for this. He agrees to the testing.

PAST MEDICAL HISTORY:	History of coronary artery disease; status-post 4 vessel CABG 5 years ago
	History of gout
	History of MI in 1992
	Multiple hospitalizations for COPD exacerbations—about once a year on average in the last 10 years
	Morbid obesity
SOCIAL HISTORY:	Lives with his new wife of 2 years, Bambi, a 28-year-old dancer
	Drinks 2 glasses of red wine every night
	Quit smoking 5 years ago; before that, he smoked 2 packs/day for 50+ years
FAMILY HISTORY:	No change from the last 20 H and P's you've done; documented well for the chart though (of course)
REVIEW OF SYSTEMS:	Occasional headache
	Occasional sore throat
	Dyspnea on exertion at 5 feet

Stable exertional chest pain; usually relieved with one nitroglycerin or rest
Cough: productive cough every morning of every day; no change in character or frequency
No nausea or vomiting
Increased difficulty initiating his urine stream

PHYSICAL EXAMINATION: BP 126/67, HR 86, RR 28, Temp 97.9°F

MS:	Oriented x 3
General:	Obese man in no distress at rest; but when you saw him walk in from the waiting room he was markedly distressed.
HEENT:	Left cataract
	Throat clear; dentures
Neck:	No masses, no bruits
Heart:	RRR without murmurs, rubs, or gallops
Lungs:	Chronic crackles throughout; no change from previous examinations; prolonged expiratory phase noted as usual
Abdomen:	+BS, soft, nontender
Neuro:	CN grossly intact; reflexes equal and symmetrical
Motor:	Full strength throughout with normal muscle tone and bulk
Sensory:	Unremarkable

LABORATORY:
ABG: 7.5 PCO_2 = 50; PaO_2 = 50; Oxygen saturation 85%

Based on your findings, which of the following should you recommend?

A. Supplemental oxygen is not indicated based on his laboratory values.
B. Supplemental oxygen is not indicated based on his physical examination.
C. Supplemental oxygen should be worn 24 hours a day by this patient.
D. Supplemental oxygen may be indicated, but you need more information.
E. Supplemental oxygen worn intermittently would be better than continuous oxygen therapy because of the concern that his respiratory drive will be too suppressed on continuous oxygen therapy.

60.

A 35-year-old Caucasian male with chronic lung disease of unknown etiology at this point presents for follow-up care. He has had episodes of sinusitis, bronchiectasis, and pancreatic insufficiency for at least 30 years. He has had recurrent pneumonias over the last 10 years. Usually his pneumonias are associated with pseudomonal infections.

PAST MEDICAL HISTORY: As above

FAMILY HISTORY:	Older brother with similar complaints
	Mother: healthy
	Father: healthy, of Scandinavian ancestry
	Has 2 sons, both healthy
SOCIAL HISTORY:	Works as a used car salesman
	Doesn't smoke
	Doesn't drink
	Listens to country western music

REVIEW OF SYSTEMS: Frequent colds
Frequent sinus infections
Frequent bloody noses because of increased blowing of nose
Chronic cough

PHYSICAL EXAMINATION:
BP 120/70, RR 18, Temp 98.5° F, P 90

HEENT:	Nasal polyps; PERRLA, EOMI
	Throat: normal tonsils
Neck:	Supple, no masses
Heart:	RRR without murmurs, rubs, or gallops
Lungs:	Coarse breath sounds; occasional expiratory wheeze anteriorly and posteriorly
Abdomen:	No HSM, nontender
Extremities:	Clubbing present, no cyanosis
GU:	Normal male genitalia; no masses

Based on your history and physical exam, which of the following does <u>not</u> support the diagnosis of cystic fibrosis (CF)?

A. Nasal polyps
B. Recurrent sinusitis
C. Recurrent pneumonias
D. Family history
E. Clubbing

61.

Yesterday a 20-year-old male presented with adult respiratory distress syndrome due to shock, and he required mechanical ventilation and positive end-expiratory pressure (PEEP). His condition gradually improves.

Which of the following would <u>not</u> be a criterion for cessation of mechanical ventilation?

A. Vital capacity greater than 15 mL/kg
B. Tidal volume 4 to 5 mL/kg
C. FiO_2 35%
D. PEEP 10 cm H_2O

62.

A 70-year-old man with a history of working in a brickyard for 50 years presents for evaluation at his granddaughter's request. He has been retired for 10 years. He is still active and plays bingo at the local church every day. He usually wins about once a week. Members of his bingo group are around his age, and recently one of his contemporaries at the bingo hall was diagnosed with tuberculosis. Your patient has been healthy and has no complaints. He denies weight loss, cough, fevers, or night sweats.

PAST MEDICAL HISTORY: Prostatic hypertrophy diagnosed 5 years ago; doing well currently
HTN for 40 years

MEDICATIONS: Propranolol 20 mg q day
ECASA q day

SOCIAL HISTORY: Widowed for 20 years
Lives alone; still drives without difficulty
Volunteers at local nursing home on occasion
Never smoked
Doesn't drink alcohol

FAMILY HISTORY: Mother died at age 80 of "old age"
Father died at age 75 of stroke
Brother alive, 68, healthy except HTN
Sister died at age 50 of stroke

REVIEW OF SYSTEMS: No sore throat
No vision changes
No chest pains
No headaches
Minor arthritis-type pain in knees in the early morning; better with movement
GU symptoms much improved; no difficulty initiating urine stream

PHYSICAL EXAMINATION:
BP 130/69, P 66, RR 15, Temp 98.8° F
Ht 6'1", 190 lbs

HEENT:	PERRLA, EOMI
	TMs clear
	Throat clear
Neck:	Supple, no masses
Heart:	RRR without murmurs, rubs, or gallops
Lungs:	Coarse breath sounds but clear
Abdomen:	Bowel sounds present in all 4 quadrants, no hepatosplenomegaly, nontender
Extremities:	No cyanosis, clubbing, or edema
GU:	Normal male genitalia, no masses

LABORATORY:
CXR: Small nodules located in upper lobes; calcified hilar lymph nodes with "hilar eggshell calcification"
PPD: 20 mm at 72 hours

3 induced sputum samples for AFB: All negative smears and cultures

Based on these findings, which of the following is the most appropriate next step?

A. Ignore +PPD in this 70-year-old man. Sputum tests are negative; therefore, it is unlikely he needs prophylaxis.
B. Initiate workup for asbestos-related disease process.
C. Start treatment for silicosis.
D. Start INH prophylaxis.
E. Initiate 4-drug therapy for tuberculosis.

63.

A 68-year-old man with a history of smoking for 50 years presents to the emergency room with acute onset of shortness of breath and right-sided chest pain, which is sharp and worse with inspiration. His wife says he has had a chronic daily cough for 30 years, but today it was worse—and then he developed this acute shortness of breath.

PAST MEDICAL HISTORY:	Negative for hospitalizations
	Hypertension for 30 years, on various agents in the past
	Diabetes insipidus diagnosed 5 years ago
SOCIAL HISTORY:	Former police officer, retired 6 years
	Lives with wife of 50 years
	Also lives with his 45-year-old unemployed son, which causes a lot of tension in the household according to the patient's wife

You diagnose a pneumothorax in the Emergency Room. His CXR also shows a "honeycomb appearance" with interstitial changes and small cystic spaces in the upper lung fields.

Putting together the pneumothorax with his CXR results, diabetes insipidus, and smoking history, which of the following are you most likely to find at lung biopsy?

  A. Plasma cells
  B. Acid-fast bacilli
  C. Chylous material
  D. Langerhans cells
  E. Fungal elements

64.

A 50-year-old African-American woman with a history of hypertension and obesity presents with a 4-month history of worsening shortness of breath. She had been able to walk up a flight of stairs without any difficulty about 3 months ago. Now she complains of shortness of breath while walking around her home. Also, at night she has a new onset of orthopnea. She denies other symptoms at this point.

PAST MEDICAL HISTORY:	Hypertension for 10 years, treated with HCTZ 25 mg daily
	Delivered 5 healthy children in her 20s; no problems during pregnancies
SOCIAL HISTORY:	Works in a daycare with 30 preschool children
	Says her job is very stressful but less stressful than her previous job, which was as a housemother for a fraternity house
	Never smoked
	Never drank alcohol
	No pets
	Widowed; lives alone
FAMILY HISTORY:	Father, 80; recent MI 1 year ago
	Mother, 79; recent admission to nursing home for Alzheimer's
	Sister, 55; healthy but obese
	Brother, 53; hypertension, on medication
	Sister, 48; with SLE

REVIEW OF SYSTEMS: No headaches
    No chest pain
    No cough
    No fever
    No sweats
    No rashes
    No joint complaints

PHYSICAL EXAMINATION:
    BP 120/85, P 90, RR 16, Temp 98.8° F
    Ht 5'2", Wt 260 lbs

HEENT:	PERRLA, EOMI, discs sharp
	Throat clear
Neck:	Supple, no masses
Heart:	RRR without murmurs, rubs, or gallops; loud pulmonic second sound
Lungs:	Clear to auscultation
Extremities:	Bilateral 2+ pitting edema; no cyanosis or clubbing noted
Skin:	No rashes
Rectal:	Heme negative

LABORATORY: Pulse oximetry on room air was 93% at rest; with walking dropped to 87%

CXR:

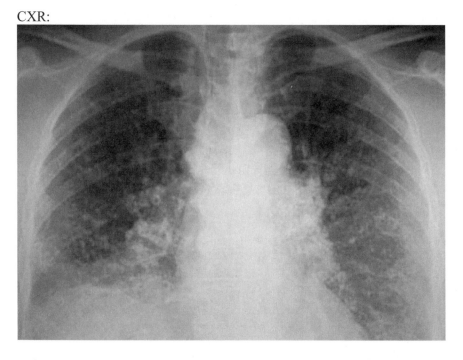

Echocardiogram: Ejection fraction of 80% and pulmonary hypertension with a PA systolic pressure of 61 mmHg. Right ventricular size and function were normal.

Pulmonary function tests: FEV_1 of 0.9 L (43% predicted) and an FVC of 1.6 L (59% predicted). High-resolution CT scan showed diffuse pulmonary nodules and hilar enlargement.

Three sputum samples for acid-fast bacilli were negative. She underwent bronchoscopy with transbronchial biopsy for evaluation of her pulmonary nodules. The bronchoscope showed hyperemia with nodular irregularities and distal concentric narrowing in the main, segmental, and proximal subsegmental bronchi.

The transbronchial biopsy is shown in the figure below. Special stains for fungi and acid-fast bacilli were negative.

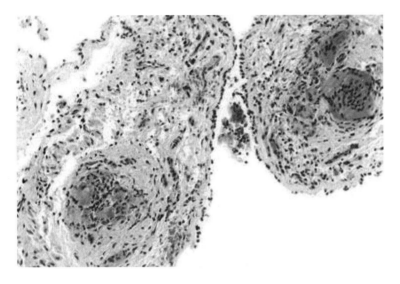

Which of the following is the most likely diagnosis?

    A. Pulmonary sarcoidosis
    B. Tuberculosis
    C. Bacterial pneumonia
    D. Asbestosis
    E. Wegener granulomatosis

65.

A 59-year-old man is seen in follow-up. He was initially evaluated for cavitating pulmonary nodules. He has a history of severe, deforming rheumatoid arthritis for 20 years that has required surgical interventions. In the past he has been on azathioprine (Imuran®), sulfasalazine, hydroxychloroquine (Plaquenil®), and methotrexate. None has been effective recently. He has been taking prednisone (varies from 5 mg to 20 mg a day) for many years. Four months ago, etanercept was begun, and his arthritic pain resolved almost completely. However, over the past 7–8 months he has developed a progressively worsening cough. It has been productive on occasion, but he denies any blood or blood-tinged sputum. Over the last 2 months, he has had increasing shortness of breath with exertion, to the point that he now cannot walk a block without being short of breath.

PAST MEDICAL HISTORY: Diabetes mellitus, adult onset at age 40; probably associated with steroids
                                   Positive PPD 30 years ago and he took INH for one year

SOCIAL HISTORY: Worked as a locksmith for 20 years before having to retire for disability
                             Stopped smoking cigarettes 30 years ago; previously smoked 1 pack/day for 10 years
                             Doesn't drink alcohol

FAMILY HISTORY: Doesn't know; he was adopted

REVIEW OF SYSTEMS: No fever
No chills
No sweats
No chest pain
No weight loss
No change in vision
No appetite changes

PHYSICAL EXAMINATION:
BP 130/82, P 69, RR 17, T 99° F, appears comfortable at rest

HEENT:	PERRLA, EOMI, developing cataract in left eye
	TMs clear
	Throat clear
Neck:	Supple, no masses
Heart:	RRR with murmurs, rubs, or gallops
Lungs:	Diffuse crackles at left base; no wheezes
Abdomen:	Bowel sounds present; no hepatosplenomegaly; no masses
Extremities:	Chronic, symmetric, deforming polyarthritis with moderate synovitis of metacarpophalangeal joints
	Joints were cool and without effusions
	Skin was without evidence of vasculitis or nodules

LABORATORY:

Sputum:	Negative for acid-fast bacilli x 3
Liver functions:	AST 30 U/L; ALT 28 U/L; total bilirubin 0.2 mg/dL; alkaline phosphatase 200 U/L; GGT 20 U/L; albumin 3.5 mg/dL
Renal function:	BUN 10 mg/dL; creatinine 0.5 mg/dL
Urinalysis:	Normal for age

Pulmonary function testing:

	Predicted	Actual	% Predicted
FVC (L)	3.8	1.9	50
FEV_1 (L)	2.6	1.5	58
FEV_1/FVC (%)	70	80	114
DLCO mL/min/mmHg	26.02	8.63	33

Which of the following do the pulmonary function findings suggest?

A. Severe obstructive lung disease, with no restrictive pattern and marked decrease in diffusing capacity
B. Restrictive ventilatory defect only
C. Restrictive ventilatory defect and normal diffusing capacity
D. Restrictive ventilatory defect and marked decrease in diffusing capacity
E. Severe obstructive disease with mild restrictive defect and normal diffusing capacity

66.

A 51-year-old man returns for follow-up. He was seen initially for cavitating pulmonary nodules. He has a history of severe, deforming rheumatoid arthritis for 20 years that has required surgical interventions. In the past, he has been on azathioprine (Imuran®), sulfasalazine, hydroxychloroquine (Plaquenil®), and methotrexate. None has been effective recently. He has been taking prednisone (varies from 5 mg to 20 mg a day) for many years. Four months ago, etanercept was begun and his arthritic pain resolved almost completely. However, over the past 7–8 months, he has developed a progressively worsening cough. It has been productive on occasion, but he denies any blood or blood-tinged sputum. Over the last 2 months, he has had increasing shortness of breath with exertion to the point that he now cannot walk a block without being short of breath.

PAST MEDICAL HISTORY:	Diabetes mellitus, adult in onset at age 40; probably associated with steroids
	Positive PPD 30 years ago and he took INH for one year
SOCIAL HISTORY:	Worked as a locksmith for 20 years before having to retire for disability
	Stopped smoking cigarettes 30 years ago; previously smoked 1 pack/day for 10 years
	Doesn't drink alcohol
FAMILY HISTORY:	Doesn't know; he was adopted
REVIEW OF SYSTEMS:	No fever
	No chills
	No sweats
	No chest pain
	No weight loss
	No change in vision
	No appetite changes

PHYSICAL EXAMINATION:
BP 130/82, P 69, RR 17, T 99° F, comfortable appearing at rest

HEENT:	PERRLA, EOMI, developing cataract in left eye
	TMs clear
	Throat clear
Neck:	Supple, no masses
Heart:	RRR with murmurs, rubs, or gallops
Lungs:	Diffuse crackles at left base; no wheezes
Abdomen:	Bowel sounds present; no hepatosplenomegaly; no masses
Extremities:	Chronic, symmetric, deforming polyarthritis with moderate synovitis of metacarpophalangeal joints.
	Joints were cool and without effusions
	Skin was without evidence of vasculitis or nodules

LABORATORY:

Sputum:	Negative for acid-fast bacilli x 3
Liver functions:	AST 30 U/L; ALT 28 U/L; total bilirubin 0.2 mg/dL; alkaline phosphatase 200 U/L; GGT 20U/L; albumin 3.5 mg/dL
Renal function:	BUN 10 mg/dL; creatinine 0.5 mg/dL
Urinalysis:	Normal for age

Pulmonary function testing:

	Predicted	Actual	% Predicted
FVC (L)	3.8	1.9	50
FEV$_1$ (L)	2.6	1.5	58
FEV$_1$/FVC (%)	70	80	114
DLCO ml/min/mmHg	26.02	8.63	33

A chest CT was performed.
Twelve discrete nodules up to 2.0 cm were identified. Margins were smooth. Eight of them (one shown in the figure below in the right upper lobe) had central necrosis or cavitation.

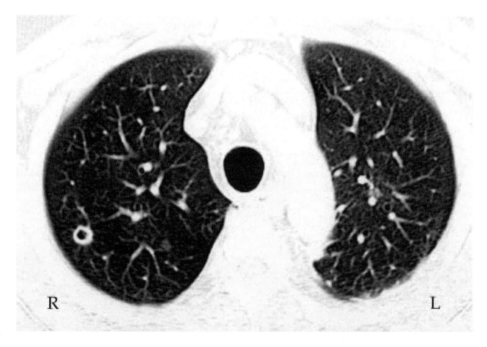

On other images, irregular posterior pleural thickening with some pleural enhancement was present. Scattered bronchiectasis was noted, especially in the posterior basal segment of the left lower lobe.

Biopsies were taken and showed progressive inflammation and necrosis in and around vessels. Arteries are seen adjacent to large nodules and are obliterated by necrosis surrounded by a granulomatous response. An obliterated vessel seen in the next figure is surrounded by granulation tissue; note the necrotic rim with multinucleated giant cell (see arrows).

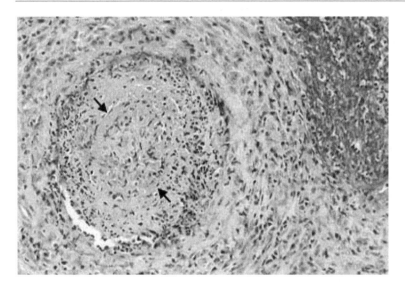

Which of the following is the most likely diagnosis at this point?

A. Tuberculosis
B. Adenocarcinoma
C. Bacterial pneumonia
D. Cavitary rheumatoid nodules
E. Wegener granulomatosis

67.

A 35-year-old woman who had a stillbirth at 25 weeks' gestation approximately 2 weeks previously presents with increasing dyspnea for 6 days, which has progressed to the point that she cannot perform daily activities without resting. Walking to the kitchen from her den causes severe dyspnea. She has no history of orthopnea or paroxysmal nocturnal dyspnea, chest pain, cough, or hemoptysis. She has no history of swelling or pain over her calves, and she has not had a history of bleeding disorder or thromboembolism. She has had 3 full-term normal vaginal deliveries 18 years, 6 years, and 3 years previously.

PAST MEDICAL HISTORY: As above; otherwise negative

SOCIAL HISTORY: Vice-President of Marketing for major computer company
Lives with husband and 3 children
Has never smoked
Drank glass of wine/week before was pregnant; none during pregnancy

REVIEW OF SYSTEMS: No fever
No chills
No productive cough
10-lb. weight loss after delivery

PHYSICAL EXAMINATION:
BP 130/90 mmHg, Pulse 125/min, RR 24/min, Temp 99.1° F

HEENT: PERRLA, EOMI
TMs clear
Throat clear

Neck:	Supple; no masses
	Right jugular venous pressure was not raised
	Wave pattern showed prominent Y collapse
Heart:	Point of maximal impulse: 5th intercostal space in the midclavicular line with a parasternal heave
	S_1 was loud; S_2 with normal splitting with a loud pulmonary component
	S_3 was present
	Holosystolic murmur over left lower sternal border; increasing with inspiration
Lungs:	Scattered rhonchi
Abdomen:	Bowel sounds present; no masses; no hepatosplenomegaly, nontender
Extremities:	No cyanosis, clubbing, or edema

LABORATORY:

ECG:	Right axis deviation, an S-wave in Lead I, and a Q-wave and inverted T-wave in lead III (S1, Q3, T3). T-wave inversion in leads V2 and V3, and S wave persistence in leads V5 and V6.
CXR:	Normal
CBC:	WBC 7100/mm^3; hemoglobin 11.5 gm/dL; platelets 375,000
ESR:	15 mm in 1 hour
Glucose:	90 mg/dL
BUN:	30 mg/dL
Creatinine:	0.8 mg/dL

Echocardiogram: Dilatation of the right ventricle and right atrium. Moderate valvular insufficiency noted (I'm not telling which valve—look up at Physical Examination…you don't need an echo for this!)

Based on your findings, which of the following is the most likely diagnosis?

A. Bacterial pneumonia
B. Sepsis
C. Pulmonary embolism
D. Myocardial infarction
E. Bacterial endocarditis

68.

A 75-year-old Caucasian male with recent fracture of his right femur 3 hours ago presents by ambulance and is seen by the local orthopedist, Dr. Dense, who places him in a cast and admits him for observation. Three hours later, you are called by Dr. Dense because his patient is now short of breath and confused. He thinks the patient might have pneumonia because he is breathing fast. He is consulting you for antibiotic choices. You tell him you will be right there and not to start anything until you evaluate the patient. It is 5:30 p.m. and he has to go because he has tickets for tonight's Universal Wrestling Federation Tournament, and he doesn't want to miss seeing Tony "the Body" in action tonight. You tell him you will take over the care for the respiratory disorder. He grunts and seems relieved.

On evaluation, you find a disheveled elderly man lying in the bed in traction. He is having some difficulty breathing. He has supplemental oxygen with a 40% FiO$_2$ facemask that is keeping his pulse oximetry at 95%. He is unable to answer any questions due to his dyspnea, and he is also quite confused. (Uh-oh; how are you going to get that extensive ROS to bill Medicare?) Eventually, he says the year is 1960 and that you are his 5th grade school teacher.

PHYSICAL EXAMINATION:
    BP 130/70, P 99, Temp 99° F, RR 24

HEENT:	PERRLA, EOMI; conjunctival petechiae
	TMs clear
	Throat clear
Neck:	Supple, no masses; petechiae on neck
Heart:	RRR without murmurs, rubs, or gallops
Lungs:	Coarse breath sounds; few basilar scattered crackles
Abdomen:	Bowel sounds present; no hepatosplenomegaly
Extremities:	No cyanosis, clubbing, some edema on the fractured leg at the ankle; exam of fractured extremity limited but neuro-vasculature looks to be grossly intact

LABORATORY: pending

Based on your history and physical findings, which of the following is the most likely diagnosis?

A. Aspiration pneumonia
B. Fat embolism
C. Cerebrovascular accident
D. Drug toxicity
E. Hospital psychosis

69.

A 50-year-old man with a history of pneumonia diagnosed 2 days ago presents for follow-up. He was seen as an outpatient and sent home on oral levofloxacin. He says he took one pill and it made his stomach hurt, so he stopped the medication. He said he meant to call and let you know, but he was too busy and thought he would get better without the medicine. Now he complains of right-sided chest pain that is pleuritic in character. He says it really hurts to take a deep breath.

PAST MEDICAL HISTORY:	Essentially negative; few office visits for sildenafil prescriptions
SOCIAL HISTORY:	Works as an attorney; prosecutes medical malpractice cases
	Lives alone
FAMILY HISTORY:	Mother alive and healthy
	Father died at age 70 of myocardial infarction
	Brother healthy 49, mechanic
REVIEW OF SYSTEMS:	Fever has been persistent and unremitting since early this morning
	Chills prominent
	Sputum production has increased markedly since yesterday
	Chest pain as described above
	Minor sore throat
	Generalized body aches and pains
	No arthritis
	No vision changes
	No rash

PHYSICAL EXAMINATION:
  BP 120/70, P 90, RR 20 (splinting), Temp 103.5° F
  HEENT: PERRLA, EOMI
      TMs clear
      Throat clear
  Neck: Supple; no masses
  Heart: RRR without murmurs, rubs, or gallops
  Lungs: Upper lung fields clear
      Left lower lung has scattered crackles
      Right lower lung has the following localized findings: Absent breath sounds; dullness to percussion; vocal fremitus is absent
  Abdomen: Bowel sounds are present; no hepatosplenomegaly
  Extremities: No cyanosis, clubbing, or edema
  Skin: No rashes noted now.

LABORATORY:
  WBC: 15,000 cells/mm^3 with 80% polys and 10% bands
     Hemoglobin/Hematocrit: 15.5 mg/dL; 52%
     Platelets: 350,000
  CXR: Marked consolidation of the Right LL with pleural effusion noted bilaterally; right much greater than left
  Pleural fluid:
     WBC 70,000 with 90% polys
     pH 7.02
     Gram stain: Few lancet-shaped Gram-positive diplococci

Based on your findings, which of the following is the most appropriate next step?

A. Admit to the hospital, start intravenous ceftriaxone plus azithromycin, and observe on therapy 24 hours before placing a chest tube.
B. Admit to the hospital, start intravenous ceftriaxone plus azithromycin; get pulmonary consult to decide if he needs a chest tube.
C. Give IM shot of ceftriaxone and oral azithromycin; observe in waiting room and discharge home if doing better in 4 hours.
D. Admit to the hospital, place a chest tube, and start intravenous vancomycin and gentamicin (for synergy).
E. Admit to the hospital, place a chest tube, and start intravenous ceftriaxone and azithromycin.

70.

A 45-year-old woman who had influenza A diagnosed last week presents today with a much worse cough and return of her fever. She was feeling better near the end of the week but now, in the last 24 hours, has become acutely ill again. She says that she has pain in her left lower chest when she takes a deep breath. Before this influenza diagnosis, she has been healthy.

PAST MEDICAL HISTORY: Negative
         Took amantadine for 5 days; finished 3 days ago

SOCIAL HISTORY: Works as a bartender in local pub; asks where you've been lately
         Doesn't drink
         Doesn't smoke but exposed to second-hand all night long, 5 days a week

FAMILY HISTORY: Non-contributory

REVIEW OF SYSTEMS: Fevers to 103° F
                                   Chills
                                   Sore throat now resolved
                                   Body achiness is severe again

PHYSICAL EXAMINATION:
      BP 110/70, P 80, RR 24, Temp 102° F
      Ill-appearing woman in moderate distress

HEENT:	PERRLA, EOMI;
	TMs clear
	Throat slightly hyperemic
Neck:	Supple, no masses
Heart:	RRR without murmurs, rubs, or gallops
Lungs:	Diffuse crackles fairly localized to the left base
Abdomen:	Bowel sounds present; no hepatosplenomegaly
Extremities:	No cyanosis, clubbing, or edema

LABORATORY: pending

Besides *Streptococcus pneumoniae*, which of the following organisms should you also consider in this patient?

A. *Staphylococcus aureus*
B. *Haemophilus influenzae*
C. *Streptococcus pyogenes*
D. *Staphylococcus epidermidis*
E. *Mycoplasma pneumoniae*

71.

A 60-year-old woman who has been on mechanical ventilation for one week due to ARDS from a pneumococcal pneumonia is slowly being weaned. Clinically she is doing well and you are pleased with her progress.

MEDICATIONS: Day 8 of ceftriaxone

Objective data from today:

HEENT:	Pupils responsive and equal
	Mild thrush of her oral mucosa
Neck:	Supple, no masses
Heart:	RRR without murmurs, rubs, or gallops
Lungs:	Still with basilar crackles right greater than left
Abdomen:	Positive bowel sounds, tolerating tube feeds well; no masses
Extremities:	No cyanosis, clubbing, or edema

LABORATORY:
      CBC shows a mild increase in WBC to 11,000 from 9,500 yesterday with 80% lymphs

Tracheal aspirate culture from 2 days ago returns today and shows *Pseudomonas aeruginosa* sensitive only to amikacin, piperacillin/tazobactam, and ceftazidime
AST 25
ALT 26
Bilirubin 0.2 mg/dL
Creatinine 0.5 mg/dL
BUN 10 mg/dL
CXR: slow improvement from admission; no new infiltrates

Based on clinical evaluation and laboratory results, which of the following is the most appropriate next step?

   A. Switch antibiotic coverage to piperacillin/tazobactam alone.
   B. Add amikacin to ceftriaxone.
   C. Switch antibiotics to piperacillin/tazobactam + amikacin.
   D. Perform bronchoscopy and then start piperacillin/tazobactam + amikacin.
   E. Continue current therapy.

72.

A 42-year-old hunter living in Arkansas presents with a 2-day history of fever and productive cough. He says that he has been so ill that he can't eat or sleep because of shaking chills. He says he has been unable to urinate for the past 12 hours because he hasn't taken in any fluids. He has had vomiting also during the past 12 hours.

PAST MEDICAL HISTORY: Hypertension for 3 years

SOCIAL HISTORY: Smokes 2 packs/day of unfiltered cigarettes
Drinks 2 martinis nightly
Eats squirrel, duck, rabbit, deer, possum, frogs, sushi
No travel history except to the northern part of the state last week

FAMILY HISTORY: Mother aged 60 and healthy
Father aged 61 and healthy
Brother 41 and healthy

REVIEW OF SYSTEMS: Fever for 2 days
Chills, shaking in nature
Sweats—soaked the bed last night
Pleuritic chest pain on occasion
No joint complaints
No rashes

PHYSICAL EXAMINATION:
   BP 150/95, RR 24, P 120, Temperature 103.4° F
   HEENT: PERRLA, EOMI
      Throat: mild erythema; no exudates
   Heart: RRR without murmurs, rubs, or gallops
   Lungs: Scattered crackles but consolidated over right middle lobe
   Abdomen: Bowel sounds present; liver edge slightly palpable below right costal margin; no spleen palpated
   Extremities: Negative for cyanosis, clubbing, or edema

LABORATORY:

WBC:	18,000 with 90% polys and 10% bands
Hemoglobin:	17.0 mg/dL
Platelets:	245,000
Electrolytes:	Sodium 145 mg/dL; chloride 110 mg/dL, K 4.0 mg/dL; CO_2 18 mg/dL
Creatinine:	1.4 mg/dL
BUN:	30 mg/dL
Blood cultures:	Taken
Sputum Gram stain:	Normal flora
CXR:	Right middle lobe pneumonia

He does not respond to ceftriaxone in the first 24 hours, and his blood culture is now growing a Gram-negative rod.

Which of the following organisms should you cover for at this point?

A. *Yersinia pestis*
B. *E. coli*
C. *Salmonella*
D. *Francisella tularensis*
E. *Haemophilus influenzae*

73.

A 50-year-old woman with a history of sore throat and cough for 3 days presents for evaluation. She lives in the San Joaquin Valley.

(OK, you can stop right there. Go to the question. Whatever more we would say in here really doesn't matter.)

Which of the following is the likely etiology of her pneumonia?

A. Coccidioidomycosis
B. Not Coccidioidomycosis
C. Not Coccidioidomycosis
D. Not Coccidioidomycosis
E. Not Coccidioidomycosis

74.

An 18-year-old college freshman developed a sore throat approximately 8 days ago that was cultured and did not grow *Streptococcus pyogenes*. However, her throat culture did grow *Staphylococcus aureus*. She presents today with complaint of fever and cough that began last night. She also describes hoarseness since she has had her sore throat symptoms. The sore throat symptoms resolved after 3 days without specific antimicrobial therapy.

PAST MEDICAL HISTORY:	Attention Deficit Disorder diagnosed at age 8; on no medication since 4 years ago
SOCIAL HISTORY:	Recently moved here from Shreveport, LA, for college Doesn't smoke or drink alcohol

Not sexually active
Has a pet parrot back in Shreveport

FAMILY HISTORY: Mother 40 y/o, healthy
Father 42 y/o, in prison for securities fraud
Sister 15 years old, pregnant

REVIEW OF SYSTEMS: Negative for other symptoms; no rash, no joint manifestations

PHYSICAL EXAMINATION:
BP 110/70, P 88, Temp 100° F, RR 18
Ill-appearing woman in no acute distress

HEENT:	PERRLA, EOMI, wears contact lenses
	TMs clear
	Throat: slightly erythematous; no exudates
Neck:	Supple, no meningismus
Heart:	RRR without murmurs, rubs, or gallops
Lungs:	Coarse breath sounds with crackles heard on the left base
Abdomen:	Bowel sounds present in all 4 quadrants, nontender; no hepatosplenomegaly
Extremities:	No cyanosis, clubbing, or edema

LABORATORY: CXR: left lower lobe infiltrate

Besides *Streptococcus pneumoniae*, which of the following is a likely etiology for her pneumonia?

A. *Chlamydophila pneumoniae*
B. *Chlamydia trachomatis*
C. *Chlamydophila psittaci*
D. *Staphylococcus aureus*
E. *Haemophilus influenzae*, type B

75.

Your receptionist asks you to see her 17-year-old daughter. She (the daughter) has had a fever and cough for 2 days and is not better with over-the-counter medications. Her cough has become productive in the past day, and last night she coughed most of the night. Her fevers have ranged up to 101.5° F. She feels bad and complains of generalized body aches.

PAST MEDICAL HISTORY: Negative

SOCIAL HISTORY: Lives with her mother and 2 brothers, ages 12 and 10
Attends high school and makes A's and B's; except a D in Art
Denies smoking or drinking or listening to rock n' roll

FAMILY HISTORY: Mother 40 years old
Father 42 years old, healthy
2 brothers, healthy

REVIEW OF SYSTEMS: Essentially negative

PHYSICAL EXAMINATION:
BP 100/60, P 90, Temp 100º F, RR 14

HEENT:	PERRLA, EOMI, wears glasses
	TMs clear
	Throat clear; non-erythematous
Neck:	Supple no masses
Heart:	RRR with ejection click; no murmurs, rubs, or gallops
Lungs:	Coarse crackles heard at the left base
Abdomen:	Bowel sounds present; no hepatosplenomegaly
Extremities:	No cyanosis, clubbing, or edema
Skin:	No rashes

LABORATORY: CXR: Left lower lobe infiltrate

Based on your findings, which of the following is the best antibiotic choice for her?

A. Gatifloxacin 400 mg q day for 10 days
B. Amoxicillin 500 mg tid for 10 days
C. Azithromycin 500 mg 2 PO today, then 1 PO q day x 4 days
D. Amoxicillin-clavulanate 850 mg PO bid for 10 days
E. Cefuroxime 250 mg PO bid for 10 days

76.

You are seeing a 50-year-old nurse, who works at a local hospital. He has had annual tuberculin skin testing for 30 years. His last PPD a year ago was 7 mm. Today he presents at 72 hours for reading of his PPD placed earlier in the week. He is healthy and denies any health problems, particularly no fevers, sweats, or weight loss.

This is an employee health check, and therefore no physical exam or other information is obtainable.

LABORATORY: PPD at 72 hours: 17 mm
CXR: Normal

Based on the data presented, which of the following is the most appropriate next step?

A. No treatment because he is older than 35 years old.
B. 4-drug therapy because he is high-risk by being in a hospital environment.
C. Start INH 300 mg daily for 12 months.
D. Start INH 300 mg daily for 9 months.
E. Repeat PPD in 2 weeks; if still positive then start therapy.

77.

Your next patient is an 18-year-old woman who is HIV-infected. Her most recent CD4 count was 10. She is moving to your area from Iowa. She says she had a TB skin test 2 years ago and some other skin tests, all of which were read as 0 mm. She remembers that the doctor there told her to tell people the number was "0 millimeters" and not "negative."

PAST MEDICAL HISTORY: She has not required hospitalization in 3 years; at that time, she was hospitalized for *Pneumocystis* pneumonia, which was when she was diagnosed with HIV and found to have AIDS

MEDICATIONS: Trizivir one PO bid, which she has been on for 3 months (she is now adherent, though she says in the past she had not been)
Bactrim DS one PO M, W, F
Azithromycin q week

SOCIAL HISTORY: Lives with her boyfriend, a welder
She works as a waitress at the local I-HOP
Smokes 3 packs/day cigarettes
Doesn't drink

FAMILY HISTORY: Unknown; ran away from home at age 13

REVIEW OF SYSTEMS: Occasional night sweats
Low-grade fevers every 3–5 days
Sore throat on occasion
Cough daily; especially in the morning
Loose stools daily; normal for her is 4–5 bowel movements daily; no blood
Vomiting on occasion
No rash
Decreased appetite

PHYSICAL EXAMINATION: Fairly well-appearing woman in no distress
BP 110/70, P 90, RR 14, Temp 99° F, Ht 5'5", Wt 110

HEENT:	PERRLA, EOMI
	TMs clear
	Throat clear
Neck:	Supple; no masses
Heart:	RRR with no murmurs, rubs, or gallops
Lungs:	Scattered rhonchi at bases; cleared with cough
Abdomen:	Bowel sounds present; liver span 10 cm; no spleen palpated
Extremities:	No cyanosis, clubbing, or edema
Skin:	Facial acne; no other rashes

LABORATORY:

WBC:	2,400 with 70% lymphs, 20% neutrophils
Hgb:	12.5 mg/dL; MCV 105
Platelets:	450,000
Electrolytes:	Normal
Albumin:	3.4 mg/dL
AST:	30 U/L
ALT:	25 U/L
Total bilirubin:	0.4 mg/dL
Viral load:	< 50 copies/mL
CD4:	50

She is due for her tuberculosis screening; which of the following do you recommend?

A. PPD containing 5 TU of tuberculin with 2 controls (mumps and *Candida*)
B. 2-step boosted PPD with 5 TU of tuberculin (place one today and repeat in 2 weeks)
C. PPD containing 250 TU of tuberculin without controls
D. PPD containing 5 TU of tuberculin without controls
E. PPD containing 250 TU of tuberculin with 2 controls (mumps and *Candida*)

78.

This is not a standard question, but rather a test of your knowledge of PPD and what is considered a positive result. It is short and to the point so you don't have to read a long drawn-out history, physical examination, and have to delve into the personal lives of patients. Just a simple and to-the-point question:

Which of the following is <u>not</u> considered an indication to place a patient on treatment for latent tuberculosis infection (assume all CXRs are normal)?

A. PPD reading at 72 hours of 11 mm in a prisoner
B. PPD reading at 48 hours of 6 mm in a patient who lives with a person who has active tuberculosis
C. PPD reading at 48 hours of 16 mm in a healthy 20-year-old
D. PPD reading at 72 hours of 7 mm in an asthmatic patient on 5 mg/day of prednisone
E. PPD reading at 72 hours of 11 mm in a diabetic

79.

A 30-year-old health care worker was recently found to have a PPD of 12 mm on his routine screen. He is about to be started on INH therapy of 300 mg daily for 9 months. He is otherwise healthy and has no complaints. His CXR was normal.

PAST MEDICAL HISTORY: Negative; except for gonorrhea at age 18

SOCIAL HISTORY: Lives with mother in a motel
Drinks on occasion; 2 beers at most on a weekend

FAMILY HISTORY: Mother 60 years old healthy; runs the motel
Father died at age 30; murdered at the motel
No siblings

REVIEW OF SYSTEMS: Negative
Denies fever, chills, sore throat
Occasionally hears voices—knows they are not real

PHYSICAL EXAMINATION:
BP 110/70, P 55, RR 14, Temp 98.5° F
Well-developed, well-nourished man in no distress

HEENT: PERRLA, EOMI
TMs: clear
Throat: clear
Neck: Supple, no masses

Heart:	RRR with S$_4$ gallop (runs marathons)
Lungs:	Scattered rhonchi; cleared with cough
Abdomen:	No masses; no hepatosplenomegaly; non-tender
Extremities:	No cyanosis, clubbing, or edema

You are about to start him on INH.

Of the following options, when should you check screening laboratory (AST, ALT, and bilirubin)?

A. Today, then q month for 3 months; none after that unless has problems
B. Today, then q month until therapy complete
C. Today, then q month for 3 months; then every other month until completes therapy
D. Today, then in 1 week; then q month until finishes therapy
E. None needed unless clinical symptoms/problems develop

80.

You are seeing a 29-year-old with documented tuberculosis. He is currently on INH, rifampin, PZA, and ethambutol. He comes in because he has noted that he cannot see colors as well. He is an interior decorator and noted that last week he tried to put two shades of teal together, and he was embarrassed when he realized what he had done. He comes in to the office dressed with an orange shirt and pink pants. You assume that he was not able to discern the colors he was wearing this morning when he put his clothes on—he relates that no, he meant to wear these today. (oops!)

PAST MEDICAL HISTORY:	Essentially negative
	Tuberculosis exposure was from his mother, who works in a nursing home
SOCIAL HISTORY:	Smokes 1 ppd for 10 years
	Drinks Rum Runners at night; quit when started on his anti-TB meds
	Lives with his mother
	Not sexually active
FAMILY HISTORY:	Mother, 55 with cavitary TB diagnosed 4 months ago
	Father died 10 years ago of massive stroke; age 60
REVIEW OF SYSTEMS:	Besides the vision changes, no other problems
PHYSICAL EXAMINATION:	Essentially normal
	Snellen office chart shows 20/30 vision in both eyes

Referral to ophthalmologist for extensive eye examination reveals loss of color discrimination.

Which of the following is the most likely etiology for his change in vision?

A. INH toxicity
B. Rifampin toxicity
C. Ethambutol toxicity
D. Tuberculous involvement of the retina
E. Combination of ethambutol and INH toxicity

81.

A 45-year-old woman with lymphoma has been neutropenic for 10 days and develops nodules in her lungs on CXR. Initially she is treated with broad-spectrum antibiotics. Amphotericin B is added on day 7, which is also the day the nodules are seen on CXR. She has been having continued fevers and now is developing respiratory distress.

A biopsy of her lung is shown in this figure:

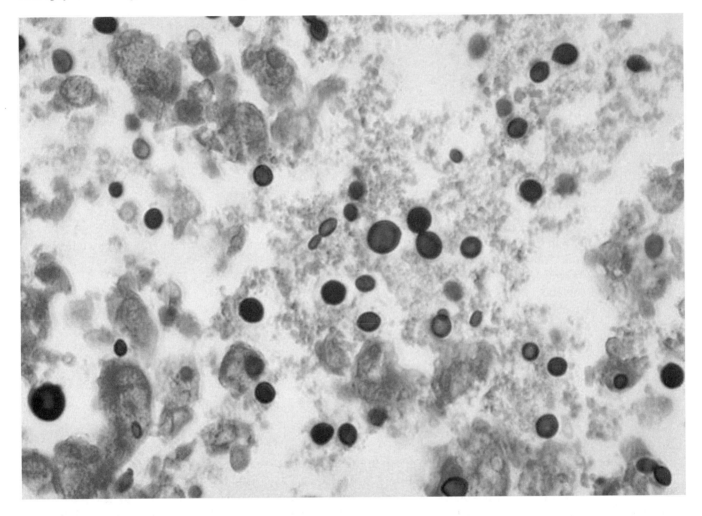

It is a methenamine silver stain. The histopathology shows numerous extracellular yeasts within an alveolar space. The yeasts show a narrow based budding and are of different sizes. A different stain would accentuate the capsule of this organism.

Based on your findings at lung biopsy, which of the following studies should you order next?

    A. Ultrasound of her liver
    B. Nothing; continue treatment with amphotericin B
    C. MRI of the mandible
    D. Lumbar puncture
    E. Upper endoscopy

82.

A 50-year-old man was placed on mechanical ventilation yesterday due to a pulmonary embolism that resulted in respiratory failure. It appears he now has developed ARDS. You have managed his ventilator settings adequately and have told the family that he will likely require prolonged mechanical ventilation before he starts to improve. He appears to be stable at 24 hours out.

PAST MEDICAL HISTORY:	Negative
SOCIAL HISTORY:	Negative
FAMILY HISTORY:	Negative
REVIEW OF SYSTEMS:	Negative (this is a rather boring case for a change)

PHYSICAL EXAMINATION:

HEENT:	PERRLA, EOMI
	TMs clear
	Intubated
Neck:	No masses
Heart	RRR with murmurs, rubs, or gallops
Lungs:	Coarse BS without other focal findings
Abdomen:	Bowel sounds present; no hepatosplenomegaly
Extremities:	No cyanosis, clubbing, or edema

Knowing that he will be on the ventilator for a prolonged period of time, which of the following would be an appropriate nutritional intervention?

A. Start parenteral TPN feeds.
B. Start peripheral TPN feeds.
C. Start enteral feeds.
D. Continue NPO status another 24 hours.
E. Continue NPO status until you are assured he is stable.

83.

An obese, 60-year-old man with diabetes mellitus complains that lately he will fall asleep during the middle of conversations and that he spends half his day asleep in front of the television set. His favorite show, he says, is the "Andy Griffith Show," and he has all of the episodes taped. He says he is proud of Opie for growing up and becoming a "famous director" but wonders why he is so bald, because Andy and Aunt Bee had no bald relatives on their side of the family. He tries to talk about how Fred the barber could help him with some tonic...but he falls asleep in mid-sentence. (You think, thank goodness; but put your professional demeanor face back on.) His wife says this happens all the time. (You secretly wonder why she complains about him sleeping).

You send him for formal sleep testing, and he is found to have moderate obstructive sleep apnea-hypopnea (OSAH).

Besides weight loss and avoidance of alcohol and sedatives, which of the following have been proven to be effective in treatment of OSAH?

A. Sleeping supine
B. Using hypnotics to induce sleep at night
C. Nasal continuous positive airway pressure (CPAP)
D. Sleeping under a fan
E. Watching "Leave It to Beaver" instead of "Andy Griffith" reruns

---

84.

A 67-year-old man with a 100-pack/year history of smoking (2 packs/day for 50 years) is essentially dragged in by his wife, who says that he has withered away to nothing and has been acting very confused lately. He says he is fine but keeps calling you his grandchild. You don't get much more information out of him.

PAST MEDICAL HISTORY: Prostatectomy 5 years ago
    HTN for 20 years on an ACE inhibitor

SOCIAL HISTORY: Retired used car salesman
    Lives with his wife of 50 years
    Doesn't drink

FAMILY HISTORY: Father died at age 75 of lung cancer
    Mother died at age 74 of lung cancer
    Brother died at age 74 of lung cancer
    Sister died at age 74 of lung cancer

REVIEW OF SYSTEMS: No fever or chills
    Has had night sweats on occasion
    30-lb weight loss in last 6 months
    No appetite
    Coughed up blood once last week (about a teaspoon, according to wife)

PHYSICAL EXAMINATION:
    Oriented only to person, place; thinks the year is 1978 (misses Disco)
    BP 110/70, P 92, RR 14, Temp 99° F, Ht 6'1", Wt 170

HEENT:	PERRLA, EOMI
	TMs clear
	Throat clear
Neck:	Supple, no masses
Heart:	RRR with II/VI systolic murmur (heard for 10 years now)
Lungs:	Coarse scattered crackles; no focal findings
Abdomen:	Bowel sounds present; no hepatosplenomegaly
Extremities:	No cyanosis, clubbing, or edema

CXR: Central/hilar mass with area of cavitation
Calcium: 11.5 mg/dL

Based on your findings, which of the following types of lung cancer does this man most likely have?

A. Large cell
B. Adenocarcinoma
C. Small cell
D. Squamous cell
E. Bronchoalveolar carcinoma

85.

A 74-year-old woman with a 100-pack year history of smoking (2 packs/day for 50 years) is essentially dragged in by her husband, who says that she has withered away to nothing and has been acting very confused lately. She says she is fine but keeps calling you her grandchild. You don't get much more information out of her.

PAST MEDICAL HISTORY: Hysterectomy 24 years ago
HTN for 20 years; on an ACE inhibitor

SOCIAL HISTORY: Retired used car salesperson
Lives with her husband of 50 years
Doesn't drink

FAMILY HISTORY: Father died at age 75 of lung cancer
Mother died at age 74 of lung cancer
Brother died at age 74 of lung cancer
Sister died at age 74 of lung cancer
Brother recently diagnosed with lung cancer

REVIEW OF SYSTEMS: No fever or chills
Has had night sweats on occasion
30-lb weight loss in last 6 months
No appetite
Coughed up blood once last week (about a teaspoon, according to husband)

PHYSICAL EXAMINATION:
Oriented only to person, place; thinks the year is 1965 (misses Elvis)
BP 110/70, P 92, RR 14, Temp 99° F, Ht 5'2", Wt 140

HEENT: PERRLA, EOMI
TMs clear
Throat clear
Neck: Supple, no masses
Heart: RRR with II/VI systolic murmur (heard for 10 years now)
Lungs: Coarse scattered crackles; no focal findings
Abdomen: Bowel sounds present; no hepatosplenomegaly
Extremities: No cyanosis, clubbing, or edema

CXR: Central mass seen in right hilum; no cavitation noted
Serum sodium: 120 mg/dL
Urine sodium: 60 mg/dL (normal should be less than 10 mg/dL with this serum sodium)

Based on your findings, which of the following types of lung cancer does this woman most likely have?

A. Large cell carcinoma
B. Adenocarcinoma
C. Squamous cell carcinoma
D. Small cell carcinoma
E. Bronchoalveolar carcinoma

86.

An otherwise healthy, 50-year-old woman presents after being discharged from the hospital with a recent diagnosis of lung cancer with a 2 cm isolated tumor. She was found to have squamous cell carcinoma, stage 1A (T1, N0, M0). She is here to find out what further therapy is indicated.

Which of the following is the next therapy for her?

A. After surgical resection, chemotherapy is indicated.
B. After surgical resection, radiation therapy is indicated.
C. After surgical resection, chemotherapy and radiation therapy are indicated.
D. After surgical resection, follow-up resection is indicated.
E. After surgical resection, no further therapy is indicated.

87.

An 18-year-old man presents for evaluation and relates that he has a herd of cattle. About 3 weeks ago, he was helping a cow deliver, and he had to assist the cow by manually removing the calf and the placenta. The cow was not ill before the delivery. He reports that he became ill about 2 days ago with a high fever, night sweats, and cough. He has noted that he also has a left upper quadrant tenderness in his belly.

PAST MEDICAL HISTORY   Negative; healthy farm boy

SOCIAL HISTORY: Lives with his mother, a widow
Has 3 cats, 2 dogs, and a pet iguana
Chews tobacco
Doesn't drink alcohol

FAMILY HISTORY: Dad died at the age of 35 in a bull-riding accident
Mother healthy, 40
Has 2 younger sisters

REVIEW OF SYSTEMS: Complains of joint aches and pains with the fever
Headache
Weakness

PHYSICAL EXAMINATION:
BP 110/80, P 110, RR 20, Temp 103° F, Ht 6'1", Wt 210 lbs
Well-developed, very muscular man in some distress
HEENT: PERRLA, EOMI
TMs clear
Throat: mild erythema

Neck:	Supple, no meningismus
Heart:	RRR without murmurs, rubs, or gallops
Lungs:	Coarse breath sounds with defined crackles at the right base
Abdomen:	Bowel sounds present; liver edge palpated 5 cm below right costal margin; spleen tip palpated 4 cm below left costal margin
Extremities:	No cyanosis, clubbing, or edema
Skin:	No rashes

LABORATORY:

WBC:	18,000 with 75% polys, 20% bands
Hgb:	16.0 mg/dL
Platelets:	150,000
Electrolytes:	Normal
AST:	100
ALT:	120
CXR:	Right lower lobe pneumonia

Which of the following is the likely etiology of his pneumonia?

A. *Coxiella burnetii*
B. *Francisella tularensis*
C. *Streptococcus pneumoniae*
D. *Staphylococcus aureus*
E. *Yersinia pestis*

88.

A 25-year-old asthmatic patient has a history of frequent exacerbations. On CXR, she frequently has lung infiltrates that migrate and do not seem to respond to antibiotic therapy. She is usually afebrile during these episodes, but it really sets off her asthma and she has a significant exacerbation. Usually she has to be admitted to the hospital and placed on systemic steroids, with aggressive pulmonary management.

PAST MEDICAL HISTORY:	Asthma since early childhood; has never required mechanical ventilation Has one child, age 2; no problems during pregnancy
MEDICATIONS:	Albuterol prn Cromolyn sodium daily Zafirlukast daily
SOCIAL HISTORY:	A 3rd year medical student (considering a career in Radiology; "doesn't really like touching patients") Married and lives with husband and 2-year-old son
FAMILY HISTORY:	Mother 50 and healthy Father 50 and has hypertension No siblings
REVIEW OF SYSTEMS:	Occasional headache Stressed by 3rd year rotations, especially when she has to "touch people"

PHYSICAL EXAMINATION:

Well-developed, well-nourished woman in moderate respiratory distress

BP 110/60, P 90, RR 30, Temp 98° F

HEENT:	PERRLA, EOMI
	TMs clear
	Throat clear
Neck:	Supple; no masses
Heart:	RRR without murmurs, rubs, or gallops
Lungs:	Scattered wheezes especially in upper lung fields
	Poor airway movement
	Few scattered crackles
Abdomen:	Bowel sounds present; no hepatosplenomegaly
Extremities:	No cyanosis, clubbing, or edema
Skin:	No rashes

LABORATORY:

WBC:	10,000 with 50% polys, 20% lymphs, 30% eosinophils
Hgb:	13.5 mg/dL
Platelets:	340,000
CXR:	Scattered infiltrates throughout all lung fields
Sputum:	Normal flora on bacterial stain
	KOH is shown in this figure:

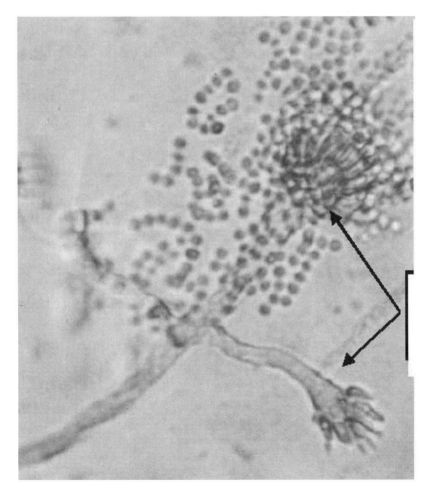

Based on your findings, which of the following is the best treatment for her condition?

A. Itraconazole 200 mg bid x 3 days, then daily thereafter
B. Amphotericin B IV 1 mg/kg IV q day
C. Amphotericin gargles with 5 mg in a 200 cc suspension
D. Systemic corticosteroids and itraconazole
E. Fluconazole 200 mg bid x 1 day then once daily thereafter

89.

You are seeing a 46-year-old man who was raised in rural Mississippi. On a routine CXR (done by another physician), a 5 mm nodule was found in his left upper lobe. The nodule has some calcifications in it. He does not smoke. He has never had a CXR before.

PAST MEDICAL HISTORY: Negative

SOCIAL HISTORY: Teaches 9th grade Art at the local high school
                    Lives alone
                    Quit smoking 20 years ago

FAMILY HISTORY: Mother 72; MI 2 years ago; doing well now
                    Father 66; MI 1 year ago; doing well
                    Brother 42; healthy

REVIEW OF SYSTEMS: No weight loss
                        No night sweats
                        No fever
                        No chills
                        No cough
                        No rashes
                        No travel history

PHYSICAL EXAMINATION:

    BP 120/70, P 90, RR 13, T 98.6° F

    HEENT: PERRLA, EOMI
                    TMs clear
                    Throat clear
    Neck: Supple
    Heart: RRR without murmurs, rubs, or gallops
    Lungs: Clear to auscultation
    Abdomen: Bowel sounds present; no hepatosplenomegaly
    Extremities: No cyanosis, clubbing, or edema
    Skin: No masses or rashes

CXR: 5 mm calcified nodule seen in mid-left upper lung field

Which of the following should you do next to work up this nodule?

A. No further workup is needed
B. Repeat CXR in one month
C. Place PPD
D. V/Q scan
E. CT of chest to evaluate the nodule

90.

A 30-year-old male is brought to the Emergency Room after being found unresponsive at home with a syringe in his arm. The patient is unresponsive, blood pressure is 120/60, and pulse is 100. His pupils are very small and unreactive. He appears cyanotic, and his respiratory rate is 8/minute. Arterial blood gas on room air shows a pH 7.22, PCO_2 of 72 and a PO_2 of 50.

Which of the following is responsible for this patient's hypoxemia?

A. Alveolar hypoventilation alone
B. Low V/Q ratio
C. Alveolar hypoventilation plus low V/Q
D. Alveolar hypoventilation plus right-to-left shunt
E. Venous blood was sampled, not arterial

91.

A 26-year-old female is admitted to the ICU after an emergency exploratory laparotomy for a ruptured ectopic pregnancy. She received 16 units of packed cells in the OR, and a Swan-Ganz catheter was placed by anesthesia because they heard rales and were concerned about volume overload. On admission, she is in shock with a blood pressure of 70/30 and a hemoglobin of 5.0 g/dL. She is on mechanical ventilation in CMV mode with FiO_2 60%, PEEP 10 cm, Rate 20, and Tidal Volume 700 cc. Two additional units of packed cells were given on arrival to the ICU, and the blood pressure came up to 100/60, and the heart rate is 120/minute. Post-transfusion labs reveal a hemoglobin of 7.0 g/dL, and the Swan-Ganz readings show a cardiac output of 10 L/min, pulmonary arterial "wedge" pressure of 12 mmHg, and a systemic vascular resistance of 600 dyne-sec-cm (low). The arterial blood gas now is PO_2 85 mmHg, PCO_2 44 mmHg, and pH of 7.26.

Which of the following therapies is the most appropriate next step in continuing the resuscitation of this patient?

A. Increase the rate of the ventilator to increase the minute ventilation and lower the PCO_2.
B. Increase FiO_2 to 70%.
C. Transfuse 2 units packed red blood cells.
D. Start dobutamine at 10 µg/kg/min to increase the cardiac output.
E. Start dopamine at 10 µg/kg/min to increase the systemic vascular resistance.

92.

A 30-year-old woman comes to your office complaining of shortness of breath. She states that she first noticed the shortness of breath 6 months ago. She is fine at rest but cannot go jogging any longer due to shortness of breath, and she is awakened at night once or twice a week with a feeling that she can't catch her breath. She denies fever, cough, sputum production, orthopnea, or chest pain. On exam, she is a well-appearing female in no apparent distress. The cardiovascular exam is normal, and auscultation of the lungs is normal. There is no leg edema, clubbing, or cyanosis. You perform routine blood work that indicates a normal CBC and chemistries. A chest x-ray is normal, and spirometry done in the office is normal. An arterial blood gas on room air shows pH 7.41, PCO_2 40 mmHg, and PO_2 of 90 mmHg.

Which of the following diagnostic tests would you perform next?

    A. High-resolution CT (HRCT) of the chest
    B. Echocardiography
    C. Full pulmonary function tests with diffusing capacity determination
    D. Flow-volume loop
    E. Exercise challenge test

93.

A 60-year-old male is sent to you by his orthopedist for pre-op clearance prior to elective hip arthroplasty. The patient has a history of asthma and is a non-smoker, though admits to smoking 1 pack a day when he was in his 20s. Previously, he had been followed by a physician at an HMO. He is new to your practice after the HMO closed in the area. He is on a steroid inhaler twice a day and reports that he uses his beta-agonist inhaler only once or twice a week. On physical exam, he is well appearing except for a limp in his right leg. His respiratory rate is 16/minute. Examination of the chest is normal with only a few scattered end-expiratory wheezes. The remainder of the physical examination is unremarkable. A peak flow done in the office is 90% of his predicted value.

Which of the following is/are the most appropriate step(s) to take prior to your clearing the patient for surgery?

    A. Spirometry before surgery
    B. Pulmonary consultation
    C. Spirometry and arterial blood gasses with a carboxyhemoglobin level
    D. You refuse to clear him for any elective surgery
    E. No pulmonary function tests prior to surgery

94.

A 30-year-old female comes to the office with complaints of dyspnea, cough, and wheezing for the past 4 months. She reports that initially the symptoms were related only to exercise, which forced her to stop her aerobic workouts. Now she has daily symptoms even at rest and awakens several nights a week with wheezing. She is a non-smoker. She denies any particular environmental factors and had no respiratory problems until now. On exam, she has a very mild end-expiratory wheeze. Office spirometry reveals a reduced FEV_1 and FEV_1/FVC at 70% predicted.

Which of the following is the best initial treatment plan?

    A. Low-dose inhaled corticosteroid alone
    B. Inhaled cromolyn, 4 times a day
    C. Inhaled beta-2 agonist, every 4-6 hours
    D. Inhaled corticosteroid plus long-acting beta agonist
    E. Sustained release theophylline, twice a day

95.

A 65-year-old male comes to the Emergency Room with increasing respiratory distress over the past two days. He is a smoker and has known COPD, for which he has been hospitalized twice in the past year for exacerbations. The patient appears cyanotic, in moderate distress utilizing accessory musculature and perched forward sitting on the stretcher. He is alert and reports feeling "better" since getting to the ER. Lung sounds are quite diminished in all lung fields, and an ABG on room air shows pH 7.30, PCO_2 63 mmHg, and a PO_2 of 44 mmHg. The respiratory therapist is awaiting your orders.

Your orders for initial oxygen therapy should be which of the following:

A. Nasal oxygen, 1-2 L/min with follow-up ABG in 20 minutes. Increase oxygen flow based on the ABG to a PO_2 of 55–60 mmHg.
B. Intubate the patient and place on mechanical ventilation with an initial FiO_2 of 100%.
C. O_2 100% by non-rebreather face mask with continuous pulse oximetry.
D. Nasal oxygen initially, 3–4 L/min with pulse oximetry to achieve a saturation of 92% or greater.
E. Withhold oxygen therapy at this time since patient is stable and you do not want to induce further respiratory acidosis.

96.

A 45-year-old man presents to your office with a 2-month history of exertional dyspnea and non-productive cough. There is no history of wheezing or prior asthma. He smoked in his early 20s but now limits himself to an occasional cigar. There is no history of chest pain, and he has a copy of an ECG done for a recent insurance physical that was normal. He works in an office with no known occupational exposure, and he is on no prescription medications.

On exam, he is a well-developed male in no apparent distress. He has no adenopathy. The cardiovascular exam is normal. On examination of the chest, you note late inspiratory crackles at the bases. He has no clubbing, cyanosis, or edema.

LABORATORY STUDIES: Hematocrit 45%; Hemoglobin 15 g/dL
CXR-PA and lateral: Increased interstitial markings at the bases
ABG: pH 7.45, PCO_2 36 mmHg, PO_2 70 mmHg on room air

You send him for full PFT testing, and this is consistent with restrictive lung disease.
Various serologic markers are sent for systemic disease and are negative.

Which of the following is the appropriate next step in this patient's workup?

A. Bronchoalveolar lavage and/or transbronchial lung biopsy.
B. CT angiography of the lung.
C. Open-lung biopsy and resection of diseased lung.
D. Follow serial pulmonary function tests at a PFT lab, which would include a determination of his total lung capacity (TLC) and diffusing capacity (DLCO).
E. Ventilation-perfusion scan.

97.

A 40-year-old female comes to your office complaining of increased dyspnea and coughing brownish sputum. She is well known to you, and has had stable asthma for the past 5 years with good control achieved with her inhaled corticosteroid and occasional use of her beta-agonist inhaler. This is her third visit to your office in the past 2 months for exacerbation of her asthma. At this visit you do a chest x-ray, which shows patchy pulmonary infiltrates, and blood work that indicates a mildly elevated WBC count with eosinophilia on the differential.

Which of the following is <u>not</u> consistent with a diagnosis of allergic bronchopulmonary aspergillosis (ABPA)?

    A. Expectoration of brown mucous plugs and airway casts
    B. Marked elevation in serum IgE level
    C. Immediate skin test reaction (Type I, wheal and flare) to *Aspergillus fumigatus*
    D. Delayed (Type IV, cell mediated) skin test reaction to *Aspergillus fumigatus*
    E. Sputum culture positive for *Aspergillus fumigatus*

98.

A surgical colleague calls you one afternoon asking if you could see him in your office. You know him to be a healthy 50-year-old male who likes to play tennis and golf. You suppress a chuckle as you surmise that he wants to talk to you about sildenafil. When he arrives at the office, you notice that he appears thinner and less tan than usual. He is carrying a large manila envelope that you see contains x-rays, and now you are regretting that sildenafil thought. He reports that he has had a dry, nagging cough for the past 4 weeks. He self-medicated himself with a quinolone antibiotic that he had at the office and after 2 weeks, he switched to azithromycin after seeing the drug rep in the halls of the hospital. He grew concerned when he developed low-grade fever, the cough became productive of clear phlegm, and he noticed that he was winded early in a set of tennis. He had a chest x-ray at the hospital today and decided to bring it to you to look at.

On physical exam you find no abnormalities, and his lungs are clear to auscultation. You walk him to the lab where a CBC is done, and you find a mild elevation in the WBC count. His chest x-ray shows diffuse bibasilar parenchymal fibrotic pattern and patchy airspace densities in the right lower lobe.

Which of the following is the most likely diagnosis?

    A. Idiopathic pulmonary fibrosis
    B. Allergic bronchopulmonary aspergillosis
    C. Loeffler syndrome
    D. Cryptogenic organizing pneumonia (COP)
    E. Hypersensitivity pneumonitis

99.

A 21-year-old woman is brought to your office, accompanied by her parents, after a "near syncope" event at home while they were carrying the daughter's trunk of dirty laundry into the house on her arrival from college. The daughter admits to feeling lightheaded while carrying the laundry and says that she is often short of breath climbing the 2 flights of stairs to her dormitory room. Upon further questioning, she admits to substernal chest pain accompanying her exertional dyspnea, but states that it isn't important because "I'm too young to have a heart attack." She denies fever, cough, hemoptysis, wheezing, orthopnea, or ankle swelling. She is on no medications and denies smoking or illicit drugs (confirmed while folks are out of the room). She says other girls in the dormitory were on diet pills, but she just avoided the late-night pizza and ice cream. She is sexually active but has never used oral contraceptives.

On physical exam, she is afebrile with a heart rate of 90 and a blood pressure of 110/60. She is of average build and in no apparent distress. Neurological exam is normal. Her lungs are clear on auscultation. Her cardiovascular exam is remarkable for a parasternal heave and an increase in the intensity of P2.

You perform a chest x-ray, which is normal, and an ECG, which reveals normal sinus rhythm with right axis deviation. CBC and basic chemistries are normal. Pregnancy test is negative.

Which of the following is the most appropriate procedure for further evaluation of this patient?

A. Pulmonary function tests
B. Echocardiogram
C. Exercise stress test
D. V/Q scan
E. Right heart catheterization

100.

An 80-year-old male is admitted to the hospital with dyspnea and a large right-sided pleural effusion. He is afebrile, complains of a cough that is productive of whitish-clear sputum and reports about a 10-lb. weight loss over the previous 6 months. He denies fever, chills, night sweats, hemoptysis, or chest pain. He has a 50-pack/year history of smoking but quit recently as a 50th anniversary present for his wife. He worked as an accountant and worked in the Brooklyn Naval Yard in World War II but denies any asbestos exposure.

On physical exam he is noted to be afebrile, without adenopathy or skin lesions. Breath sounds are diminished at the right side, and he has dullness to percussion posteriorly to the inferior border of the scapula. There is no clubbing, cyanosis, or edema; his nails and fingertips on his right hand are discolored from nicotine.

CBC: WBC count of 5000 with 50% neutrophils, 3% bands, 24% lymphs, 17% monocytes, and 6% eosinophils

Serum chemistries indicate: Glucose 84 mg/dL; protein 7.8 g/dL; LDH 162 U/L

Review of the chest x-rays (PA, lateral, decubitus) shows a large, free-flowing effusion with no discernible underlying lung or mediastinal pathology.

Sputum Gram stain has a few WBCs, no organisms
Sputum cytology: negative for malignant cells

You perform a right-sided thoracentesis and remove almost 1 liter of dark, straw-colored fluid. Pleural fluid is sent for routine studies:

Cell count:	RBCs 8100μL			
	WBC 3600/μL	Differential:	88% lymphocytes	
			1% neutrophils	
			11% monocytes	
Fluid Chemistries:	Glucose	45 mg/dL		
	Protein	5.9 mg/dL		
	LDH	332 U/L		
Cytology: Negative				

Which of the following is the most likely etiology of this patient's pleural effusion?

A. Tuberculosis
B. Parapnemonic effusion
C. Lymphoma
D. Bronchogenic carcinoma
E. Malignant mesothelioma

101.

A 40-year-old female patient comes to your office with complaints of a "flu-like" illness that began 4 days ago. She has just returned from Ohio, where she remembers there was a flu going around the neighborhood. While in Ohio, she helped her parents and neighbors shovel out an old barn that had been used as a bird roost.

Which of the following would you recommend?

A. Cultures for *Histoplasma capsulatum*
B. A histoplasmin skin test
C. Acute and convalescent serologic testing and treatment with amphotericin B
D. Empiric trial of amphotericin B
E. No testing or therapy

102.

A 55-year-old male mail carrier is referred to your office from the hospital Emergency Room. He had been seen there after a fall on the ice, which left him with right-side pain. In the ER he had a chest x-ray done to look for rib fractures. No rib fractures were found, but a 2.5 mm smooth, well-demarcated peripheral lesion was seen in the left lower lobe. He is a non-smoker and reports to be in good health. He denies any occupational exposures and enjoys the long walks while delivering the mail. His father is alive with hypertension; his mother died of breast cancer. He had a prior chest x-ray 1 year ago for a "rule-out" pneumonia office visit.

Which of the following is the most appropriate next step?

A. Bronchoscopy
B. Transthoracic needle biopsy
C. Thoracic surgery
D. Obtain prior chest x-rays for comparison
E. Order sputums for AFB and fungus

103.

A 50-year-old male patient is brought to your office at his wife's insistence. You have seen him in the past for borderline hypertension, but when you last saw him 2 years ago, he was on no medications.

His wife has insisted that he come today because she says that he is always sleeping. She adds that he fell asleep parking the new car in the driveway and crashed through the garage wall. She states that his snoring has gotten so bad that she has moved to another bedroom. You reassure the patient's wife and steer her to your waiting room.

The patient admits to being even sleepier during the daytime, though he thinks that he gets a good night's sleep. He knows he snores, but it doesn't bother him. He admits to waking up tired and often with morning headaches. He is concerned about his performance at work, where he sometimes operates heavy equipment. He denies that he is depressed and states that he doesn't use drugs or alcohol.

On physical exam, you note that he has gained 20 lbs since his visit 2 years ago and that he now weighs 230 lbs. He is 5'8" tall. Blood pressure on repeated measurement is 170/105. On examination of his throat, you notice for the first time his large uvula. Cardiopulmonary as well as neurological exams are within normal limits.

Which of the following would you recommend?

A. Order polysomnography.
B. Order polysomnography with trial of nasal continuous positive airway pressure (CPAP).
C. Advise weight loss, exercise regimen, and follow-up visit in one month.
D. Ear, nose, and throat consultation for uvulopalatopharyngoplasty.
E. Recommend an initial trial of acetazolamide and theophylline before more invasive testing is performed.

104.

A 74-year-old male with a known history of COPD presents to the Emergency Room cyanotic and in severe respiratory distress. He is a thin man weighing 70 kg. An arterial blood gas indicates severe respiratory acidosis and hypoxemia on room air (pH 7.00; PCO_2 120 mmHg; and PO_2 40 mmHg). He is intubated immediately and placed on mechanical ventilation in the assist/control mode at the following settings:

Rate: 25/min   Tidal Volume: 1000cc   Peak inspiratory flow rate: 50 L/min

When you arrive in the ER to see your patient, you note that his blood pressure is 60/30 and his heart rate is 140/min. His pulse is thready, his neck veins are full, and his trachea is midline. There are equal breath sounds bilaterally. There are many alarm lights going off on the ventilator. You yell for someone to page Respiratory Therapy, disconnect the patient from the ventilator for a few minutes, and watch his blood pressure and heart rate improve.

The respiratory therapist arrives.

Which of the following orders do you give the respiratory therapist for mechanical ventilation:

A. T-bar with 80% oxygen on blow by
B. Assist/control mode, Rate 12/min, Tidal Volume 700cc, Peak flow 80 L/min.
C. Assist/control mode, Rate 28/min, Tidal Volume 600cc, Peak flow 40 L/min
D. Assist/control mode, Rate 18/min, Tidal Volume 1000cc, Peak flow 60 L/min

105.

A 42-year-old woman with a history of end-stage renal disease on hemodialysis presents to the Emergency Room with fever of 103° F, shaking chills, hypotension 70/50, tachypneic, and tachycardic. Her dialysis graft site is erythematous, warm to the touch, and has purulent drainage at a prior access site. A diagnosis of septic shock is made, and the patient is given intravenous antibiotics, IV fluids, and arrangements are made to transfer the patient to the ICU with a vascular surgery consult to remove the hemodialysis graft. The intensivist meets the patient in the ER and immediately places a Swan-Ganz catheter out of concern of volume overloading this patient with end-stage renal disease and now a non-functioning dialysis catheter.

The initial hemodynamic profile for this patient would most resemble which of the following:

	Cardiac Output L/min	Systemic Vascular Resistance dynes-sec/cm5	Wedge Pressure mmHg
A.	High	Low	Low
B.	Low	High	Low
C.	Low	High	High
D.	Low	High	Normal/Low

106.

A 29-year-old man is brought to the ER by friends. The patient was at a party with his friends when he became confused and then unresponsive. On exam: BP 60/30, P 140, T 97° F, O_2 saturation 88%. Extremities with marked cyanosis. Mouth – cyanosis of lips. Labs: Hb 14, HCT 42, WBC 1,000, ABG-pH 7.32, PO_2 46, PCO_2 44, Na 136, K 4.0, Cl 105, HCO_3 20.

The patient is placed on 100% O_2 by mask without improvement in his cyanosis.

Which of the following therapies should he receive?

  A. Methylene blue
  B. Amyl nitrite
  C. Bicarbonate drip
  D. Narcan
  E. IV alcohol

107.

A 60-year-old male patient is found to have a 4 cm lung mass in his right upper lobe on CXR. CT scan confirms that it is suspicious for malignancy, but there are no other lesions or significant adenopathy. Bullous lung disease is noted in the apices, particularly on the right. A fine-needle aspiration of the mass reveals non-small cell carcinoma. A thoracic surgery consult is requested, but the surgeon refers him back to you for pre-op clearance. The patient has a history of asthma and admits to at least a 30 pack/year history smoking, though he has cut back to "a few a day." He reports that he uses his beta-agonist inhaler only once or twice a week because it only makes him cough.

On physical exam, he is well appearing except for a limp in his right leg. His respiratory rate is 16/minute. Examination of the chest is normal with only few scattered end-expiratory wheezes. The remainder of the physical examination is unremarkable. Pulmonary function tests (with bronchodilators held prior to testing) reveal an obstructive pattern with FEV_1 of 1.6 liters. There is minimal response to bronchodilators in the lab. ABG on room air show pH 7.41, $PaCO_2$ 38, and PaO_2 of 87.

In addition to initiating a smoking-cessation program, which of the following do you recommend?

  A. Refer him to an oncologist for non-surgical treatment of his tumor.
  B. Refer him for a pulmonary consultation.
  C. Order a quantitative ventilation scan.
  D. Start inhaled steroids and repeat PFT in 4 months.

108.

A 75-year-old male is admitted to the hospital with an exacerbation of COPD. He is treated with oxygen, antibiotics, and bronchodilators. On the fourth day, he is feeling better and he wants to go home. A pulse oximetry on room air today reveals a saturation of 89%, which was confirmed by a simultaneous ABG on room air, which demonstrated a PaO_2 of 58 and a saturation of 89%. With ambulation, the oxygen saturation falls to 86%, and the patient becomes dyspneic. His HCT on admission was elevated to 52%. You request a referral from Social Services for home oxygen for your patient, and you are told that "he doesn't qualify but he could pay for it himself." Your patient, and his family, are quite distressed to learn that they will have to pay for the oxygen out of their own pockets. You are determined to see if you can get your patient qualified for home oxygen.

Which of the following is the best plan of action?

A. Secretly tell your patient to ambulate and repeat the ABG.
B. Order an ECG and echocardiogram to evaluate for cor pulmonale.
C. Resubmit the application on the basis of his erythrocytosis.
D. Take up a collection for your patient.

109.

A 40-year-old female comes to your office complaining of increased dyspnea and coughing accompanied by fever and night sweats. She is well known to you and has had stable asthma for the past 10 years, with good control achieved with her inhaled corticosteroid and occasional use of her beta-2 agonist inhaler. This is her third visit to your office in the past 2 months for "exacerbation of her asthma." CBC indicates a mildly elevated WBC count with 15% eosinophils.

Which of the following would a chest x-ray most likely reveal?

A. No infiltrates
B. Bilateral peripheral infiltrates
C. Segmental atelectasis
D. Right upper lobe cavity

110.

A 52-year-old man presents to your office with a 2-month history of exertional dyspnea and non-productive cough. There is no history of wheezing or prior asthma. He has a 10 pack/year smoking history but quit 10 years ago. There is no history of chest pain, and he has a copy of an ECG done for a recent insurance physical that was normal. He works in an office with no known occupational exposure, and he is on no prescription medications.

On exam, he is a well-developed male in no apparent distress. He has no adenopathy. The cardiovascular exam is normal. On examination of the chest, you note late inspiratory crackles at the bases. He has no clubbing, cyanosis, or edema.

LABORATORY STUDIES: Hematocrit 45%; Hemoglobin 15 g/dL
CXR – PA and Lateral: Normal
ABG: pH 7.45; PCO_2 36 mmHg; PO_2 70 on room air
Office spirometry: reduced FVC, reduced FEV_1, but FEV_1/FVC normal

Which of the following should be the next step in this patient's workup?

A. Pulmonary function tests at a PFT lab, which would include a determination of his Total Lung Capacity (TLC) and Diffusing Capacity (DLCO)
B. Transbronchial biopsy
C. Open lung biopsy
D. High-resolution CT of the chest

CARDIOLOGY

111.

A 45-year-old man being evaluated for ischemic heart disease has had chest pain with exertion for about 5 months and finally came to see you this week for evaluation. He says the pain occurs only with exertion and is a pressure-like feeling in his chest. The pain does not radiate, and he has no sweating or shortness of breath with the pain. The pain mainly occurs when he is running on his treadmill, although lately he has had chest pain occur while having sexual intercourse (Ah-ha!, the real reason why he comes to see you!). Pain subsides after resting for a few minutes. He does not have any chest pain except with exertion and has never had pain at rest.

PAST MEDICAL HISTORY: Hypertension for 4 years treated with fosinopril 20 mg q day
                                     Hernia repair 10 years ago

SOCIAL HISTORY: Lives with his wife of 2 years; his 3rd marriage
                          Works as a librarian by day; bartender by night
                          No children
                          Doesn't smoke or drink

FAMILY HISTORY: Father 70; s/p CABG at age 60
                          Mother 70; Alzheimer disease
                          Brother 50; angioplasty a year ago for left main coronary artery disease

REVIEW OF SYSTEMS: Negative for any other symptoms

PHYSICAL EXAMINATION:
   Ht 5'10, Wt 180, BP 120/70, P 85, RR 14, Temp 98.8° F

HEENT:	PERRLA, EOMI
	TMs clear
	Throat clear
Neck:	Supple; no thyromegaly
Heart:	RRR without murmurs, rubs, or gallops
Lungs:	CTA
Abdomen:	Bowel sounds present; no masses; no hepatosplenomegaly
Extremities:	No cyanosis; clubbing, or edema
Rectal:	Heme negative; no masses

LABORATORY: Normal for age

You decide to perform an exercise stress test on him.

Which of the following should make you stop the test urgently?

A. Sinus tachycardia of 130 bpm
B. ST segment depression of 1.5 mm
C. Mild cramping in his left calf
D. Decrease in systolic BP > 15 mmHg
E. Respiratory rate of 30

112.

A 60-year-old man with recent inferior myocardial infarction is 1-day status-post his infarction and has been doing well. This afternoon, however, he develops recurrence of his chest pain. You quickly get him to the cath lab, and there he has a markedly decreased cardiac output, as well as decreased PCWP of 10. His RA pressure is elevated at 15 with a PA pressure of 20/11. He continues to deteriorate and becomes more hypotensive with a BP of 75/50.

Based on these findings, which of the following describes what has happened and how you should treat him?

    A. Pericardial tamponade; perform emergent pericardial tap.
    B. RV infarction with secondary failure; administer normal saline.
    C. Biventricular failure; give diuretics, preload and afterload reducers, and inotropic agents.
    D. Mitral stenosis with secondary RV failure; refer for valvuloplasty.
    E. Pulmonary hypertension; oxygen.

113.

A 30-year-old graduate student is brought in by ambulance to the Emergency Room, clutching his chest and looking very ill. He denies any prior medical history and says this has never happened before. The symptoms began at home while watching reruns of his favorite television show, "Queen for a Day."

PAST MEDICAL HISTORY: Negative

SOCIAL HISTORY: Lives with his two brothers
                        Works as a television repairman when he is not in graduate school
                        Stopped smoking 10 years ago; before that, ½ pack/day for 10 years
                        Drinks martinis daily (one/day)

FAMILY HISTORY: Father 60 y/o with MI 3 years ago
                        Mother 59 y/o with MI 2 years ago
                        Uncle died at age 30 of "blood clot" to lung
                        Aunt died at age 35 of "blood clot" to brain
                        Two brothers are healthy

REVIEW OF SYSTEMS: Essentially unremarkable

PHYSICAL EXAMINATION:
    Ht 5'10, Wt 190, BP 90/40, Pulse irregular and 100 to 150, RR 24, afebrile

HEENT:	PERRLA, EOMI
	TMs clear
	Throat clear
Neck:	Supple, no thyromegaly
Heart:	Irregular without murmurs, rubs, or gallops
Lungs:	CTA
Abdomen:	Bowel sounds present; no masses palpated
Extremities:	No cyanosis, clubbing, or edema

An ECG is obtained in the ER and is shown below:

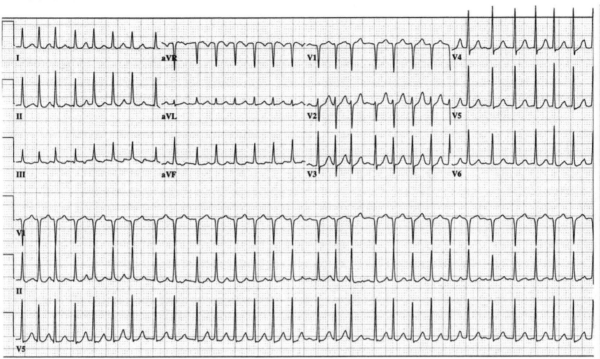

Which of the following is the correct interpretation of the arrhythmia that he is suffering from at the moment?

A. Sinus arrhythmia
B. Ventricular tachycardia
C. Atrial flutter
D. Atrial fibrillation
E. Sick sinus syndrome

114.

A 55-year-old man collapses while playing tennis and is brought to the Emergency Room. The EMTs found him in cardiopulmonary arrest, performed CPR, applied a 200-joule shock to his chest, and inserted an endotracheal tube and IV. He has been bagged, and chest compressions continued on the way to the ER. At the time you see him, you get a rhythm strip that shows ventricular tachycardia. He has received epinephrine 1 mg IV push.

Which of the following antiarrhythmics would be reasonable to administer now?

A. Bretylium tosylate
B. Phenytoin
C. Sodium bicarbonate
D. Procainamide
E. Amiodarone

115.

A 70-year-old man has been having recurring episodes of dizziness over the last several months. You admit him to the hospital because of a fainting spell that occurred earlier today. Initial laboratory and ECG are normal. There is no evidence of acute myocardial infarction by history or laboratory. He says that he notices the dizzy spells, and that is about it. He has no prodrome and no other symptoms with them. This fainting spell is the first one that he has had. He was not aware that it was about to happen.

PAST MEDICAL HISTORY: Prostatic hypertrophy diagnosed 5 years ago
                                   Colon polyp removed 3 years ago

MEDS: ECASA qd
     Nifedipine 30 mg qd

SOCIAL HISTORY: Former logger, retired for 20 years
                        Lives with 4th wife
                        Chews tobacco for 60 years
                        Doesn't smoke
                        Drinks a beer every now and then; none in 6 weeks

FAMILY HISTORY: "Outlived everyone in my family"
                        Mother died at age 67 of stroke
                        Father died at age 50 of MI
                        Brother died at age 60 of stroke
                        Sister died at age 60 of MI
                        Son died at age 30 of motor vehicle accident

REVIEW OF SYSTEMS: Negative

PHYSICAL EXAMINATION: at admission:
     Well-developed, well-nourished man in no distress
     Ht 6'1, Wt 190 (unchanged in 2 years), BP 120/70, RR 18, P 76 regular, T 97.9° F

     HEENT: PERRLA, EOMI, Discs sharp
                     TMs: Clear
                     Throat: Clear
     Neck: Supple
     Heart: RRR with II/VI systolic murmur heard for 20 years
     Lungs: CTA
     Abdomen: Bowel sounds present; no masses; no hepatosplenomegaly
     Extremities: No cyanosis, clubbing, or edema
     Rectal: No masses; heme negative

LABORATORY:
     CBC: Normal
     Electrolytes Normal
     ESR 12
     Thyroid function tests normal

The next morning, when the nurse's aide comes in to take vitals, he tells her that 5 minutes ago he had another dizzy spell. She notifies the nurse who is on her coffee break. The charge nurse comes in and looks at the monitor and sees that he is in Normal Sinus rhythm. You come in on rounds and he relates this story to you. You go back and look at the rhythm strip from the approximate time this event happened. You note absent QRS complexes every third beat. The PR interval is slightly prolonged **but** is constant from beat to beat. P waves are present at regular intervals.

Which of the following is the most appropriate action to take at this point?

A. Insertion of an unspecified catheter into the charge nurse
B. Administration of atropine, one-time dose 2 mg IV
C. Administration of isoproterenol at a constant infusion rate 2 mg/min
D. Insertion of a permanent cardiac pacemaker
E. This is a benign arrhythmia; therefore, no specific therapy is indicated

116.

A 50-year-old woman comes in for her routine checkup. She has not had any problems and relates that she is doing well, except she says that her feet swell frequently and that this has just started to occur.

PAST MEDICAL HISTORY: Essentially negative; delivered 3 children by normal, spontaneous vaginal delivery at 28, 30, and 35 years ago

MEDS: "menopause pill"

SOCIAL HISTORY:	Lives with her husband and 35 y/o son in Divide, CO
	Drinks a 6-pack of beer/week
	Smokes 2 packs/cigarettes daily
	Works as a weather forecaster

FAMILY HISTORY:	Mother with CHF diagnosed at age 50
	Father with CHF diagnosed at age 50
	Brother 51 y/o good health

REVIEW OF SYSTEMS:	No shortness of breath
	Chronic cough especially in the morning for years
	No edema of the hands or elsewhere noted
	No orthopnea
	No dyspnea on exertion or at rest
	No weight gain or weight loss

PHYSICAL EXAMINATION:
   Ht 5'5", Wt 120
   BP 110/80, Temp 98° F, RR 12, P 88

HEENT:	PERRLA, EOMI Discs sharp
	TMs clear
	Throat clear
Neck:	Supple, no masses
	Jugular venous pulse is 3 cm H_2O
	Hepatojugular reflux is negative
Heart:	RRR without murmurs, rubs, or gallops
Lungs:	CTA

Abdomen:	Bowel sounds present; no ascites; no masses
Extremities:	2+ pitting edema to just past the ankle area bilaterally
	No cyanosis, clubbing noted

Which of the following should <u>not</u> be considered in the differential?

A. Right heart failure
B. Pelvic thrombophlebitis
C. Venous varicosities
D. Cyclic edema
E. Hypoalbuminemia

117.

An 18-year-old man lives on a military base in Germany and presents to you with complaints of fever (102.2° F) and complains of lower back, knee, and left wrist pain. The pain is not localized to any one joint. He had a severe sore throat about 3 weeks ago for which he did not seek treatment.

PAST MEDICAL HISTORY:	Up to date on all his immunizations, including anthrax and yellow fever
	Treated for syphilis on arrival to base 8 months ago

SOCIAL HISTORY:	Works as a dishwasher in the mess hall
	Smokes 1 pack/day of cigarettes
	Drinks 6-pack of beer nightly

FAMILY HISTORY: Negative

REVIEW OF SYSTEMS: Negative except for above

PHYSICAL EXAMINATION:
    Ht 6', Wt 220, BP 120/50, Temp 102° F, P 99, RR 18

HEENT:	PERRLA, EOMI, Discs sharp
	TMs clear
	Throat now clear
Neck:	Supple; no masses
Heart:	RRR without murmurs, rubs, or gallops
Lungs:	CTA
Abdomen:	Bowel sounds present, no masses, no hepatosplenomegaly
Extremities:	Multiple swellings noted on his elbows and wrists; each approximately 0.5 cm
Skin:	2 erythematous pinkish areas on the anterior trunk, each about 4–6 cm in diameter

LABORATORY:
    CBC: Normal
    Blood cultures: negative
    Throat culture: negative
    ESR 93
    ASO (antistreptolysin-O) titer is elevated

Based on your working diagnosis, which of the following therapeutic interventions should you order at this point?

A. Parenteral penicillin and steroids
B. Parenteral penicillin and aspirin
C. Parenteral penicillin and aspirin and steroids
D. Supportive care only
E. Aspirin only

118.

A 25-year-old man has had recent syncope that appears to be exercise-induced. He has developed progressive shortness of breath for the past few days and increasing pedal edema. He tried increasing his usual dose of furosemide without relief.

PAST MEDICAL HISTORY: Hypertension for 5 years; currently on nifedipine 30 mg qd and furosemide 20 mg qd

SOCIAL HISTORY: Lives alone in a trailer
Drinks 2 six-packs/beer a week
Smokes ½ pack a day of cigarettes; occasional cigar

PHYSICAL EXAMINATION:
Well-developed, well-nourished man in mild distress
BP 160/80 mmHg, P 80, RR 18, Temp 98.4° F

HEENT:	PERRLA, EOMI, bilateral cataracts (mild)
	TMs clear
	Throat clear
Neck:	Supple, +JVD to 8 cm
Heart:	RRR with III/VI harsh systolic murmur
Lungs:	Bilateral crackles to mid lung fields
Abdomen:	Bowel sounds present; no fluid wave; liver down about 5 cm below right costal margin
Extremities:	No cyanosis; mild clubbing present; 3+ pitting edema to knee
GU:	Mild scrotal edema

LABORATORY:
Echocardiogram: Disproportionately thickened ventricular septum and systolic anterior motion of the mitral valve

Based on your findings, which of the following is likely to be present?

A. Delayed carotid upstroke
B. Radiation of the murmur to the carotids
C. Decrease of the murmur with handgrip
D. Signs of mitral stenosis
E. Reduced left ventricular ejection fraction

119.

A 35-year-old Caucasian male living in northern Louisiana has been having sharp, pleuritic chest pains that are relieved by sitting upright. He has reported some fever for several days and a non-productive cough.

PAST MEDICAL HISTORY: Essentially negative; came in 3 years ago for URI

SOCIAL HISTORY:
Works as a policeman
Doesn't smoke
Drinks 2 beers on the weekends when he plays poker with his buddies

FAMILY HISTORY:
Mother with depression
Wife is a manic-depressive and steals things all the time from local department stores

REVIEW OF SYSTEMS:
No weight loss
No chills
No nausea or vomiting

PHYSICAL EXAMINATION:
Ht: 6'1, Wt 190 (very muscular), BP 120/70, RR 10 and splinting, P 110, T 100.5° F

HEENT:	PERRLA, EOMI
	TMs clear
	Throat: clear
Neck:	Supple; no meningismus
Heart:	RRR without murmurs and gallops
Lungs:	CTA
Abdomen:	+BS, soft, No organomegaly
Extremities:	No cyanosis, clubbing, or edema
Skin:	No rashes

Which of the following findings would <u>least</u> support a diagnosis of acute pericarditis?

A. Frequent atrial premature beats
B. A pericardial rub is not present
C. Diffuse T-wave inversion with ST-segment elevation
D. PR-segment depression, especially in lead II
E. Serum creatine phosphokinase concentrations of 2x normal

120.

A 27-year-old Caucasian male who lives in Jackson, MS, presents to his local Emergency Room complaining of dizziness over the past few days. (OK, isn't this everyone's dreaded question—not another dizzy young person!) However, he reports that over the past 4 days he has had 3 episodes of syncope followed by periods of unresponsiveness! (Oops, OK this is not just some dumb blond guy with "dizziness.") He has always been in excellent health and is a personal trainer to the "stars" of Jackson. His last illness was about 4–5 months ago when he developed fever, chills, and generalized weakness while he was spending a month as a guest personal trainer in a spa off of Long Island, NY.

PAST MEDICAL HISTORY: Negative except for above
                                 Denies use of steroids; says he is "natural"

SOCIAL HISTORY: Lives with wife of 3 years; she is a plastic surgeon in town—they refer each other clients all the time (nice setup, eh?)
                        Doesn't smoke
                        Doesn't drink alcohol
                        Denies drug use

FAMILY HISTORY: Father 60 y/o with HTN
                        Mother 55 y/o with HTN
                      Brother 32 y/o with severe obesity

REVIEW OF SYSTEMS: Essentially negative

PHYSICAL EXAMINATION:
    Ht; 5'8", 230 lbs
    BP 110/80, P 30 (yes that is not a typo—thirty), RR 18, Temp 98.6° F

    HEENT: PERRLA, EOMI
                    TMs clear
                    Throat: clear
    Neck: Supple
    Heart: RRR with severe bradycardia
    Lungs: CTA
    Abdomen: Bowel sounds present; abs of steel; no rebound; no hepatosplenomegaly
    Extremities: No cyanosis, clubbing, or edema
    GU: Normal male genitalia; rectal heme negative

LABORATORY:
    CXR: Normal

    Serum Chemistries: Normal

    ECG: Complete heart block with nonspecific ST- and T-wave changes; no findings consistent with prior myocardial infarction

    ER (did a drug screen): + for cocaine (hmm…maybe he isn't so "natural" after all)

Which of the following is the most likely cause of his complete heart block?

A. Infection transmitted by a bite from a tick
B. Infection caused by HIV
C. Myocardial infarction from cocaine use
D. Myocardial infarction from coronary artery embolus
E. Infection transmitted by a bite from a louse

121.

A 60-year-old man with negative past medical history presents for his annual physical examination. He reports no problems.

PAST MEDICAL HISTORY: Really, really negative!

SOCIAL HISTORY: Works as a minister in local community church
Not married
Doesn't smoke
Doesn't drink

FAMILY HISTORY: Father died at age 78 of MI
Mother died at age 55 of MI

REVIEW OF SYSTEMS: Negative

PHYSICAL EXAMINATION:
BP 130/76, P 110, RR 18, Temp 99° F

HEENT:	PERRLA, EOMI
	TMs clear
	Throat clear
Heart	RRR without murmurs, rubs, or gallops
Lungs	CTA
Abdomen:	Bowel sounds present, no hepatosplenomegaly
Extremities:	No cyanosis, clubbing, or edema
GU:	Normal male genitalia

LABORATORY:
CBC normal; no anemia
Lytes normal
ECG: 12 lead tracing; shows 2 premature ventricular complexes (PVCs)

Which of the following statements about premature ventricular complexes is true?

A. Less than 40% of males have PVCs on a 24-hour Holter monitor.
B. PVCs such as these can cause symptoms.
C. His PVCs predict a higher incidence of cardiac mortality.
D. The frequency and nature of PVCs cannot be correlated with increased mortality in patients with known coronary artery disease.
E. The frequency of isolated PVCs decreases with age.

122.

You are asked to evaluate a 76-year-old woman admitted to the orthopedic service for a left hip fracture after suffering a fall earlier this morning. She was getting up to go to the bathroom early this morning and says that she "just passed out." Essentially, no further history or physical exam has been done except by anesthesia, who noted that her pulse is 40.

PAST MEDICAL HISTORY: Hypertension for 30 years, for which she is taking:
Low-dose atenolol 25 mg qd
Thiazide 25 mg qd
Diltiazem long-acting 240 mg qd

SOCIAL HISTORY: Never married
Lives alone in 40-room mansion, the "Perkins' House"
Smokes 2 packs/day of cigarettes
Doesn't drink alcohol

REVIEW OF SYSTEMS: Dizziness has been going on for several weeks
No syncope before this episode
Some paraesthesias of her fingers
Headaches on occasion
Tongue "itchy"
Eyes watery
Throat scratchy
Neck "swells" up
Palpitations all the time
Dyspnea on occasion at rest and at exertion
Taste different now; has metallic taste
Abdominal pains every day…sharp like a knife, move around a lot
Leg cramps all the time
Skin itches a lot
Increased forgetfulness
Hair loss noted on forearms
Teeth itch
Stools glow in the dark

After 45 minutes of positives, especially the last two, you decide to move on.

PHYSICAL EXAMINATION:
BP 90/50, HR 42, Temp 98.5° F, RR 18
Well-developed, well-nourished woman in mild distress

HEENT: PERRLA, EOMI
Discs sharp
TMs occluded by cerumen
Throat clear
Neck: Supple, no thyromegaly or masses
No bruits
Heart: RRR without murmurs, rubs, or gallops, but bradycardic
Lungs: CTA
Abdomen: Bowel sounds present, no hepatosplenomegaly, no masses

Extremities:	No cyanosis, clubbing, trace pedal edema
GU/Rectal:	Heme-negative stool, no masses; normal female external genitalia

ECG: Sinus bradycardia at 45 bpm; occasional sinus pauses lasting 3 seconds; no ST-T wave changes; no Q waves or other abnormalities; axis is normal

Which of the following would be the best next step in treatment for her arrhythmia at this point?

A. Placement of a permanent pacing wire.
B. Placement of a temporary pacing wire, and stop her diltiazem and atenolol.
C. Stop diltiazem and atenolol and observe.
D. Place temporary pacer now and schedule for permanent placement with her hip repair.
E. Give atropine q hour until heart rate returns to normal; stop atenolol and diltiazem.

123.

A 17-year-old high school student is referred by his high school basketball coach to you for a physical examination. He is healthy and has no complaints.

PAST MEDICAL HISTORY: No immunizations since age 12 (had Td booster then); has received 2 MMRs; no hepatitis B vaccination

SOCIAL HISTORY: A/B honor roll student
Works afternoons at the movie theater; runs the popcorn machine
Sleeps about 4 hours a night after getting all his homework done
Doesn't smoke or drink
Is sexually active with girls; always wears a condom
Wears seatbelts

FAMILY HISTORY: Mother 44, healthy
Father 44, healthy
Brother 16, healthy
Brother died suddenly while playing basketball at age 19; no autopsy obtained
Sister 15, healthy

REVIEW OF SYSTEMS: Negative

PHYSICAL EXAMINATION:
6'3", 210 lbs
BP 120/70, P 65, RR 18, Temp 98.5° F

HEENT:	PERRLA, EOMI
	TMs clear
	Throat clear
Neck:	Supple; no murmurs heard in neck
	Brisk carotid upstroke
Heart:	RRR with III/VI harsh systolic murmur
	Murmur increased with Valsalva
	Murmur decreased with passive leg-raising
Lungs:	CTA
Abdomen:	Bowel sounds present; no hepatosplenomegaly

Extremities:	No cyanosis, clubbing, or edema
GU:	Tanner V pattern hair growth and gonadal development
Skin:	Acne on face and back

Based on your findings in the history and physical examination, which of the following is your most likely diagnosis?

A. Anomalous coronary artery disease
B. Severe mitral stenosis
C. Constrictive pericarditis
D. Upper arch aortic aneurysm
E. Hypertrophic cardiomyopathy (idiopathic hypertropic subaortic stenosis)

124.

A 16-year-old high school student is referred by his high school wrestling coach to you for a physical examination. He is healthy and has no complaints.

PAST MEDICAL HISTORY: No immunizations since age 12 (had Td booster then); has received 2 MMRs; doesn't know about hepatitis B vaccination

SOCIAL HISTORY: C student
Sleeps about 10 hours a night
Smokes marijuana on occasion
Smokes a cigarette on occasion
Drinks beer on occasion
Is not sexually active
Doesn't wear seat belts

FAMILY HISTORY: Mother 44, healthy
Father 44, healthy
Brother 16, healthy
Brother died suddenly while skiing at age 17; no autopsy obtained

REVIEW OF SYSTEMS: Negative

PHYSICAL EXAMINATION:
5'11", 250 lbs
BP 130/70, P 72, RR 18, Temp 98.7° F

HEENT:	PERRLA, EOMI
	TMs clear
	Throat clear
Neck:	Supple; no murmurs heard in neck
	Brisk carotid upstroke
Heart:	RRR with III/VI harsh systolic murmur
	Murmur increased with standing
	Murmur decreased with squatting
Lungs:	CTA
Abdomen:	Bowel sounds present; no hepatosplenomegaly
Extremities:	No cyanosis, clubbing, or edema

GU: Tanner IV pattern hair growth and gonadal development
Skin: Acne on face and back

Which of the following diagnostic tests will confirm your diagnosis?

A. Treadmill stress test
B. Echocardiogram
C. Doppler ultrasound of his scrotum
D. Biopsy of cervical lymph node
E. ECG

125.

A 30-year-old man presents to the Emergency Room with 18 hours of left precordial pain that is worse when lying supine and relieved when sitting upright. He is afraid he is having a heart attack because his grandma (age 92) died last week of an MI. He had a viral illness about a week ago.

PAST MEDICAL HISTORY: Negative

SOCIAL HISTORY: Works as a psychic on the psychic hot line (says he didn't predict this)
                       Married with children
                       Doesn't smoke or drink

FAMILY HISTORY: Grandma mentioned above died at age 92 of MI
                       Grandpa died at age 92 of stroke
                       Father 65 y/o and mother 70 y/o, alive and well

REVIEW OF SYSTEMS: Low-grade fevers
                           Occasional cough
                           He says his psychic abilities have been diminished the last 2 days

PHYSICAL EXAMINATION:
    BP 130/70, P 110, RR 20, Temp 99.5° F

    HEENT: PERRLA, EOMI
                  Throat: slight erythema
    Neck: Supple, no masses; no bruits
    Heart: RRR with faint friction rub when he leans forward
    Lungs: CTA
    Abdomen: +BS; no masses; no hepatosplenomegaly
    Extremities: No cyanosis, clubbing, or edema

LABORATORY: ECG reveals diffuse concave-up ST elevation with sinus tachycardia

Your likely next steps would include all of the following <u>except</u>:

A. Thrombolytics for treatment of an acute MI
B. Non-steroidal antiinflammatory agents
C. Supplemental oxygen by mask or nasal cannula
D. Admission for serial ECGs and observation
E. Echocardiogram

126.

A 17-year-old woman with diagnosis of coarctation of the aorta by a local cardiologist is following up with you for further treatment. She has not had menses yet. Otherwise, she is healthy and did not have any problems until her family noted that she was not growing properly.

PAST MEDICAL HISTORY: Negative

SOCIAL HISTORY: Lives with mom and dad in an apartment
A senior in high school
Denies smoking or drinking

FAMILY HISTORY: Grandfather with hypertension
Grandmother with hypothyroidism

REVIEW OF SYSTEMS: No menses

PHYSICAL EXAMINATION:
BP 110/70 upper extremities; 80/50 lower extremities; P 90; RR 18; Temp 98.6° F

HEENT: PERRLA, EOMI
TMs clear; low-set ears
Low posterior hairline
High-arched palate
Neck: Marked webbing of the neck
Heart: RRR without murmurs, rubs, or gallops
Lungs: CTA
Abdomen; Bowel sounds present, no hepatosplenomegaly
Extremities: Short digits; no cyanosis or clubbing; hands look edematous
GU: Minimal breast development
Normal external genitalia
No secondary hair development

Which of the following other cardiac abnormalities is associated with the presence of her coarctation of the aorta?

A. Bicuspid aortic valve
B. Mitral stenosis
C. Patent ductus arteriosus
D. Sinus venosus
E. Ventricular septal defect

127.

Here is a straightforward knowledge question. Occasionally, they will throw something like this at you, particularly if they are testing something like a non-Internal Medicine concept. This question would be important if you worked in an ER and a newborn was brought in with cyanosis.

Which of the following is the most common cyanotic heart defect manifesting in newborns?

    A. Tetralogy of Fallot
    B. Total anomalous pulmonary venous return
    C. Transposition of the great vessels
    D. Tricuspid atresia
    E. VSD

128.

A 2-year-old child comes into the Emergency Room with severe cyanosis. The parents say the child has a congenital heart defect. You note that the child is squatting when left alone.

PAST MEDICAL HISTORY: Negative except for knowledge of congenital heart defect

SOCIAL HISTORY:
    Attends daycare
    Lives with mother and father; neither smoke

FAMILY HISTORY:
    Non-contributory
    No siblings with congenital heart disease

REVIEW OF SYSTEMS: Decreased appetite recently

PHYSICAL EXAMINATION:
    BP 80/40 (normal), P 120 (tachycardic), RR 30 (tachypneic), Temp 98.5° F
    Cyanosis is evident
    Heart: Relatively quiet sounds; right ventricular impulse is noted
    Pulmonary closure is not heard
    Rest of exam normal

Well, let's make this easy for you. This is an older child with congenital heart disease and cyanosis. The most common etiology for this is tetralogy of Fallot. His physical exam and the squatting that you note are consistent with this diagnosis.

Which of the following correctly describes the 4 components of tetralogy of Fallot?

    A. Large VSD, left ventricular outflow tract obstruction, overriding aorta, LVH
    B. Large VSD, right ventricular outflow tract obstruction, overriding aorta, LVH
    C. Large VSD, right ventricular outflow tract obstruction, overriding aorta, RVH
    D. ASD, VSD, patent ductus arteriosus, LVH
    E. ASD, right ventricular outflow tract obstruction, overriding aorta, RVH

129.

A 24-year-old woman presents to your office complaining of palpitations. These occur most often when she drinks coffee. She has never had syncope. The palpitations can last up to 3–5 minutes and spontaneously resolve.

PAST MEDICAL HISTORY: Negative

SOCIAL HISTORY:
    Works as a cross-country truck driver
    Married with 1 child
    Smokes 2 packs/day of cigarettes
    Drinks 1/5 of vodka on the weekends

FAMILY HISTORY:
    Mother 60 with HTN
    Father 50 with HTN

REVIEW OF SYSTEMS: Negative

PHYSICAL EXAMINATION:
    BP 110/70, P 90, RR 16, Temp 98.8° F, Ht. 6'1", Wt 230 lbs

HEENT:	PERRLA, EOMI
	TMs clear
	Throat clear
Neck:	Supple
Heart:	RRR without murmurs, rubs, or gallops
Lungs:	CTA
Abdomen:	Benign
Extremities:	No cyanosis, clubbing, or edema
GU:	Normal female external genitalia

Which of the following would be the next most useful test in evaluating this patient?

  A. Stress test
  B. Left heart catheterization
  C. Right heart catheterization
  D. Holter study
  E. Echocardiogram

130.

A 45-year-old man with diabetes and severe knee arthritis is referred to you by his rheumatologist. He has chest pain with typical and atypical features for angina. Sometimes the pain is a "pressure" in his mid-chest, but mostly he describes sharp stabbing pain at the right upper sternal border. He denies any lung disease. He cannot walk very far due to his arthritis.

PAST MEDICAL HISTORY:	Severe arthritis; takes ibuprofen 800 mg three times daily; occasionally has to take narcotic agents to relieve the pain Diabetes for 10 years—takes insulin 30 U NPH in a.m.
SOCIAL HISTORY:	Lives alone in an apartment with modern conveniences Smokes ½ pack of cigarettes daily Doesn't drink alcohol
FAMILY HISTORY:	Father 70 with HTN Mother died at age 72 of stroke Brother 42 with diabetes
REVIEW OF SYSTEMS:	No radiation of pain No shortness of breath with pain No headaches No dyspnea on exertion—but can't walk so difficult to assess

PHYSICAL EXAMINATION:
   BP 120/80, RR 20, Temp 98.7° F, P 88

HEENT:	PERRLA, EOMI TMs clear Throat clear; poor dentition
Neck:	Supple
Heart:	RRR without murmurs, rubs, or gallops
Lungs:	CTA
Abdomen:	Benign
Extremities:	Severe osteoarthritis of the knees

Which of the following is the most appropriate next step to evaluate this patient?

A. Electrophysiologic study.
B. Treat the patient for an ulcer because of all the non-steroidals he is taking.
C. Routine stress test.
D. Dobutamine stress echo.
E. Proceed to left heart catheterization.

131.

A 60-year-old man presents with a large anterior myocardial infarction. He is hypotensive and tachycardic. Vital signs are tenuous at best with a BP of 90/50 mmHg and a heart rate of 120. He begins to become unresponsive and appears to be deteriorating on arrival to the ER.

Which of the following treatments would <u>not</u> be appropriate?

    A. Placement of an intraaortic balloon pump
    B. Getting the patient to the cardiac cath lab immediately
    C. Starting nitroprusside or nitroglycerin IV for afterload reduction
    D. Placement of a Swan-Ganz catheter to monitor pressures and output
    E. Starting inotropic agents (dopamine or dobutamine)

132.

You are seeing a new patient who is a 65-year-old man with a history of poorly controlled hypertension. Three months ago, he developed shortness of breath, increased fatigue, and two-pillow orthopnea. Last month while he was traveling in Eureka Springs, Arkansas, he consulted a physician about these symptoms and was started on digoxin (0.25 mg/day), hydrochlorothiazide (50 mg a day), and potassium supplementation. At that time, he weighed 190 lbs with a blood pressure of 150/80 mmHg. He said his doctor said something about "JVD" of 4 cm. He had swelling of his ankles at that time also. An ECG from the visit one month ago showed left ventricular hypertrophy. CXR at that time showed cardiomegaly without effusion. Routine lab then showed BUN of 28 mg/dL and serum creatinine of 1.4 mg/dL.

PAST MEDICAL HISTORY: Poorly controlled hypertension

SOCIAL HISTORY:
    Lives with wife and dog
    Smokes ½ pack/day of cigarettes
    Drinks 1 beer a week

FAMILY HISTORY:
    Father died of MI at age 67
    Mother died of MI at age 66

REVIEW OF SYSTEMS:
    No fever
    Morning cough—clears with persistent coughing
    Weight loss of 7 pounds
    Still fatigued but a little better

PHYSICAL EXAMINATION:
    BP 130/79, P 96, RR 18, Temp 99° F, Weight 183 lbs

HEENT:	PERRLA, EOMI
	TMs clear
	Throat clear
Neck:	Supple; neck veins flat; no JVD
Heart:	RRR without murmurs, rubs, with an S₃ gallop
Lungs:	Few scattered crackles in bases
Abdomen:	Bowel sounds present; no hepatosplenomegaly
Extremities:	No cyanosis, clubbing, or edema

Lab today:

    BUN 45 mg/dL

    Serum creatinine 1.6 mg/dL

    Serum sodium 136 mEq/L

    Serum potassium 3.6 mEq/L

    Serum digoxin 1.8 ng/mL (therapeutic 1.0–2.0)

Which of the following is the best course to take at this time?

    A. Add nothing at this point and follow up in one month.

    B. Increase digoxin dose.

    C. Add an ACE inhibitor.

    D. Change hydrochlorothiazide to furosemide.

    E. Add calcium channel blocker.

133.

A 65-year-old man presents for surgical repair of bilateral inguinal hernias that he has had for over 3 years. He denies chest pain or dyspnea on exertion. He says he feels healthy as a horse.

PAST MEDICAL HISTORY:	Inferior myocardial infarction 3 months ago
	Hypertension for 15 years
MEDICATIONS:	Isosorbide dinitrate 20 mg tid
	Captopril 25 mg tid
	Atenolol 20 mg qd
	Enteric-coated aspirin qd
SOCIAL HISTORY:	Works as a carhop at a local drive-in
	Returned to work 6 weeks after his MI
	Roller-skates to work, which is about 3 miles away
	Mows his lawn on the weekend
	Quit smoking in 1972
	2 glasses of red wine once a week
FAMILY HISTORY:	Father died of MI at age 70
	Mother died of MI at age 67
	Brother died of MI at age 56
REVIEW OF SYSTEMS:	Negative

PHYSICAL EXAMINATION:

    BP 120/70, P 60, RR 18, Temp 99.2° F

HEENT:	PERRLA, EOMI, developing cataract in left eye
	TMs clear
	Throat: clear
Neck:	Supple, no bruit
Heart:	RRR without murmurs, rubs, or gallops
Lung:	CTA
Abdomen:	Bowel sounds present, no hepatosplenomegaly

Extremities: No cyanosis, clubbing, or edema
Laboratory: CXR normal
              ECG: Q waves in leads II, III, and AVF; otherwise normal

Which of the following is most appropriate at this point?

A. Proceed to surgery now.
B. Approve for surgery now, depending on results of echocardiogram.
C. Approve for surgery in 3 months, depending on the results of a radionucleotide stress test.
D. Schedule surgery in 3 months, if clinically unchanged.
E. Wait 9 months before proceeding to surgery.

134.

A 67-year-old Chinese-American is seen in follow-up after an anterior myocardial infarction. He is doing well and has no complaints.

PAST MEDICAL HISTORY: Negative before the MI

MEDICATIONS: ECASA one qd
                        Propranolol 40 mg PO tid
                        Isosorbide dinitrate 20 mg tid

SOCIAL HISTORY: Retired history professor
                        Lives with wife
                        Has never smoked cigarettes
                        Drinks occasional beer on weekend

FAMILY HISTORY: Unknown; adopted

REVIEW OF SYSTEMS: Unremarkable

PHYSICAL EXAMINATION:
    BP 120/70, RR 18, P 42, Temp 98.3° F

    HEENT: PERRLA, EOMI
                TMs clear
                Throat clear
    Neck: Supple, no JVD
    Heart: RRR without murmurs, rubs, or gallops
    Lungs: CTA
    Abdomen: Bowel sounds present, no masses
    Extremities: No cyanosis, clubbing, trace pedal edema

Which of the following is the next best step in his management?

A. Order thyroid function tests.
B. Schedule for electrophysiologic testing.
C. Decrease the propranolol dose.
D. Insert temporary pacemaker.
E. Discontinue aspirin therapy.

135.

A 50-year-old woman is referred to you for evaluation of a pulsatile abdominal mass. Her history is remarkable for long-standing hypertension as well as smoking for 30 years (1 pack/day). She has had some mild abdominal pain that brought her initially to her local physician.

PAST MEDICAL HISTORY: Negative as above

SOCIAL HISTORY: Works in Sun City, Arizona, as a transcriptionist (notes she has been more
                                                  forgetful lately and leaves her transcription equipment in odd places—
                                                  like the bathroom)
                                                  Married with 2 children
                                                  Smoking history as above

FAMILY HISTORY: Essentially unremarkable

REVIEW OF SYSTEMS: No intermittent claudication
                                                  No peripheral edema
                                                  No chronic stasis changes
                                                  No fevers
                                                  No cough
                                                  No chills
                                                  No weight loss

PHYSICAL EXAMINATION:
     BP 120/70, Temp 38.7° F, P 70, RR 18
     She is in no acute distress.

          HEENT: PERRLA, EOMI
                                 TMs clear
                                 Throat: clear
          Neck: Supple
          Heart: RRR without murmurs, rubs, or gallops
          Lungs: CTA
          Abdomen: Bowel sounds present; there is an ill-defined mid-epigastric pulsatile mass without bruit
          Extremities: No cyanosis, clubbing, or edema

LABORATORY: Ultrasound of the abdomen shows a 5.6 cm infrarenal abdominal aortic aneurysm

Which of the following is the next best step in his management?

A. Repeat abdominal ultrasound every 6 months until the aneurysm reaches 6 cm.
B. Observation is best until she develops symptoms, then proceed to repair.
C. Place her on warfarin.
D. Vascular surgery consultation for aneurysm repair.
E. Have her wear a tight-fitting corset.

136.

A 46-year-old woman presented initially to the hospital with acute substernal chest pain. She described no previous cardiac history. Her initial ECG showed acute ST-segment elevation of 5 mm and Q waves in the inferior-lateral leads. Subsequently her CPK increased to 3,300. It is now the fourth day post-MI and you are seeing her for daily rounds.

She says that in the last few hours, she has become short of breath and feels like she is not feeling as well as yesterday. She has not had any syncopal episodes.

Significant aspect of the physical examination:

She now has a holosystolic murmur, which is loudest at the apex.
No signs of cardiac tamponade are present.

You order a stat echocardiogram.

At the same time as ordering the echocardiogram, which of the following do you do next?

A. Notify your cardiovascular surgeon to come right away and evaluate her for emergent repair of VSD.
B. Notify your cardiovascular surgeon to come right away and evaluate her for emergent mitral valve replacement.
C. Notify your cardiovascular surgeon to come in the next day or two to evaluate her for elective repair of post-MI VSD.
D. No surgery is indicated; this is non-surgical emergency only, and she will respond to pressor agents quickly.
E. Schedule her for cardiocentesis.

137.

You are called to evaluate a 35-year-old man who is to undergo significant tooth extraction.

PAST MEDICAL HISTORY: Non-significant

SOCIAL HISTORY: Works as a clown on the rodeo circuit; frequently gets hit in the belly by bulls, horses, and women he dates

FAMILY HISTORY: Unremarkable

PHYSICAL EXAMINATION: Essentially unremarkable

For which of the following would antimicrobial prophylaxis for endocarditis be indicated?

A. History of acute rheumatic fever but no cardiac murmur
B. History of coronary artery bypass grafting
C. History of ventricular septal defect repaired 3 years ago without residual murmur
D. History of previous endocarditis
E. Ostium primum atrial septal defect

138.

A dentist calls wanting to know about endocarditis prophylaxis for his patients. He gives you a list of items he is concerned about and asks your opinion if they require prophylaxis.

Which of the following require prophylaxis for dental procedures?

- A. Atrial septal defect
- B. History of coronary artery surgery
- C. Hypertrophic cardiomyopathy
- D. Presence of an implanted defibrillator with epicardial leads
- E. None of these choices requires prophylaxis

139.

A dentist calls wanting to know which dental procedures require prophylaxis. She gives you a list that she is concerned about.

Which of the following dental procedures require prophylaxis for endocarditis?

- A. Orthodontic appliance adjustment
- B. Initial placement of orthodontic bands
- C. Suture removal
- D. Impressions
- E. Placement of removable orthodontic appliances

140.

A 70-year-old woman had a prosthetic hip joint placed 6 years ago. She has not been to the dentist in years and has decided that maybe she should make a visit. She read on the Internet that some people need to take antibiotics before they go to the dentist. She is penicillin-allergic (anaphylaxis).

Based on her history so far, which of the following is correct about whether prophylaxis is warranted?

- A. Yes, she should take amoxicillin 2 grams 1 hour before her visit.
- B. Yes, she should take cephalexin 2 grams 1 hour before her visit.
- C. Yes, she should take clindamycin 600 mg 1 hour before her visit.
- D. No, presence of prosthetic joints does not require antibiotic prophylaxis.
- E. The answer depends on which device she had implanted—a porcine or mechanical hip.

141.

A 60-year-old man is about to undergo a cystoscopy and has a prosthetic valve. He is not allergic to any medications.

Which of the following antibiotic(s) is/are appropriate for infective endocarditis prophylaxis?

A. Ampicillin 2 grams IM or IV plus gentamicin 1.5 mg/kg
B. Vancomycin 1 gm IV over 1–2 hours plus gentamicin 1.5 mg/kg
C. Amoxicillin alone 2 grams PO 1 hour before procedure is sufficient
D. Vancomycin alone 1 gram IV over 1–2 hours
E. None of the choices is correct

142.

A 17-year-old senior at HubCap High in Snake Pit, Arizona, is the starting guard on the state basketball championship team. He has been offered a full scholarship at Duke of Earl University after never missing a game in four seasons and setting the all-time school record in both total points and assists. Seated in the stands for the final game of the season, you are summoned when he collapses at mid-court after a thunderous game-ending dunk shot. You assist in his full resuscitation from ventricular fibrillation, accompanied in this effort by the local paramedics who were there in 3½ minutes.

With an opportunity to examine him in the hospital, you are struck by his bifid carotid impulses—which are mirrored in his apex cardiogram, the latter of which you are able to both palpate and project via shadows on the bed clothing. He has a harsh holosystolic murmur at the lower left sternal border that accentuates with the upright posture as well as the Valsalva strain. Occasional premature contractions are followed by radial artery impulses, which are diminished relative to the apparent sinus cycle pulsations.

You feel certain that the young man has which of the following?

A. Hypertrophic obstructive cardiomyopathy (HOCM)
B. Myxomatous mitral valve prolapse (MVP)
C. Ostium secundum atrial septal defect (ASD)
D. Ostium primum atrioventricular septal defect (AVSD)
E. Acquired (muscular) ventricular septal defect (VSD)

143.

Mr. Crankshaft works in the local auto-reclaiming yard where coworkers have been stunned to observe unusual "spells" in their boss. He is 56-years-old and has been well all of his life but is now having episodes of crashing headache, sweating, irritability, and ashen pallor... "Farley, you look like you seen a ghost!" During one such episode, the coworkers cajole him into making an immediate Emergency Room (ER) visit while you are on duty and find his blood pressure to be 228/136 mmHg. With further questioning, you learn that Aunt Ethel had a "tumor taken off her thyroid gland" and that Uncle Clem has had a "tumor removed from on top of one of his kidneys." You notice further that your patient has a neat row of small nodules along the leading edge of his protruded tongue.

You know not only his diagnosis but also the nature of the familial associations, realizing that chromosomal analyses might very well lead, in selected family members, to prophylactic removal of which of the following?

    A. Kidneys
    B. Pituitary glands
    C. Adrenal glands
    D. Thyroid glands
    E. Parathyroid glands

144.

A 61-year-old man presents for evaluation. He weighs 205 lbs (body mass index [BMI] = 31 kg/M^2 @ height of 5' 8"), and smokes 2½ packs daily of unfiltered Prairie Dogs. His latest serum cholesterol was 326 mg/dL with low- and high-density (LDL & HDL) sub-fractions of 236 and 32, respectively, and triglycerides of 290. He engages a patron in a shouting match, whereupon he is seen to clutch his chest in horror with what he describes as "crushing, heavy, smothering" chest discomfort. The local Emergency Medical Service (EMS) personnel are summoned and arrive promptly; they administer oxygen and nitroglycerin after documenting a systemic arterial blood pressure of 190/110 mmHg.

At the hospital, he is found to have completely normal "cardiac markers," and his electrocardiogram reveals deep symmetrical T-wave inversions across all of the precordial leads.

You write "unstable angina" as your impression on the chart, knowing that the most likely acute pathophysiology of this event has been which of the following?

    A. Mural thrombus formation on a ruptured or eroded atherosclerotic plaque
    B. Dissection of the thoracic aorta at the left coronary ostium
    C. Intense vasospasm of the left anterior descending coronary (resulting in total occlusion)
    D. Myocardial oxygen demand due to accelerated hypertension
    E. Adverse rheologic properties of the coronary circulation (via hyperlipidemia)

145.

A 63-year-old, retired, second-grade English teacher presents to the ER with the local EMS after she suffered 40 minutes of crushing chest pain at home. You note her ashen skin color with moist clammy features and a BP of 80/60 mmHg with a heart rate of 122/min. Her systemic venous pressure appears to be elevated, and there is no murmur.

Her ECG reveals 6–8 mm ST-segment elevation in leads I, aVL, and V1-V6 with hyperacute T-wave changes in the same leads and developing deep Q waves.

Without an apparent mechanical complication of her acute event, you know that her prognosis may be improved by which of the following?

    A. Acute mitral valvuloplasty
    B. Surgical resection of the myocardial infarction segment
    C. Urgent revascularization
    D. Immediate high-dose adrenolytic therapy (e.g., propranolol 80 mg every 6 hr)
    E. Chronic subcutaneous home infusion of dobutamine

146.

Your next patient is the shipping agent at your local Gigantic Falcon Food Store, where he works a vigorous 60-hour week. He will consume 24 packs of unfiltered cigarettes during such a week and, indeed, you have already recognized his developing (emphysematous) chronic obstructive pulmonary disease (COPD). He has mentioned to you that if he tries to walk with any vigor, he develops squeezing calf pain that interrupts his exercise. His BP has inched up to 152/94 mmHg despite efforts at both weight loss and reduced salt intake.

You are now seeing him in the office for what you feel sure is exertional angina pectoris. You order a stress exercise evaluation that confirms an apparent ischemic response. The patient declines your suggestion of diagnostic coronary catheterization, and you now contemplate empiric therapy.

You will select sublingual nitrates, daily aspirin, and which of the following?

A. Enalapril maleate
B. Atenolol
C. Pindolol
D. Propranolol HCl
E. Losartan K^+

147.

A 42-year-old machinist presents to the clinic with a history of 6 weeks of nagging mid-abdominal pain. He has not been previously ill. You discover that his peripheral eosinophil count is 4% and that his urine sediment is "telescopic" with red cells, white cells, and granular casts. Visceral angiography suggests the correct diagnosis, which is confirmed by biopsy that demonstrates involvement of medium-sized vessels showing the characteristic ring of acellular azurophilic fibrinoid necrosis. All tests for anti-neutrophil cytoplasmic antibody (ANCA) markers are negative, as is a hepatitis screen.

Which of the following is the most likely diagnosis?

A. Classic polyarteritis nodosa (PAN)
B. Microscopic polyarteritis (MPA)
C. Churg-Strauss syndrome
D. Wegener granulomatosis
E. Kawasaki disease

148.

You are on duty in the ER when a group of four companions present their friend, a 21-year-old woman who works for the local escort service. She is acutely ill with a temperature of 104° F, HR 130/min, respirations 18/minute, and apparent distress. Her systemic venous pressure is elevated, and the jugular venous pulse contour is dominated by large "cv" waves that swell with each inspiration. Your auscultatory examination reveals a Grade III/VI holosystolic murmur heard best at the lower left (and right) sternal border(s), and which accentuates to Grade IV/VI intensity with inspiration. The liver seems to pulsate with each systole.

A chest x-ray reveals scattered focal white fluffy opacities. You recognize what is no doubt a complication of her intravenous heroin usage.

Which of the following is the most likely diagnosis, manifested as acute?

A. Mitral regurgitation
B. Aortic valvular regurgitation
C. Tricuspid regurgitation
D. Ruptured sinus of Valsalva aneurysm
E. Bleeding pulmonary arteriovenous (AV) fistula

149.

A 41-year-old used car salesman comes to see you in the ER after developing one of his "spells," during which his heart feels as if it will "jump out of (his) chest." These episodes begin abruptly, particularly if he doubles his normal daily caffeine intake (which usually consists of 3 cups of coffee and 2–3 cans of cola). He is concerned that he will pass out with today's episode, although he has never done so before.

You quickly establish that the patient's HR is 150/min and supine BP 110/70 mmHg, and the patient is placed on a monitor, which confirms the presence of a "wide complex tachycardia."

A 12-lead ECG is obtained **during tachycardia** and reveals a precisely regular rhythm without discernible P-waves, QRS-duration of 185 milliseconds, a mean electrical QRS axis of –110 degrees in the frontal plane (toward the patient's right shoulder), and a rather monomorphic QRS configuration with large dominant R-waves in V_1.

You would surmise which of the following?

A. A calcium antagonist given intravenously (IV) **cannot** be selected safely as the initial treatment.
B. This could **not** be ventricular tachycardia with the apparent preservation of hemodynamic stability.
C. This could **not** be antidromic WPW because the QRS complexes are too wide.
D. The patient **must** be cardioverted emergently.
E. Either digitalis or adenosine IV **may** be given with impunity as the drugs most likely to convert the tachycardia.

150.

You staff the ER of your local hospital one afternoon when parents present with their 6-year-old son. They are concerned that he has not been able to start school. He appears to them to have "weak muscles" that have resulted in a "funny way of walking," as well as frequent falls and difficulty in rising from a chair or ascending the stairs at night at bedtime. They describe a curious method of rising from the floor wherein he "walks up" his torso (using a hands-to-knees sequence, etc.—which you recognize as Gowers sign). On your examination, you are struck by the apparent hypertrophy of his calf muscles.

Which of the following would you say to the parents?

A. They may expect a normal life span for their son.
B. They must be aware of the risk of sudden death.
C. Happily, his children will have little or no chance of the disease.
D. Sadly, should they decide to have additional children, all of his sisters theoretically could be similarly affected.
E. He is at risk for premature myocardial infarction.

151.

You are called to the ER to be introduced to a retired 66-year-old high school English teacher who has been sitting up at night for the past week, unable to lie flat for more than 15 minutes. Your examination in the ER reveals a HR of 100/min, respirations of 20/min, jugular venous distension to the angle of the jaw with the patient sitting bolt upright, hepatomegaly with a vertical expanse of percussive dullness of 15 cm in the mid-clavicular line, pitting ankle edema, and a murmur of tricuspid regurgitation that is holosystolic at the lower left sternal border and which increases from Grade I/VI to III/VI on inspiration (known as the Rivero-Carvallo maneuver—[editor's note—OK you can tell a cardiologist wrote this one so don't blame me!]). Careful auscultation further reveals gallop sounds early in diastole from both ventricles (RVS_3 & LVS_3). The lung fields are filled with diffuse inspiratory rales and crackling noises.

Your patient is clearly suffering from which of the following?

A. Acute pulmonary thromboembolism
B. Cor pulmonale heart disease
C. Biventricular congestive heart failure
D. Pericardial effusion with pericardial tamponade
E. Eisenmenger transformation

152.

A 61-year-old patient seen in the ER presents with hypotension (88/60 mmHg), tachycardia (122/min), distended neck veins dominated by the "x" descents, and a globular cardiac silhouette on the chest x-ray. Careful analysis of her blood pressure reveals that the systolic Korotkoff sounds are first heard **in exhalation only** at 110 mmHg, whereas they are heard **throughout the respiratory cycle** only after further lowering the cuff pressure to 88 mmHg. You are well acquainted with this remarkable physical finding and immediately suspect the proper diagnosis.

Which of the following interventions is most likely to benefit this patient's care?

A. Pleurocentesis
B. Transfusion of two units of packed, washed red blood cells
C. IV administration of propranolol
D. IV infusion of 1.5 million units of streptokinase over 60 minutes
E. Catheter pericardiocentesis

153.

An 18-year-old ballet dancer seeks your consultation in the outpatient clinic because of cardiac consciousness (manifested as an intermittent "skipping" and "flipping" inside her chest). You are struck by her graceful physiognomy and measure her height as 70" and arm span as 71.5". Her joint laxity permits easy apposition of her thumbs to her forearm surfaces and, indeed, she reports the childhood ability to "touch her elbows together behind her back."

Her physical examination includes the following: There is a mid-systolic click and a Grade II/VI late-systolic murmur. There is murmur augmentation with both standing and Valsalva strain. There is murmur diminution with prompt squatting, followed (often) by dramatic augmentation of the murmur with resumption of the standing posture, occasionally to Grade VI intensity (e.g., audible in the room without a stethoscope).

Based on your findings, you are certain that she has which of the following?

  A. Myxomatous mitral valve prolapse (MVP)
  B. Ostium secundum atrial septal defect (ASD)
  C. Ostium primum atrioventricular septal defect (AVSD)
  D. Acquired (muscular) ventricular septal defect (VSD)
  E. Hypertrophic obstructive cardiomyopathy (HOCM) (IHSS)

154.

A 56-year-old automobile mechanic presents to the ER with extreme dyspnea accompanied by a stabbing right thoracic pain that increases with each inspiration. The respiratory rate is 28/min; systemic arterial pressure is 100/84 mmHg. The jugular pulsations are noted to be elevated nearly to the earlobes with the patient sitting bolt upright; no clear pattern is discerned, although they seem to pulsate at a rate equal to the patient's arterial pulse of 110/min. A pleural rub is heard at the site of the chest discomfort. A right ventricular lift is apparent, and the pulmonary artery is palpable. S_2 is split widely and P_2 is loud and palpable. The patient reports having just completed a nearly non-stop 4,300-mile round-trip solo drive of an 18-wheeler to another garage on the West Coast and back. He is also known to have recently diagnosed unresectable adenocarcinoma of the colon, for which he refused further treatment. The patient admits to smoking 2½ packs per day of cigarettes since he was 15 years old (i.e., > 100 pack years).

This patient has an acute version of which of the following disorders?

  A. Tricuspid regurgitation due to ruptured chordal apparatus
  B. Tricuspid stenosis due to malignant carcinoid syndrome
  C. Cor pulmonale due to pulmonary thromboembolism
  D. Pericardial constriction due to previous blunt chest trauma (steering wheel injury via motor vehicle accident)
  E. Pericardial tamponade resulting from metastatic pericardial disease via bronchogenic carcinoma

---

155.

Your next patient is a 32-year-old African-American attorney who has been under extraordinary stress in the midst of a high-profile courtroom drama. He asked to see you because of chest pains. Your review of his ECG shows ST-segment elevations in multiple leads with prominent J-points and T-wave magnitudes that exceed the magnitude of the ST-segment elevations in those leads bearing the ST abnormalities. The patient's BP is (and has been) normal, as is his physical examination. Fortunately, the patient's life insurance evaluations had included an ECG tracing that you are able to obtain for comparison, and you note the static nature of these changes.

You know that the most likely explanation of the ST-segment findings is which of the following?

  A. Normal repolarization variant
  B. Prinzmetal's variant angina pectoris
  C. Chronic pericarditis
  D. Recording artifact
  E. Hypothyroidism (and hypothermia)

156.

Your new patient today is a 64-year-old retired coal miner from Fancy Gripp, West Virginia, who presents with progressive dyspnea and peripheral edema. He has sought compensation for "black lung" and has smoked non-filter cigarettes up to 3½ packs daily for 52 years. He begins each day with a 90-minute coughing session productive of "from ½ to ¾ of a coffee cup" of dark sputum ("almost like tar"). His P_aO_2 on room air is 53 mmHg with a P_aCO_2 of 52 mmHg, HCO_3 of 32 mmol/L and pH of 7.37. His ECG reveals maximum positive-amplitude R waves in limb lead III and isoelectric QRS complexes in lead aVR.

The most likely cause of QRS frontal plane axis deviation in this patient is which of the following?

A. Systemic arterial hypertension, "essential" of long-standing
B. Pulmonary arterial hypertension, acquired via cor pulmonale
C. Severe calcific valvular aortic stenosis, acquired
D. Severe non-calcific valvular pulmonic stenosis, congenital
E. Coarctation of the thoracic aorta, post-ductal (adult type)

157.

A 61-year-old shop foreman gets off work at 3:30 p.m. and decides to stop at the local bar to share a few cold ones with the Friday crowd. After his third mug of beer, each followed by a double shot of whiskey, he lurches off the back of the stool landing on the floor, apparently unconscious. Trained in the basics of Advanced Cardiac Life Support (ACLS), the bartender quickly confirms that he indeed has a pulse with an apparent rate of 145/min. As the EMS team arrives on the scene, the patient has regained consciousness, though very intoxicated. They use their "quick-look" paddle electrodes and demonstrate clearly a wide complex tachycardia, which is quite regular and continues at the rate of 145/min. The QRS duration is 0.185 sec, and there appear to be P waves at a much slower rate. As the medics prepare to administer protocol-driven treatment, they call you in the ER describing all of the above.

You tell them that this indeed is most likely which of the following?

A. AV nodal re-entry tachycardia (AVNRT)
B. Multifocal atrial tachycardia (MAT)
C. Sinus tachycardia with bundle branch block (BBB)
D. Ventricular tachycardia (VT)
E. Ventricular fibrillation (VF)

158.

A 52-year-old CEO sits down for dinner with his family but is reluctant to eat because of an overpowering feeling of "indigestion." As a registered nurse, his wife is insistent on a "911" call, and the patient is transported to your ER. His BP is 90/70 mmHg, HR 50/min, and his general appearance is characterized by sweating and ashen pallor.

The ECG shows 2–3 mm ST-segment elevation in leads II, III, and aVF accompanied by "hyperacute" (tall peaked) T waves but no Q waves at this point.

Which of the gentleman's coronary arteries listed below is likely occluded?

A. Left anterior descending (LAD)
B. Diagonal branch of the LAD
C. Posterior circumflex branch of the left coronary
D. Proximal right coronary artery (RCA)
E. Right ventricular branch of the RCA

159.

A 19-year-old college student seeks a pre-employment physical from you in preparation for applying for the position of lifeguard at the local country club. You note his tall, thin habitus and obtain height and arm-span measurements of 72" each. Your examination documents a Grade II/VI systolic ejection "flow" murmur in the pulmonary outflow tact and apparent fixed splitting of the second heart sound. His ECG demonstrates a mean electrical QRS axis of 115 degrees in the frontal plane, and there are prominent R waves in Lead V1 with a R:S ratio of (1.3:1).

You recognize that his apparent right ventricular hypertrophy (RVH) is surely a result of which of the following?

A. Ostium secundum atrial septal defect (ASD)
B. Cystic fibrosis
C. Primary pulmonary hypertension
D. Membranous ventricular septal defect (VSD)
E. Type A Wolff-Parkinson-White syndrome (WPW)

160.

A 27-year-old used car salesman presents with his latest episode of palpitations and rapid heart action. He relates countless such episodes since his late teens and one episode of syncope. He felt as if he would lose consciousness with today's episode, but did not. You confirm a heart rate of nearly 220/min and succeed in obtaining a 12-lead ECG **during tachycardia** showing **no** R-R interval variability, narrow QRS complexes (100 msec), and discernible P waves hidden in the succeeding ST segments with a QP interval of 110 msec. The patient produces a previous routine tracing from his billfold; it reveals a PR interval of 0.07 sec (70 msec) and slurred sluggish upstrokes as the initial portion of the QRS complexes in multiple leads.

Your best diagnosis is which of the following?

A. First-degree AV block with Mobitz I progression (Wenckebach's)
B. WPW with orthodromic tachycardia (AVRT)
C. AV nodal re-entrant tachycardia (AVNRT)
D. Multifocal atrial tachycardia (MAT)

161.

Your next new patient admitted to your team on the Inpatient Service is a 62-year-old man who has suffered from congestive heart failure for the last 7 years. He has attempted to take his medications faithfully, but the complexity of his regimen and his failing eyesight have sometimes resulted in inadvertent errors. In the ER, he is noted to have a narrow complex tachycardia at a rate of 88/min with apparent retrograde P waves hidden in the ST segments. You recognize non-paroxysmal junctional tachycardia (NPJT) and understand this rhythm to reflect a nonspecific acceleration (to within the range of 70–130/min) of what would otherwise represent the normal rate range of the junctional tissues (40–60/min) in a resting adult.

The best descriptor for this known mechanism of arrhythmia is which of the following?

A. Re-entry
B. Early after-depolarizations
C. Enhanced automaticity
D. Delayed after-depolarizations
E. Atrio-ventricular bypass (via a congenital anomalous pathway)

162.

Your next patient is a 29-year-old with known phenylketonuria (PKU) and for whom you have attempted to provide general care for the last 10 years. Maintenance of a low-protein diet has been sporadic at best, in part because of her constant mobility. She found herself unexpectedly pregnant last year, since which she has given birth to a child who has been evaluated by one of your pediatrician colleagues. She reports the pediatrician's observation of brachio-femoral delay and an upper:lower limb BP asymmetry of 100 systolic in both arms as compared to 80 mmHg in the legs. All pressures were obtained by careful Doppler measurements.

You recognize that the child has which of the following?

A. Kawasaki disease
B. Takayasu disease
C. Tetralogy of Fallot
D. Coarctation of the aorta

163.

The lead singer of a grunge rock band comes to your Emergency Room complaining of severe dyspnea, fever, and chills for the last 3 days. She admits to using intravenous heroin.

On examination, her temperature is 102.3° F, heart rate is 125 beats/min, and blood pressure 100/60 mmHg. She has large *v* waves in her jugular pulse. The carotid pulses are normal. She has a faint systolic murmur heard along the lower left sternal border, which becomes louder on inspiration. A third heart sound is present in the same area. She has scattered rhonchi and wheezes on lung examination. There are no splinter hemorrhages or other manifestations of endocarditis in the extremities, although there are several pustules present over the antecubital veins in both arms.
Laboratory data show a white blood count of 15,600 with a preponderance of neutrophils. Hemoglobin is 12.2 gm/dL; serum electrolytes, AST, and ALT are normal. Blood samples are sent for bacterial and fungal cultures, as well as hepatitis and HIV screening.

Which of the following is most likely to be present on an imaging study?

A. A chest x-ray showing pulmonary edema
B. A chest x-ray showing left ventricular enlargement
C. An echocardiogram showing a large vegetation on the aortic valve
D. An echocardiogram showing a large perforation in the anterior mitral valve leaflet
E. A ventilation/perfusion lung scan showing multiple perfusion defects

164.

A 19-year-old female collapses and dies during a sprint at a track meet. She was previously healthy and had no abnormalities on her school's routine physical examination for athletes.

Unfortunately, of autopsies done on individuals like this woman, a majority show no abnormalities.

If an abnormality is found at autopsy, which of the following is most likely?

   A. Large mitral valve leaflets with infiltration of myxomatous material on microscopic examination
   B. An anomalous origin of the left anterior descending coronary artery from the right coronary cusp
   C. Hypertrophic cardiomyopathy
   D. Severe pulmonic stenosis

165.

A certain young actress played the part of one of four sisters who lived in Boston during the Civil War. In the movie, she takes some bread to some starving immigrant neighbors, one of whom has scarlet fever. A few years later, she is shown dying of a cardiac-related illness.

If this had been a real case, which of the following would she most likely have on physical examination?

   A. A soft S_1
   B. A soft, decrescendo blowing murmur heard at the lower left sternal border in the sitting position.
   C. A sound heard with the diaphragm at the apex shortly after S_2
   D. A midsystolic click followed by a systolic murmur heard at the left sternal border
   E. A sound heard best with the bell at the apex after S_2

166.

An elderly actor with known severe coronary artery disease played a part in a movie alongside his real-life actress daughter, having to do with a certain pond. His elevated neck veins could easily be seen on the screen. He had known advanced left and right heart failure from previous myocardial infarctions.

Which of the following patterns would these neck veins most likely have?

   A. Large *a* waves and slow *y* descents
   B. Large *a* waves and very large *v* waves
   C. Rapid *x* and *y* descents
   D. Regular cannon *a* waves
   E. Distended neck veins with no pulsatile activity

167.

A 45-year-old Caucasian male CIA agent stationed in a Middle Eastern country develops the acute onset of severe dyspnea. He has no prior cardiac history and denies having chest pain. By the time he is taken to a hospital, he is in acute respiratory distress and requires intubation and mechanical ventilation. He has a very abnormal chest x-ray with total unilateral opacification. A preliminary diagnosis of acute pneumonia is made, blood cultures are drawn, and he is started on antibiotics.

After 48 hours, however, he is hypoxic on 100% FIO_2 and is becoming progressively hypotensive. You are the CIA's best internist, on call at all times for just such an emergency, and you are immediately flown halfway around the world in the back seat of an F14 fighter.

Upon arrival at the hospital, you are escorted to the bedside of a man identified to you only as "Joe." You learn from your colleagues on site that Joe has no known medical problems and does not smoke. He was completely well prior to the onset of symptoms.

On examination, you find a fit-appearing man who, at the moment, is obviously extremely ill. His blood pressure is 70 mmHg systolic, his heart rate is 120 beats/minute, and he is afebrile. His neck veins are elevated to the jaw with his torso inclined to 30°. He has a very prominent apical impulse. He has a rapid rate with a soft apical S_3. At times, through the respiratory noise, you think you hear a soft, early systolic decrescendo murmur near the apex. There are coarse breath sounds throughout the left lung and diminished breath sounds on the right. You confirm the chest x-ray findings. His white blood count is normal. The blood cultures are not growing anything, and tracheal cultures show normal flora. An ECG shows sinus tachycardia, but is otherwise normal.

You have brought along a new miniaturized echocardiogram machine, but the echo is extremely difficult technically because of his supine position and being on a mechanical ventilator.

Which of the following is the likely cause of this man's severe illness?

  A. Unilateral pneumonia
  B. An acute myocardial infarction with cardiogenic shock
  C. An acute myocardial infarction with a new ventricular septal defect
  D. Acute aortic regurgitation from infectious endocarditis; "Joe" was a closet IV drug abuser
  E. Acute mitral regurgitation from rupture of a myxomatous chordae

168.

You are a physician moonlighting in a small town hospital. A severely ill man shows up at the front door. You determine that he has acute mitral regurgitation from rupture of a myxomatous chordae.

Which of the following should you do as soon as possible?

  A. Transfer him via emergency air ambulance for urgent coronary angiography and probable coronary bypass grafting.
  B. Transfer him emergently for mitral valve repair or replacement.
  C. Start him on low-dose intravenous dopamine and, cautiously, on intravenous nitroprusside.
  D. Change the antibiotic coverage to the broadest possible spectrum and add positive end-expiratory pressure to his ventilator settings.
  E. Transfer him emergently for aortic valve replacement.

169.

You have been transported back in time to Paris in 1839. You have arrived on the scene in the palatial home of the French playwright and poet, Louis-Charles-Alfred de Musset. M. de Musset is having an argument with his companion, the romantic writer George Sand, pseudonym of Amandine-Aaurore-Lucile Dudevant, with whom he has had a torrid love affair for the past 7 years. Mme. Dudevant is outraged by the statement of her somewhat debauched friend, who has told her that he could tell where the prostitutes were in Paris by listening to their earrings tinkle as they constantly bobbed their heads. These prostitutes had chronic aortic regurgitation.

De Musset is one of the very few non-physicians for whom a physical examination finding is named. The origin of this honor is not clear, but it may have had to do with the illnesses contracted by de Musset and George Sand during their time together.

If one were to examine one of the ladies of the evening to whom the great poet referred, you would find which of the following?

A. A decreased rise time and volume in the carotid pulses
B. A late-peaking systolic ejection murmur in the second right intercostal space
C. Rapid y descents in the neck veins
D. A low-pitched, mid-diastolic rumble at the apex
E. Cyanosis and clubbing of the fingertips

170.

You have a 65-year-old neighbor who has just told you that he has been having intermittent chest pain that began 6 months ago. He has no history of heart disease and, other than hypertension, has no known medical problems. He describes a pressure-type sensation in his mid chest that occurs when he takes his 5-mile walk every day. You live in the foothills of the mountains and have seen your neighbor going up and down some fairly serious grades on his walk. The chest pain occurs usually when he is walking up the last steep hill. He has discovered that if he rests for 10 minutes before attempting this climb, he does not get the pain.

You, being the concerned internist that you are, convince him to come to your office for an evaluation. On examination, his blood pressure is 140/95, but otherwise there are no abnormalities. You happen to have a treadmill in your office, and he exercises for 11 minutes on a Bruce protocol (13.4 METs). He develops mild chest pain at peak exertion and has 1 mm of horizontal ST-segment depression in leads II, III, and aVF, which return to normal within 3 minutes into the recovery phase.

Of the following, what should you recommend?

A. Prescribe sublingual nitroglycerin as needed and begin secondary prevention for coronary artery disease.
B. Immediate hospitalization and cardiac catheterization with the intention of revascularization by your cardiologist partner.
C. Medical therapy with amlodipine and aspirin.
D. Repeat the exercise study with thallium scintigraphy.
E. Prescribe sublingual nitroglycerin and an angiotensin-converting enzyme inhibitor.

171.

A patient has been transferred to your hospital because of an episode of syncope and chest pain. At the other facility, a myocardial infarction was ruled out with cardiac markers, and they are at a loss to know why he had this episode. Upon arrival, he is resting comfortably and has had no more chest pain since the event 2 days ago. He had never had a similar episode. He recalls the sudden onset of sharp chest pain while sitting watching television and then waking up with his wife leaning over him. She tells you that he lost consciousness for about 30 seconds and did not have any tonic-clonic movement or loss of bowel or bladder control. He was immediately aware of his surroundings on awakening. He denies any other medical problems except a tibial fracture of his right leg 2 years ago, when he fell off his lawn tractor while negotiating a tight turn on a hillside.

On examination, his blood pressure is 130/70 mmHg, and heart rate is 67 beats/min and regular. There are no orthostatic changes. His neck veins are moderately elevated with prominent *v* waves. He has a prominent left parasternal lift and a third heart sound along the left sternal border. He has a positive Küssmaul sign in the neck veins and a pulsatile liver. His apical impulse is in the normal location and has a normal diameter. There are no murmurs, and his lungs are clear to auscultation. His right leg is mildly edematous below the knee, but not painful.

All of his laboratory data is normal except his chest x-ray and ECG. The former shows a prominent right heart border and large proximal pulmonary arteries. The left heart configuration is normal. His ECG shows sinus rhythm, a QRS axis of 80°, tall peaked P waves in the inferior leads, and deeply inverted T waves across the precordial leads. You have been provided with an ECG from 2 years ago. At that time, the axis was 30°, the P waves were normal, the axis was 15°, and the T waves were upright in the precordial leads.

You ask for a cardiology consult, and your colleague is concerned about the chest pain, syncope, and the newly inverted precordial T waves. She strongly recommends cardiac catheterization and coronary angiography to rule out a recent coronary event, possibly causing ventricular tachycardia as a cause of the syncope. She does not understand, however, how to correlate the physical examination findings with this diagnosis, so she plans to do a right heart catheterization as well.

Rather to her surprise, his coronary arteries are completely normal, and contrast left ventriculography shows no wall motion abnormalities.

Hemodynamics from the left and right heart catheterization are as follows:

Right atrial pressure (mmHg)	18
Right ventricular pressure	70/20
Pulmonary arterial pressure	72/35
Pulmonary capillary wedge pressure	10
Left ventricular end-diastolic pressure	8

She, being an excellent cardiologist, immediately schedules another test.

Which of the following will she most likely order?

    A. A transthoracic echocardiogram
    B. A transesophageal echocardiogram
    C. An arterial blood gas
    D. A ventilation/perfusion lung scan
    E. A carbon monoxide-diffusing lung study (DL_{CO})

172.

The chief of cardiology at a major university teaching hospital is generally agreed among the house staff to be manic and have a 5-minute attention span. You have the privilege of being the senior resident in the coronary care unit while he is your attending physician. You are minding your own business on rounds, listening to the medical student drone on with his presentation. You notice that the chief is becoming restless, always a bad sign. The student says something about the patient's neck veins being elevated when the attending suddenly launches into an impromptu lecture on the causes of neck vein elevation.

He turns to the white board and draws 2 figures: See below:

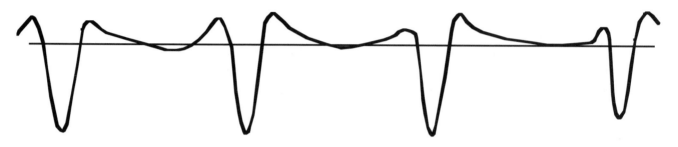

Patient A, right atrial pressure (the horizontal line presents 20 mmHg)

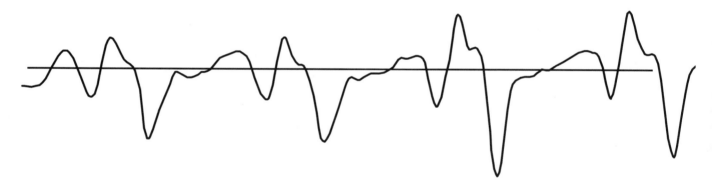

Patient B, right atrial pressure (the horizontal line represents 20 mmHg)

The chief then makes some statements about these drawings to the medical student and asks which of them are true.

Which of the following is your most likely answer?

    A. Patient A is more likely than patient B to have pulsus paradoxus.
    B. Patient A is more likely than patient B to have an early diastolic sound.
    C. Patient A is more likely than patient B to have calcification of the pericardium on chest x-ray.
    D. Patient A is more likely than patient B to have had symptoms for months.
    E. Patient A is more likely than patient B to have a Küssmaul sign.

173.

A 56-year-old woman comes to your Emergency Room complaining of the acute onset of chest pain 2 hours ago. She is in so much discomfort that it is hard to obtain a history, but she says she had been doing well until the onset of this pain, except for a mild upper respiratory infection for the past few days. She describes the pain as a sharp, stabbing feeling in the center of her chest. She has no history of cardiac disease, but does have risk factors of hypertension, hyperlipidemia, Type 2 diabetes, and substantial obesity.

On physical examination, her blood pressure is 160/96 and her heart rate is 115 beats/min. Her cardiac examination is extremely difficult because of her obesity and her constant movement as she tries to find a comfortable position. At least she has no pedal edema.

According to the ACC/AHA guidelines on the management of acute chest pain, she is given an aspirin to chew, blood is drawn for cardiac markers, and an electrocardiogram is obtained. Her ECG appears here:

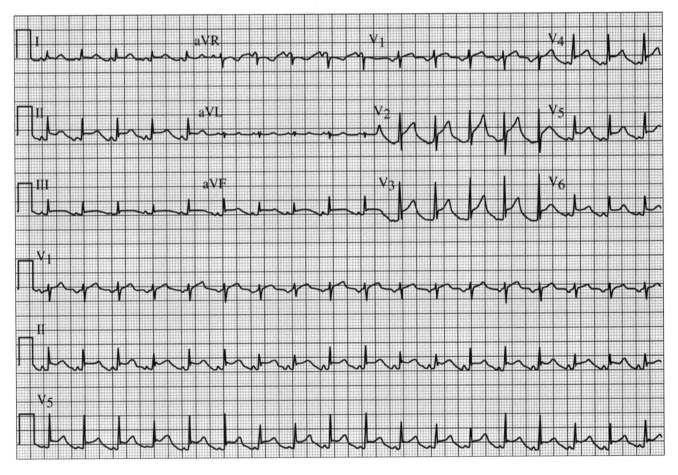

You should immediately do which of the following?

    A. Start an appropriate dose of tissue plasminogen activator (tPA) and intravenous heparin.
    B. Although the transportation time is 90 minutes, arrange immediate transfer to a tertiary care medical center for acute coronary angiography and probable coronary intervention.
    C. Start intravenous heparin, clopidogrel, and a GP IIb/IIIa inhibitor.
    D. Have the cardiologist come to the hospital and perform a transesophageal echocardiogram to rule out an acute thoracic aortic dissection.
    E. Treat the immediate pain with an intravenous narcotic and start ibuprofen 2400 mg/day.

174.

The history and electrocardiographic findings of various patients are listed below.

Which of these patients is likely to benefit the most from thrombolytic therapy?

A. A 46-year-old man with the onset of chest pain 4 hours ago, who has small Q waves and 3 mm of ST-segment elevation in leads II, III, and aVF

B. An 80-year-old woman with a recent onset of mild right hemiparesis and 2 hours of chest pain with an ECG showing no Q waves and 4 mm of ST-segment elevation from leads V1 to V6, and 2 mm of ST-elevation in leads I and aVF

C. A 75-year-old man with the onset of chest pain 5 hours ago and a new left bundle branch block

D. A 65-year-old man with 2 previous coronary bypass surgeries and 2 hours of chest pain, who has 3 mm of ST-segment depression and new T wave inversion in leads V1 to V4

E. A 72-year-old woman with the onset of chest pain 3 hours ago with tall R waves and ST-segment depression in leads V1 and V2

175.

You are a passenger on an Antarctic cruise. You have just attended a grand soirée in the main dining room, and you and your spouse have walked up to the front deck to catch a breath of fresh air. Immediately ahead of the mighty ship looms a towering white mass. The ship is slowly turning to the left, but strikes what is obviously an iceberg. A large chunk of ice breaks off and falls onto the chest of a young woman who is standing nearby. She crumples to the deck and you rush to assist her. One of the ship's crew runs over to help you, and together you move her unconscious form to Captain Smith's cabin. The ship's surgeon arrives moments later.

He is immediately concerned upon palpating the woman's pulse. It seems that her blood pressure is very low. The surgeon examines her chest and notes a large mid-sternal hematoma. He palpates her sternum and tells you that it is obviously fractured. You, being the observant person you are, point out her extremely distended neck veins. The surgeon examines the neck closely and remarks about the single collapse of the veins during each heartbeat. He pulls out his stethoscope and listens to her heart and lungs. Captain Smith enters the cabin to inquire about the young lady's condition. He assures you that his initial impression is that the ship has received only minor damage from the collision.

You continue to observe the actions of the surgeon. Which of the following is he most likely to do next?

A. Call for the ship's chaplain to read the last rites to her

B. Insert a large trocar through her left lateral chest wall

C. Insert a long, large bore needle into her left chest toward her cardiac apex

D. Apply rotating tourniquets to her arms and legs

E. Apply a tight wrap to her chest to stabilize the sternum

176.

A 70-year-old man is admitted to another hospital with an acute anterolateral myocardial infarction and is transferred to your tertiary care medical center 2 days later for further management. He had coronary bypass surgery 8 years ago. Because he continues to have mild chest pain, you refer him to your colleague for coronary angiography. The procedure shows occlusion of the left anterior descending and the right coronary arteries and a high-grade stenosis in the proximal circumflex artery. His internal mammary artery is a small vessel that is grafted to the distal left anterior descending. There is very slow flow through the graft, and a 90% stenosis of the left anterior descending distal to the insertion of the graft. The saphenous vein graft to the obtuse marginal branch of the circumflex is widely patent. The vein graft to the distal right coronary has a 95% irregular stenosis in its mid portion. The cardiologist successfully deploys a stent in the right coronary graft.

The patient recovers without further complications. He exercises for 7 METs on a treadmill prior to discharge without chest pain or ECG changes. He is placed on secondary prevention medications and discharged to home.

Four days later he is readmitted to your service complaining of atypical chest pain, nausea, vomiting, and diarrhea. His neck veins are not elevated; he has a few wheezes in both lungs, and some mild abdominal tenderness. His laboratory data show a white blood count of 15,800 and a bicarbonate of 20 mEq/L. You make a diagnosis of possible viral gastroenteritis and treat him with intravenous fluids.

The next morning he is clearly worse, now with severe dyspnea, audible wheezing, and confusion. On examination, his blood pressure is 140/85 mmHg, heart rate is 125, and his temperature is 102.2° F. He has prominent *a* and *v* waves in the neck, and the veins are elevated to the jaw at 30°. He has diffuse rales and wheezing in both lungs, and he is using his accessory muscles of respiration. His heart is very difficult to hear through the respiratory sounds. He groans as you palpate his abdomen, but his belly is soft and there are a few scattered bowel sounds. His extremities are cold and somewhat mottled. There is a bluish-black appearance to the end of one of his toes.

The impressive parts of his laboratory data are his metabolic acidosis, high white blood count, and an arterial blood gas that shows a pH of 7.15, pO_2 of 50, pCO_2 of 40, and a bicarbonate of 12. He is transferred to the critical care unit, where he is intubated and placed on mechanical ventilation. An emergency echocardiogram is obtained.

Which of the following is the most likely finding?

   A. Extremely poor left ventricular function with an ejection fraction of 10% and elevated right heart pressures
   B. A large, lobulated, mobile mass in the apex of the left ventricle
   C. Rupture of the tip of the posterior papillary muscle and severe mitral regurgitation
   D. A ventricular septal defect
   E. Rupture of the anterior wall of the left ventricle with a large pericardial effusion and signs of tamponade

---

177.

A very tall, thin young man comes to your clinic complaining of mid-back pain. He says 3 days ago, he began having a sharp, non-radiating, continuous pain between his scapulae. The pain has been severe enough that he has been unable to sleep. He has not had any similar symptoms previously, and has no other known medical problems.

His examination is remarkable for his 6' 8" height, long, spindly fingers, and pectus excavatum. There is no palpable tenderness in his back. His femoral pulses seem somewhat diminished. On neurological examination, he has some mild weakness to dorsiflexion of his right foot.

Expecting bad things, you consult your cardiologist colleague and she elects to perform a transesophageal echocardiogram.

Which of the following statements concerning this disorder is true?

A. Dissection of the ascending aorta should be treated with aggressive medical therapy and close observation.
B. Appropriate medical therapy for an aortic dissection is intravenous nitroprusside alone.
C. Lowering the aortic systolic pressure is the most important aspect of medical therapy.
D. All descending thoracic aortic dissections require immediate surgery.
E. Aortic dissection can occur in the third trimester of pregnancy without any obvious predisposing factors.

178.

Which of the following cardiac conditions tolerates exercise well?

A. Aortic regurgitation
B. Aortic stenosis
C. Mitral stenosis
D. Hypertrophic cardiomyopathy
E. Eisenmenger syndrome

179.

A 76-year-old man was shooting pool when he collapsed to the floor. His friends report that he was lining up a shot when he suddenly lost consciousness, was unarousable for about 20 seconds, had no jerking movements, and did not lose control of his bowel or bladder. When he woke up, he was completely aware of his surroundings and was ready to resume his game, but his friends insisted that he come to your Emergency Room. Upon questioning, the man denies any cardiac symptoms or history, although he admits to having three previous episodes of syncope. His risk factors for coronary artery disease include age, male sex, and hypertension.

On examination, his blood pressure is 110/65 mmHg, and heart rate is 165 beats/min. He has prominent regular cannon *a* waves in the neck veins. His cardiac and neurological examination is otherwise normal. His basic electrolytes, complete blood count, and cardiac markers are all normal. His electrocardiogram shows a narrow QRS tachycardia at a rate of 168.

Since he is hemodynamically stable, you decide to admit him to the telemetry unit and observe his course. He does well, still at the same heart rate, until 2 hours later when he gets up to use the bedside commode. He then climbs back into the bed and faints. A rhythm strip of the whole event is captured by the monitoring equipment.

Which of the following most likely describes the findings on the rhythm strip?

A. Sudden cessation of the narrow QRS complex tachycardia followed by a 15-second period of asystole
B. A 30-second episode of rapid ventricular tachycardia
C. A 30-second episode of 3rd degree AV block with a slow ventricular escape rhythm
D. A 30-second episode of *torsade de pointes*
E. An acceleration of the ventricular rate to 330 from 165, indicating that the initial rhythm was atrial flutter with 2:1 A:V block

180.

A 59-year-old man comes to your office because of a history of "congestive heart failure." He reports increasing dyspnea over the past 2 years to the point where he can now only walk about 50 feet before having to stop. He also complains of being somewhat light-headed when he stands up. He denies chest pain, orthopnea, or paroxysmal nocturnal dyspnea. He shows you the pills that he was prescribed by his previous physician and, after a quick consultation with the "Physician's Desk Reference," you conclude that they are digoxin and furosemide. His risk factors for coronary artery disease include age, male sex, and hypertension.

On examination, his blood pressure is 180/110 mmHg and his heart rate is 85 while sitting. Upon standing, his blood pressure is 145/85 and his heart rate is 105. His neck veins are not elevated. His lungs have moderate bibasilar crackles. He has a very prominent apical impulse and a low-pitched sound heard best at the apex just before the first heart sound. The remainder of the examination is normal.

Laboratory data are all normal except for a BUN of 38 mg/dL and a creatinine of 2.2 mg/dL. His chest x-ray shows cardiomegaly with moderate pulmonary vascular redistribution. His electrocardiogram shows sinus rhythm with voltage criteria for left ventricular hypertrophy. There are nonspecific ST segment and T wave changes, particularly in the precordial leads.

For a better understanding of his heart failure, you obtain an echocardiogram.

Which of the following is the most likely finding?

- A. Concentric left ventricular hypertrophy and severe aortic stenosis
- B. Concentric left ventricular hypertrophy, segmental wall motion abnormalities, and a left ventricular ejection fraction of 15%
- C. Concentric left ventricular hypertrophy and a left ventricular ejection fraction of 80%
- D. Normal-sized, non-hypertrophied ventricles with a strange speckled pattern, huge atria, and a left ventricular ejection fraction of 45%
- E. Minimal left ventricular hypertrophy, four chamber cardiac enlargement, and a left ventricular ejection fraction of 10%

181.

A hypertensive patient with concentric left ventricular hypertrophy and a left ventricular ejection fraction of 80% presents to you in referral on digoxin and furosemide.

Which of the following is the best therapy for such a patient?

- A. Stop digoxin, decrease the dose of furosemide, and start beta-blockers.
- B. Continue digoxin and furosemide and schedule coronary angiography.
- C. Continue digoxin and furosemide; add an angiotensin-converting enzyme inhibitor, low dose carvedilol, and spironolactone.
- D. Admit him for infusion of intravenous amrinone.
- E. Continue digoxin and furosemide; add an angiotensin-converting enzyme inhibitor, low-dose carvedilol, and spironolactone, and schedule him for intermittent outpatient dobutamine infusion.

182.

A 35-year-old woman is referred to you because of episodes of palpitations. She brings with you a copy of her electrocardiogram, which is shown below. Before doing anything else, you decide to look at it.

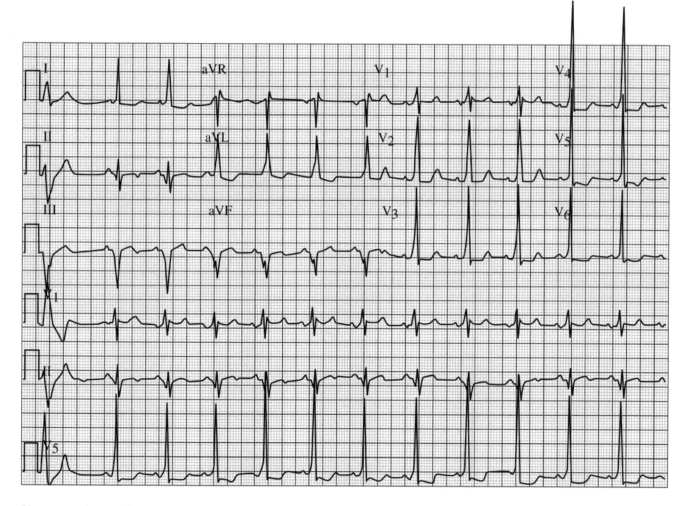

Your eyes immediately bug out and, without further ado, you order which of the following tests?

- A. An echocardiogram
- B. A chest x-ray
- C. An electrophysiology study
- D. Coronary angiography
- E. Implantation of a cardio defibrillator

183.

A 39-year-old male has sudden onset of severe chest pain. It radiates into both arms and is associated with diaphoresis. By the time he arrives in the Emergency Room, the pain has resolved. He reports his father died of a heart attack at home at age 45. The patient has a history of mild hypertension. He has a high arched palate on physical examination.

Cholesterol: 245, ECG: 1st degree AV block/no ischemic changes.

Which of the following would you do next?

A. Contrast chest CT scan
B. Cardiac catheterization
C. Admission to ICU to obtain serial enzymes to rule out MI
D. Administer TPA
E. Upper endoscopy

184.

A 70-year-old male, status post AVR replacement 2 years ago for aortic stenosis, presents with widespread ecchymosis on his back and legs and some bruising on the back of both hands. His last INR was 3 weeks ago and was 3. He states he saw an M.D. 6 days ago for a cough and was put on a medication described as a "white tablet."

His chronic medications include: warfarin 5 mg qd, albuterol inhaler 2 puffs 4 times a day, and nortriptyline 25 mg q hs.

Which of the following medications was he placed on?

A. Trimethoprim/sulfamethoxazole
B. Amoxicillin
C. Codeine
D. Cefixime

185.

A 39-year-old woman with a prosthetic aortic valve presents with bruising. Her last INR 6 weeks ago was 2.4; today's INR is 6.5. She has not taken any extra warfarin.

Which of the following, when taken on a daily basis, could explain her increased INR?

A. Calcium carbonate
B. Acetaminophen
C. Oral contraceptive pills (OCP)
D. Ranitidine
E. None of the answers is correct

186.

A 73-year-old man with prosthetic aortic valve presents for primary care. He has been well controlled on warfarin 3 mg q hs for 6 years with INR 2.5–3.0. He is concerned about his prostate, memory problems, and heart disease, and would like to take supplements recommended by his niece who works at a health food store.

Which of the following would you specifically recommend <u>against</u>?

    A. Gingko biloba
    B. Cat's claw
    C. Saw palmetto
    D. Folate

INFECTIOUS DISEASES

187.

A 25-year-old man comes to the ER complaining of weakness in both legs. He reports that he started to have a tingling sensation in his toes about a day ago. Next, he noticed a foot-drop sensation developing. On awakening this morning, he had problems grasping objects and noted some weakness in his upper legs. He has had no fever, diplopia, dysphagia, or dyspnea. He had a "cold" one week prior to his current symptoms. He removed a tick from his waist about a week and a half ago. He eats homegrown vegetables and fruits that his mother cans for him back in West Virginia.

PAST MEDICAL HISTORY: Negative
                                    Immunizations up to date

SOCIAL HISTORY: Works as a truck driver in the Washington, D.C., area
                                    Smokes 2 packs/day of cigarettes
                                    Doesn't drink alcohol

FAMILY HISTORY: Negative

PHYSICAL EXAMINATION:
    BP 120/76, RR 18, Temp 97.9° F, P 86

HEENT:	PERRLA, EOMI
	Discs sharp
	TMs clear
	Throat clear
Neck:	Supple
Heart:	RRR with I/VI systolic flow murmur
Lungs:	CTA
Abdomen:	Bowel sounds present; no hepatosplenomegaly
Extremities:	No cyanosis, clubbing, or edema
Neuro:	Symmetrical weakness of lower extremities—distal muscles more affected than proximal muscles
	Bilateral foot drop
	Weakness of both hands noted
	Cranial Nerves II-XII tested and intact
	Sensory perception is normal
	Patellar and Achilles reflexes are absent bilaterally

Which of the following is the most likely diagnosis?

    A. Botulism (food-borne)
    B. Poliomyelitis
    C. Tick paralysis
    D. Guillain-Barré syndrome
    E. Rabies

188.

A 30-year-old man with AIDS presents for worsening fatigue. He was found to be HIV-infected about 12 years ago. His CD4 count at that time was 180/cu mm, and he began taking trimethoprim-sulfamethoxazole and zidovudine (AZT). During the last several years, he has not wished to take any antiretroviral therapy and takes only monthly aerosolized pentamidine for *Pneumocystis* prophylaxis. Five months ago, his hemoglobin level started to decrease. A workup for gastrointestinal bleeding revealed nothing. Laboratory for iron, B_{12}, and folate were all normal. A serum erythropoietin level was 700 mU/mL (normal is 4–26). He received a red cell transfusion about 3 months ago.

His physical examination is unremarkable.

LABORATORY STUDIES:

Hemoglobin:	8.0 gm/dL
Hematocrit:	23%
WBC:	5,000/cu mm
CD4 count:	62/cu mm
Reticulocyte count:	0%

A bone marrow aspirate and biopsy reveal red blood cell aplasia with giant pronormoblasts.

Which of the following is the likely etiology for his anemia?

A. Parvovirus B19
B. HTLV-I from his transfusion 3 months ago
C. *Campylobacter jejuni*
D. Pentamidine-induced anemia
E. Prior zidovudine use

189.

A 35-year-old woman works as a forester in Southern Arkansas. She comes to you with a 3-month history of cough and recent development of hemoptysis. While talking to her, you discover that she has lost 10 pounds in the last 3 months. She has been smoking cigarettes for 20 years and smokes up to 2 packs a day.

PAST MEDICAL HISTORY: Negative

SOCIAL HISTORY: Lives in Camden, Arkansas, with her husband of 3 years
                      4 children ages 20, 18, 16, 1
                      Drinks 6-pack of beer on the weekend
                      No illicit drug use

FAMILY HISTORY: Father died at age 67 of lung cancer
                      Mother died at age 64 of lung cancer

PHYSICAL EXAMINATION:
              BP 110/70, P 88, Temp 100° F, RR 25, Weight 130 lbs
              HEENT: PERRLA, EOMI
                            TMs clear
                            Throat clear

Neck:	Supple
Heart:	RRR without murmurs, rubs, or gallops
Lungs:	Scattered crackles in the bases
Abdomen:	No hepatosplenomegaly
Extremities:	Draining lesion on her left leg (she forgot to tell you about that)
	Has been there for 3 months; puts "poultice" on it, and it gets better but then gets worse again

LABORATORY:

CXR:	Pulmonary mass noted at right base
Gram stain of lesion fluid:	Gram-positive cocci in clusters
KOH of lesion fluid:	Small budding yeasts
Acid-fast smear of lesion fluid:	No organisms seen

Based on your findings, which of the following is the most likely diagnosis?

A. Coccidioidomycosis
B. Histoplasmosis
C. Blastomycosis
D. Tuberculosis
E. Lung carcinoma

190.

A 55-year-old man has fever and cough. He has AIDS and a history of disseminated histoplasmosis 2 years ago. He was treated initially with amphotericin B and had been maintained on itraconazole since. Last month, he started having fever and chills. Histoplasmosis was suspected again and amphotericin B was restarted. Blood cultures, however, grew *Mycobacterium intracellulare,* and he was started on appropriate medications for that. He was restarted on his itraconazole maintenance therapy last month. Today, he comes in with recurrence of his fever and chills.

MEDICATIONS:	Combivir and efavirenz for 6 months
	Rifabutin 600 mg/day for 1 month
	Azithromycin 500 mg daily for 1 month
	Ethambutol 1200 mg daily for 1 month
	Itraconazole 200 mg daily for 2 weeks
	Ranitidine 150 mg bid for 2 weeks for gastric reflux symptoms
	Trimethoprim-sulfamethoxazole DS 1 daily

PHYSICAL EXAMINATION:
Temp 103° F, BP 120/70, RR 24, P 100

HEENT:	PERRLA, EOMI
	TMs clear
	Throat: clear
Neck:	Supple
Heart:	RRR without murmurs, rubs, or gallops
Lungs:	Diminished breath sounds at left base
Abdomen:	Liver down about 3 cm below the right costal margin
	Spleen tip palpable
Extremities:	No lesions noted

LABORATORY:

WBC:	1200 cells/cu mm
Hgb:	10 gm/dL
Platelets:	100,000

Yeast forms seen on peripheral smear.

Which of the following is most likely correct?

A. A serum cryptococcal antigen will be positive.
B. The patient has itraconazole-resistant *Histoplasma*.
C. Blood cultures will grow *Candida krusei*.
D. The yeast forms are likely contaminants.
E. Itraconazole and its metabolites are below therapeutic levels.

191.

A 30-year-old woman with negative past medical history presents to you with a 1-week history of pain in her wrists and hands. She has been afebrile and has not had a rash. She lives in New Lyme, Connecticut. She lives in a city complex and does not go into wooded areas. She has no pets and has not had any tick bites.

Recently, her 8-year-old son had an erythematous rash on his face and arms. His rash got worse if he took a warm bath or was out in the sun. He also was afebrile.

PHYSICAL EXAMINATION:
Essentially normal except for her wrists and hands, which are moderately tender. No effusions of the joints are noted. She has no conjunctivitis or scleral changes on examination.

Which of the following is the likely etiology for the symptoms in these two patients?

A. Human herpesvirus 6
B. Parvovirus B19
C. Measles
D. *Borrelia burgdorferi*
E. *Neisseria gonorrhoeae*

192.

A 19-year-old chicken farmer comes to your office with a 2-week history of non-productive cough with low-grade fever. Additionally he has had sore throat and hoarseness associated with these symptoms. He has not had diarrhea, rigors, sweats, or chills. He owns a pet cockatoo and several parakeets. He is sexually active and uses condoms with every episode of intercourse. He denies IV drug use or other risk factors for HIV. He does not smoke.

PAST MEDICAL HISTORY: Negative

SOCIAL HISTORY: On further questioning, he admits to smoking marijuana in the past—but says he never inhaled. Lives alone on his farm called the "Chicken Coupe"

PHYSICAL EXAMINATION:
Vitals are normal except for a temperature of 99.8° F

HEENT:	PERRLA, EOMI
	Sclera anicteric
	Throat: red and inflamed; no exudates
Neck:	Supple
Heart:	RRR without murmurs, rubs, or gallops
Lungs:	Fine crackles heard at the right lung base
Abdomen:	Bowel sounds present
	No hepatosplenomegaly
Extremities:	No cyanosis, clubbing, or edema
Skin:	No rash

LABORATORY:

Leukocyte count:	12,000/cu mm; 60% neutrophils, 25% lymphocytes, 10% monocytes, 2% eosinophils
ESR:	57 mm/hr
TB Skin test:	0 mm

CXR: Patchy infiltrate in the right lower lobe

Which of the following organisms is most likely to be causing his illness?

A. *Chlamydophila pneumoniae*
B. *Chlamydophila psittaci*
C. *Legionella pneumoniae*
D. *Coxiella burnetii*
E. *Streptococcus pneumoniae*

193.

A 30-year-old woman presents in her 32nd week of pregnancy. She initially sees her obstetrician with complaints of fever and myalgias without any localizing symptoms. She denies any other problems. Her OB sends her to you for evaluation.

PAST MEDICAL HISTORY: 1st pregnancy; no problems until now

SOCIAL HISTORY: Doesn't smoke or drink
                          Works as a pharmaceutical rep

FAMILY HISTORY: Non-contributory

REVIEW OF SYSTEMS: Really quite uninteresting (hmm, guess that isn't "codeable"—too bad)

PHYSICAL EXAMINATION: Normal except for a temperature of 102.5° F

LABORATORY:
WBC is 10,000/cu mm with 70% neutrophils, 10% bands
Urinalysis is normal

Blood cultures are growing a Gram-positive diphtheroid-like organism.

Which of the following is the most appropriate antibiotic for this organism?

    A. Intravenous ceftriaxone
    B. Intravenous clindamycin
    C. Intravenous gentamicin
    D. Intravenous penicillin G or ampicillin
    E. Oral penicillin or amoxicillin

194.

A short and to-the-point question: You diagnose *C. difficile* (non-severe) diarrhea in a patient. You treat the patient with oral metronidazole and the patient's diarrhea resolves. The patient returns 3 weeks later with diarrhea again due to *C. difficile*.

Which of the following is the best next plan?

    A. Treat with oral vancomycin.
    B. Treat with oral vancomycin and clindamycin.
    C. Treat with oral clindamycin.
    D. Treat again with oral metronidazole.
    E. Do not treat with antibiotics.

195.

You are seeing a 30-year-old man with AIDS whom you have been following for years and recently have noticed that his CD4 count has continued to fall. He has not had any opportunistic infections and has done well with his antiretroviral therapies. You feel that he has most likely developed a more resistant HIV infection. He is taking trimethoprim/sulfamethoxazole for *Pneumocystis* prophylaxis. His physical examination is unremarkable.

LABORATORY:
    CD4 lymphocyte count is 28/cu mm.
    Viral load is 350,000 copies/mL.

Because of his worsening immunosuppression, which of the following do you recommend he start today?

    A. Clarithromycin weekly
    B. Azithromycin weekly
    C. Rifampin daily
    D. Rifabutin and clarithromycin daily
    E. Nothing

196.

Marla Ferguson is a 39-year-old woman with a recent history of otitis media treated with amoxicillin. She presents with a 12-hour history of severe headache, nausea, and vomiting—and is now lethargic.

PAST MEDICAL HISTORY: Negative except for recent otitis 2 weeks ago; did not take all of her amoxicillin; stopped after 4 days. (The weekend came and she didn't want to mix her prescribed drug with margaritas.)

SOCIAL HISTORY: Former Ms. USA Winner
Now a talk show host for local TV station; has her own show "Ms. Marla Loves Detroit"
Doesn't smoke
Drinks a margarita on the weekend

FAMILY HISTORY: Non-contributory

PHYSICAL EXAMINATION:
     T 102.6° F, P 110, RR 24, BP 130/65 mmHg

HEENT:	PERRLA, EOMI
	Disc sharp
	TMs clear
	Throat clear
Neck:	Mild nuchal rigidity
Heart:	RRR without murmurs
Lungs:	Scattered crackles throughout; greatest in left lower lobe
Abdomen:	Benign
Extremities:	Normal
Neuro:	Lethargic
	No papilledema
	Cranial nerves tested intact
	No focal deficits

LABORATORY:

WBC:	20,000 cu mm; 76% segs; 10% bands
Electrolytes:	Normal
CSF WBC:	3000 WBC/cu mm; 95% neutrophils
CSF Glucose:	20 mg/dL (serum glucose 100 mg/dL)
CSF Protein:	176 mg/dL
CSF Gram stain:	Loaded with neutrophils and a few Gram-positive, lancet-shaped diplococci

Which of the following is/are the best empiric antibiotic choice(s) for her?

A. Ceftazidime alone
B. Vancomycin alone
C. Ceftriaxone and vancomycin
D. Ampicillin and ceftazidime
E. Penicillin

197.

A 60-year-old man is evaluated because of a 1-week history of lower extremity weakness, new onset of difficulty speaking, and decreased attention span. He has had occasional diarrhea and abdominal pain in the last year. Of significance is that he has lost about 25 lbs during the past year. He complains of joint pains, particularly in his knees. He has had low-grade fever but no chills during the last year. He reports occasional night sweats. He has noted no other neurologic findings like seizures. His wife reports that areas of his skin are becoming darker—particularly those exposed to light.

PAST MEDICAL HISTORY: Healthy before this episode

SOCIAL HISTORY:	Lives in Michigan
	Works in the auto industry

FAMILY HISTORY:	Negative

REVIEW OF SYSTEMS:	Pretty much covered in the HPI

PHYSICAL EXAMINATION:
    Bp 130/80, T 99.9° F, P 84, RR 18

General:	Alert, but oriented only to person and place!
HEENT:	PERRLA, EOMI
	Mild facial droop
	Throat clear
Neck:	Scattered lymphadenopathy in the anterior and posterior cervical chains; most nodes are 1 x 1 cm but a few are 2 x 1 cm
Heart:	RRR without murmurs, rubs, and gallops
Lungs:	CTA
Abdomen:	Spleen tip palpated; no hepatomegaly
	A questionable abdominal mass discerned with deep palpation
Extremities:	No cyanosis, clubbing, or edema
Neuro:	Right lower extremity with increased tone and 4/5 muscle strength
	Sensation is normal
	Deep tendon reflexes are symmetrical

LABORATORY:

Hemoglobin:	15.2 gm/dL
Hematocrit:	50%
WBC:	30,000/cu mm; 65% neutrophils, 28% lymphs
ESR:	13 mm/hr
Glucose	200 mg/dL
Albumin	3.5 gm/dL
ALT	30 U/L
AST	25 U/L

CT of the head shows a hypodense left frontal lobe lesion. A stereotactic brain biopsy is taken and shows acute inflammation and necrosis with **no** malignant cells. Gram stain shows 1+ WBCs but **no** organisms. However, a specimen stained with periodic acid-Schiff (PAS) shows multiple PAS-positive foamy macrophages.

This last little tidbit is your clue to this complicated problem. If you don't know it, that is fine—that is what CME and learning is for. **However**, learn this today; because this little organism has received a lot of medical press and likely is fair game for the Boards.

Which of the following organisms is likely responsible for his condition?

    A. *Coxiella burnetii*
    B. *Mycobacterium tuberculosis*
    C. *Trophermyma whippleii*
    D. *Nocardia asteroides*
    E. *Actinomyces israelii*

198.

A 28-year-old woman, who is a health care worker in Memphis, Tennessee, is being evaluated for a 2-week history of progressive shortness of breath, dry cough, fever, and weight loss. She lives with her boyfriend who has a history of IV drug abuse in the 1960s and hung out with Elvis. She denies use of IV drugs and says that her boyfriend has been "clean" since the late 1980s. She does not know his HIV status, however.

PAST MEDICAL HISTORY: Negative

SOCIAL HISTORY: Works as a nurse's aide in local hospital
                         Doesn't smoke or drink
                         Lives with current boyfriend for the past 3 years, monogamous

FAMILY HISTORY: Negative

PHYSICAL EXAMINATION:
   BP 120/70, P 80, RR 28, Temp 101° F

   HEENT: PERRLA, EOMI
                 TMs clear
                 Throat: oral thrush
   Neck: Mobile, nontender lymph nodes noted in the posterior cervical chain
   Heart: RRR with I/VI systolic flow murmur
   Lungs: Scattered crackles especially prominent in left base
   Abdomen: Liver is 4 cm below right costal margin; mildly tender
                 Spleen tip palpable
   Extremities: No cyanosis, clubbing, or edema
   Neuro: No deficits noted

LABORATORY:
   WBC: 3200/cu mm; 80% lymphocytes
   Hemoglobin: 9.8 mg/dL
   Platelets: 110,000/cu mm
   AST: 100 U/L
   ALT: 89 U/L
   HIV ELISA: Positive
   Western blot: Pending
   CD4 lymphocytes: 37/cu mm

Which of the following is the most likely diagnosis?

   A. Disseminated *Pneumocystis* infection
   B. Disseminated *Histoplasma* infection
   C. Lymphoma
   D. Disseminated *Mycobacterium tuberculosis*
   E. Disseminated coccidioidomycosis

199.

A 19-year-old college student is brought into the Emergency Room by his roommates because they were unable to awaken him this morning. They report that he has not had any alcohol for the past 3 months and is a model student. During the past 2 to 3 days, however, they say that he has exhibited bizarre behavior and has been intermittently confused. He takes no medications, and his friends adamantly deny that he has ever used any type of illicit drug.

PAST MEDICAL HISTORY: Several visits to the ER for "the drip"

SOCIAL HISTORY: Majoring in Interior Design
                         Works as a stripper at the local "men's bar"

PHYSICAL EXAMINATION:
    T 102° F, P 100, RR 22, BP 120/70, Ht: 5'3", Wt: 260 lbs

General:	Responds only to deep pain
HEENT:	PERRLA, EOMI
	TMs clear
	Throat clear
Neck:	Supple
Heart:	RRR without murmurs, rubs, or gallops
Lungs:	CTA
Abdomen:	Bowel sounds present, no hepatosplenomegaly
Extremities:	No cyanosis, clubbing, or edema; **no** rash
Neuro:	No focal neurologic signs

LABORATORY:
    Lumbar puncture:

WBC	80 WBC/cu mm (50% neutrophils, 50% lymphocytes)
RBC	10 RBC/cu mm
Protein	73 mg/dL (normal)
Glucose	60 mg/dL (plasma glucose 80 mg/dL)
Gram Stain:	Negative

CBC:	Normal
Electrolytes:	Normal

MRI of head: Focal lesion at the base of the left temporal lobe with mild edema
CXR: Normal

Based on your findings, which of the following is the likely diagnosis?

A. Neurosyphilis
B. *Bartonella henselae* infection
C. Varicella meningoencephalitis
D. *Streptococcus pneumoniae* meningitis
E. Herpes simplex meningoencephalitis

200.

A 45-year-old man lives in Nevada and comes in with a chief complaint of urinary frequency and burning. He has never had these symptoms. He has had fever for 2 days and now has chills.

PAST MEDICAL HISTORY: Negative

SOCIAL HISTORY: Smokes 2 packs a day
Drinks 2 whiskey shots daily

FAMILY HISTORY: Mother died of alcoholic liver disease at age 50
Father died of alcoholic liver disease at age 50
Brother died of alcoholic liver disease at age 50
Sister died of alcoholic liver disease at age 50
Cousin died of alcoholic liver disease at age 50

PHYSICAL EXAMINATION:
BP 90/70, R 25, Temp 104° F, P 120

General:	Severely ill-appearing man in some distress
HEENT:	PERRLA, EOMI
	TMs clear
	Throat clear
Neck:	Supple
Heart:	RRR without murmurs, rubs, or gallops
Lungs:	CTA
Abdomen:	Bowel sounds present, liver span 16 cm
Extremities:	Trace pedal edema
GU:	No lesions
	Suprapubic tenderness noted
	Rectal exam heme negative; nontender prostate

LABORATORY:
Blood cultures positive for *E. coli*; sensitive to ciprofloxacin, amikacin, and piperacillin only

You start therapy with intravenous ciprofloxacin, and he responds nicely. It is day 5 of admission, and you are ready to send him home to complete oral antibiotics.

Which of the following agents should you <u>not</u> use with his ciprofloxacin?

    A. Cimetidine
    B. Ranitidine
    C. Sucralfate
    D. Loratadine
    E. Disulfiram

201.

A 65-year-old man with non-insulin-dependent diabetes mellitus is seen in your office because of severe pain and tenderness of his right ear. He has been doing well before this.

PAST MEDICAL HISTORY: Essentially negative except for his NIDDM for 30 years
           Currently takes metformin 1000 mg daily

SOCIAL HISTORY: Lives alone
           Doesn't smoke or drink
           Retired college math professor

PHYSICAL EXAMINATION:
    BP 130/70, P 100, RR 20, Temp 103° F

HEENT:	PERRLA, EOMI
TMs:	Examination extremely painful and shows marked edema, erythema, and purulent material in the external auditory canal
	External ear is markedly swollen
	Throat clear
Neck:	Supple; no meningismus
Heart:	RRR without murmurs, rubs, or gallops
Lungs:	CTA
Abdomen:	Benign
Extremities:	No cyanosis, clubbing, or edema

Which of the following is the likely etiology for his infection?

    A. *Pseudomonas aeruginosa*
    B. *Staphylococcus aureus*
    C. *Streptococcus pneumoniae*
    D. *Candida albicans*
    E. *Streptococcus diabeticus*

202.

A 65-year-old salt water fisherman in Galveston, Texas, is brought to the ER with fever and lethargy. He was well until 3 days ago, when he started having fever and shaking chills. He took acetaminophen and ibuprofen but did not get any better. Today he became confused, and so he was brought in by his wife, Missy. He has chronic hepatitis C but has refused therapy to date. His diagnosis was made when he had an acute attack of jaundice 3 years ago.

PAST MEDICAL HISTORY: Vietnam Veteran; had malaria in 1961

SOCIAL HISTORY: Lives with wife in a small apartment
                         Drinks a fifth of vodka a week
                         Smokes 2 packs of cigarettes daily

PHYSICAL EXAMINATION:
     BP 100/60, Temp 104° F, P 120, RR 25

     General: He is lethargic and confused
     HEENT: PERRLA, EOMI
                   TMs clear
                   Throat: clear
     Neck: Supple; no meningismus
     Heart: RRR with I/VI systolic ejection murmur
     Lungs: CTA
     Abdomen: Liver down 4 cm
     Extremities: Scratches noted on legs and arms
     Skin: Numerous spider angiomas noted on trunk
                   Several 2-cm bullous lesions noted on the trunk; appear to contain fluid

Which of the following is the most likely diagnosis?

   A. Invasive *Streptococcus pyogenes* infection
   B. *Staphylococcus aureus*
   C. Malaria
   D. *Vibrio vulnificus*
   E. Leptospirosis

203.

A 30-year-old man comes to the ER with increasing ataxia. He says that the room spins all of the time, and he cannot walk without holding on to something. He denies any other complaints.

PAST MEDICAL HISTORY: Negative

SOCIAL HISTORY:
Works as a bellhop in a local hotel
Admits to having multiple sexual partners (both male and female)
Smokes 2 packs/day of cigarettes
Drinks a 6 pack of beer daily

FAMILY HISTORY: Non-contributory

PHYSICAL EXAMINATION:
BP 130/70, P 90, Temp 99° F, RR 18

HEENT:	PERRLA, EOMI
	TMs clear
	Throat clear
Neck:	Supple; no meningismus
Heart:	RRR without murmurs, rubs, or gallops
Lungs:	CTA
Abdomen:	Bowel sounds present, no hepatosplenomegaly
Extremities:	Benign
GU:	No lesions
Neuro:	Romberg sign is present. Possible decreased position sense in lower extremities

LABORATORY:

MRI of head:	Normal
WBC:	2500/cu mm; 60% polys, 30% lymphs
CD4:	160/cu mm
HIV ELISA:	Pending
Electrolytes:	Normal

Renal panel including creatinine and BUN: Normal
Serum VDRL: Positive at 1:32
Serum fluorescent treponemal antibody test (FTA-ABS): Positive
LP Results are below:

CSF WBC:	50 WBCs/cu mm; 65% lymphocytes
CSF Protein:	150 mg/dL
CSF Glucose:	60 mg/dL (plasma glucose 90 mg/dL)
CSF VDRL:	Negative

Based on your findings, which of the following is the appropriate treatment?

A. Benzathine penicillin G, 2.4 million units IM, single dose
B. Benzathine penicillin G, 2.4 million units IM, q week x 3 weeks
C. Penicillin G, 3 million units intravenously q 4 hours
D. Penicillin G, 1 million units intravenously q 6 hours
E. Vancomycin, 1 gram intravenously q 12 hours and ceftriaxone, 2 grams IV q 24 hours

204.

A 60-year-old woman with AML is undergoing chemotherapy. She finished her current round of chemotherapy 2 weeks ago and has been neutropenic for about a week. She was admitted last week with fever and has been on piperacillin/tazobactam and ciprofloxacin for this time period. Today, a blood culture from 3 days ago is growing a yeast subsequently determined to be *Candida krusei*. CT of the abdomen shows no lesions. She had a central venous catheter placed 2 weeks ago with her chemotherapy.

PHYSICAL EXAMINATION:
BP 130/70, P 80, RR 18, Temp 102° F
General: Well appearing; mild distress with fevers and chills

HEENT: PERRLA, EOMI
Discs examined by ophthalmologist and are normal
Throat: clear; no thrush
Heart: RRR without murmurs, rubs, or gallops
Lungs: CTA
Abdomen: Bowel sounds present; no hepatosplenomegaly
Extremities: No rashes; no cyanosis, clubbing, or edema
GU: Normal; no rectal abscesses
Skin: Insertion site for central venous catheter looks clean and nontender; no evidence of infection

Which of the following do you recommend?

A. Change the catheter site; add intravenous fluconazole.
B. Change the catheter site; add caspofungin.
C. Do not change the catheter site; add caspofungin.
D. Do not change the catheter site; add intravenous fluconazole.
E. Continue current therapy; *Candida krusei* is a contaminant.

205.

A 35-year-old man underwent a heart transplant 5 days ago. He is receiving immunosuppressive therapy with methylprednisolone, cyclosporine, and azathioprine. Today, he develops a temperature of 102° F.

PHYSICAL EXAMINATION: Ill-appearing man on the ventilator since surgery
BP 130/50, Temp 102° F, RR 30, P 100

SIGNIFICANT FINDINGS:
Chest: Crackles heard over both lung fields

LABORATORY:
Tracheal secretions are now yellow
FiO_2 requirements have increased from 35% to 50%
Pulmonary artery wedge pressure is 15 mmHg (normal 6–12)
WBC: 17,000/cu mm with 90% neutrophils
CXR: Extensive and widespread bilateral alveolar and interstitial infiltrates

Both the donor and the recipient are CMV-positive.

Which of the following is most likely the etiology for his pneumonia?

  A. *Legionella pneumoniae*
  B. *Pneumocystis jiroveci*
  C. CMV
  D. *Pseudomonas aeruginosa*
  E. *Cryptococcus neoformans*

206.

A 40-year-old man is followed for tuberculosis. He began therapy about 1 month ago and is taking the standard 4-drug regimen of INH, rifampin, pyrazinamide, and ethambutol. He is in for routine screening lab, because he had some abnormal liver function tests at the time of his initial diagnosis. Everything is normal except for a uric acid of 11 mg/dL.

Which of the following drugs is most likely responsible for this finding?

  A. INH
  B. Rifampin
  C. Pyrazinamide (PZA)
  D. Ethambutol
  E. None of these is responsible

207.

Ted Nougat is a 20-year-old man who came to you with a 1-week history of fever, chills, and left eye conjunctivitis with an associated pre-auricular lymph node. He reported that he was well until this episode. He lives at home with a dog and 3 cats. None of the pets have been ill.

PAST MEDICAL HISTORY: Negative

SOCIAL HISTORY: Works as a veterinarian's assistant; recently was bitten by a turtle and a rabbit

PHYSICAL EXAMINATION: Besides the lymph node and the non-purulent conjunctivitis, everything else is normal.

He was started on oral cephalexin. He returns 3 days later with no improvement. A surgery colleague sees him and performs a biopsy, which shows necrotizing granuloma without organism. Acid-fast stains are negative.

The most likely organism causing this picture is which of the following?

  A. *Borrelia burgdorferi*
  B. *Bartonella henselae*
  C. Herpes simplex I virus
  D. *Staphylococcus aureus,* methicillin resistant
  E. *Aeromonas hydrophilia*

208.

A 28-year-old woman has a history of AIDS for the past 3 years. She presents to you with a 1-week history of "floaters" in her right eye. She came today because she noted blurred vision in that eye since awakening this morning.

PAST MEDICAL HISTORY: Diagnosed with HIV 3 years ago with PCP presentation; currently on zidovudine, lamivudine, efavirenz, and trimethoprim/sulfamethoxazole prophylaxis; has not had any problems since her diagnosis 3 years ago

SOCIAL HISTORY: Works as a cafeteria worker at the local elementary school
Former boyfriend was an IV drug abuser

PHYSICAL EXAMINATION:
BP 110/70, P 80, RR 18, Temp 98.8° F

HEENT:	PERRLA, EOMI
	Discs: Normal on undilated examination
	Central visual acuity is preserved
	Anterior chamber appears clear
Heart:	RRR without murmurs, rubs, or gallops
Lungs:	CTA
Abdomen:	Bowel sounds present; no hepatosplenomegaly

LABORATORY:
CD4: 30/cu mm
Viral Load 50,000 copies/mL

A photo taken by the ophthalmologist is shown in this figure:

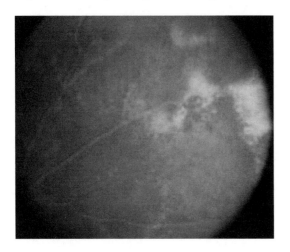

Which of the following is the most likely diagnosis?

A. *Pneumocystis jiroveci* retinitis
B. *Toxoplasma* chorioretinitis
C. Cytomegalovirus retinitis
D. Neurosyphilis
E. HIV retinopathy

209.

A 45-year-old man underwent prosthetic mitral valve replacement 6 weeks ago. He comes in today with fever and chills.

Which of the following is the likely organism that would cause endocarditis in this patient?

A. *Staphylococcus aureus*
B. Methicillin-sensitive *Staphylococcus epidermidis*
C. Methicillin-resistant *Staphylococcus epidermidis*
D. Viridans-type *Streptococci*
E. HACEK organisms

210.

An 18-year-old man lives in rural Arkansas. He is not a hunter. He works on a farm and has numerous animals, including rabbits, chicks, ducks, chinchillas, and sheep. He presents with a 2-week history of fever, night sweats, and malaise. He has noted a painful swelling in his right axilla for the past week. He had some "leftover" dicloxacillin and started taking it about 3 days ago but has not improved.

PAST MEDICAL HISTORY: Negative; 1st visit to the doctor since he was 12 for a broken collarbone
                                Due for Tdap now

SOCIAL HISTORY: As above
                                  Lives on the farm with his 2 brothers
                                  Doesn't drink or smoke
                                  Chews tobacco

PHYSICAL EXAMINATION:
    BP 110/70, P 110, RR 18, Temp 103° F

    HEENT: PERRLA, EOMI
                      TMs clear
                      Throat clear
    Neck: Supple
    Heart: RRR without murmurs, rubs, or gallops
    Lungs: CTA
    Abdomen: No hepatosplenomegaly
    Extremities: No cyanosis, clubbing, or edema
                      4 x 3 cm left axillary lymph node; tender
                      No skin lesions

LABORATORY:
    WBC: 17,000 with left shift

To confirm your diagnosis, which of the following is the best course?

A. Biopsy of lymph node
B. Gram stain of lymph node aspirate
C. Culture of lymph node aspirate
D. Assay for acute and convalescent titers
E. Febrile agglutinins

211.

A 72-year-old Caucasian male presents with a 3-day history of fever, malaise, and myalgias. He recently returned from a trip to Missouri, where he reports being bitten by a tick approximately 10 days ago. He was there on a fishing trip (he did quite well—20 lbs of fresh trout, and he brings you 2 of his best filets). He is healthy otherwise and reports that he was doing well.

PAST MEDICAL HISTORY: No medications

SOCIAL HISTORY:
Retired from a medical publishing firm
Never smoked
Drinks 2 glasses of wine on the weekends

FAMILY HISTORY: Negative

REVIEW OF SYSTEMS:
No rash
No joint manifestations
No conjunctivitis
No lymphadenopathy

PHYSICAL EXAMINATION:
BP 120/70, P 100, RR 18, Temp 103° F

HEENT:	PERRLA, EOMI
	TMs clear
	Throat clear
Neck:	Supple
Heart:	RRR without murmurs, rubs, or gallops
Lungs:	CTA
Abdomen:	Bowel sounds present; no hepatomegaly; spleen tip 2 cm below left costal margin
Extremities:	No cyanosis, clubbing, or edema

LABORATORY:

WBC:	2,200 with 60% polys, 20% bands
Hemoglobin:	12.5 mg/dL
Platelets:	140,000/cu mm
AST:	150 IU/L
ALT:	140 IU/L

Based on your history, physical, and laboratory values, which of the following is the most likely etiology?

   A. Tularemia
   B. Ehrlichiosis
   C. Histoplasmosis
   D. Blastomycosis
   E. Lyme disease

212.

A previously healthy 24-year-old Caucasian woman comes to your office for evaluation of joint pain and fever. She had been well until 3 days ago, when pain and swelling developed in the left knee and right ankle. Skin lesions also appeared, primarily on the extremities. The patient has a dozen sexual partners, who are reported to be healthy. (At least she is honest!)

On physical examination, temperature is 38.2° C (100.8° F). Approximately 5 papulopustular skin lesions are present on the extremities; a few are also noted on the lower torso. There is arthritis with effusion in the right ankle and left knee, and the left wrist and the base of the right thumb are tender.

Based on your findings, which of the following is the most likely organism responsible?

   A. *Neisseria gonorrhoeae*
   B. *Chlamydia trachomatis*
   C. HIV
   D. *Streptococcus pyogenes*
   E. *Borrelia burgdorferi*

213.

A 50-year-old Hispanic man comes to your office because of a 2-week history of fever, sore throat, shortness of breath, nonproductive cough, and vague pleuritic chest discomfort. He also has had swelling in the neck and night sweats for 3 months. He has not consumed unpasteurized milk products. He has 15 healthy pet cats. Twenty-five years ago, he immigrated to Miami from Cuba.

PAST MEDICAL HISTORY: Negative

SOCIAL HISTORY:
                  Denies IV drug use
                  Admits to homosexual activity
                  Drinks tequila—a ½ pint daily
                  Doesn't smoke

PHYSICAL EXAMINATION:
     T 102° F, P 110, RR 28, BP 135/90 mmHg

       HEENT: PERRLA, EOMI
                      TMs clear
                      Throat: oral candidiasis
       Neck/Lymph: 5 x 5 cm firm, rubbery, non-fixed lymph nodes in the right supraclavicular fossa; 1 cm
                      nodes are noted in the anterior and posterior cervical chains, axillae, and inguinal areas
       Heart: RRR with I/VI flow type murmur

Lungs:	Bibasilar crackles
Abdomen:	Bowel sounds present; liver span 15 cm
Extremities:	No cyanosis, clubbing, or edema

LABORATORY:

Chest X-Ray:	Bilateral lower lobe interstitial infiltrates and right paratracheal and bilateral hilar lymph node enlargement
Hemoglobin:	13 gm/dL
WBC:	4500/cu mm

| HIV Elisa: | Positive |
| HIV Western blot: | Pending |

CD4 Lymphocyte:	45/cu mm
Serum bilirubin:	1.8 mg/dL
AST:	250 U/L

pH:	7.43
PO$_2$:	64 mmHg
PCO$_2$:	33 mmHg

Which of the following is most likely responsible for his illness?

A. *Bartonella henselae*
B. *Pneumocystis jiroveci*
C. *Rhodococcus equi*
D. *Mycobacterium tuberculosis*
E. Coccidioidomycosis

214.

A 65-year-old woman has a 30-year history of insulin-dependent diabetes mellitus. She is currently in the hospital for pneumonia due to *Streptococcus pneumoniae*. A colleague admitted her, and you are covering the weekend. You notice that she still has an indwelling Foley catheter that has been in since her admission 5 days ago through the ER. You remove the catheter and send a urinalysis. She complains of dysuria but is afebrile.

PAST MEDICAL HISTORY: Negative except for above

SOCIAL HISTORY:
Works as a librarian in the medical school library
Lives with her partner, Louise
Drinks 1 beer a day for 40 years
Doesn't smoke

PHYSICAL EXAMINATION: Improving pneumonia with decreased crackles in right base; otherwise unremarkable

LABORATORY: | Urinalysis: | 100 WBCs/hpf |
| | Gram stain shows numerous neutrophils with budding yeast; no bacteria |
Serum creatinine is 1.5 mg/dL

Which of the following is the most appropriate management?

A. Oral fluconazole
B. Intravenous fluconazole
C. Re-insertion of the indwelling urethral catheter for bladder irrigation of amphotericin B
D. Intravenous amphotericin B
E. Oral amphotericin B

215.

A 16-year-old comes to the ER because of dysphagia and respiratory distress. This morning, he had acute onset of fever and a severe sore throat. He is now drooling. His voice is raspy, and he has stridor.

He is in obvious distress and leaning forward with the "I am going to die" look.

Which of the following should you do next?

A. Call for immediate ENT or anesthesia consult and start erythromycin now.
B. Call for immediate ENT or anesthesia consult and start vancomycin and ceftriaxone now.
C. Call for immediate ENT or anesthesia consult and start penicillin now.
D. Call for immediate ENT or anesthesia consult and start linezolid now.
E. Take culture of back of throat; notify ENT/anesthesia and then start ceftriaxone and vancomycin.

216.

A 25-year-old man with a history of IV drug abuse is admitted with fever, malaise, headache, and weakness. He denies other symptoms at this time. He has not been in the hospital before.

PAST MEDICAL HISTORY: Negative; admits to using IV drugs for 5 years and currently still using

SOCIAL HISTORY: Works at a local restaurant as a cook
                        Drinks two 6-packs of beer on the weekends
                        Smokes 1 pack of cigarettes daily

FAMILY HISTORY: Father 50 and healthy
                        Mother 50 and healthy

REVIEW OF SYSTEMS: Weight loss of 10 lbs noted for the past 2 months
                        Chronic "smoker" morning cough
                        Occasional night sweats

PHYSICAL EXAMINATION:
    BP 98/70, RR 30, Temp 102° F, P 110

    HEENT: PERRLA, EOMI
                TMs clear
                Throat slightly erythematous
    Neck: Supple; no lymphadenopathy noted
    Heart: RRR without murmurs, rubs, or gallops

Lungs:	Coarse breath sounds; clear with cough
Abdomen:	Bowel sounds present; no hepatosplenomegaly
Extremities:	No cyanosis, clubbing, or edema

LABORATORY: Blood cultures grow *Salmonella typhimurium*

You start him on intravenous ceftriaxone initially and then change him to oral ciprofloxacin 750 mg twice daily to complete a 2-week course. He follows up as an outpatient at the end of therapy and is doing well. However, 4 weeks later, he returns with the same symptoms, and again blood cultures grow *Salmonella typhimurium*.

Which of the following diagnostic tests should you order at this time?

   A.   Quantitative serum immunoglobulins
   B.   CT scan of the head
   C.   HIV ELISA
   D.   Intravenous urography
   E.   Bone marrow biopsy

217.

An 84-year-old man comes to the ER because of jaw tightness and neck stiffness. About a week ago, he had a minor injury to his left thigh—his grandson jabbed a pitchfork into his thigh while cleaning out the barn. He applied local care and pretty much ignored the wound as it healed. He takes no medications.

PAST MEDICAL HISTORY: Pneumonia at age 36
                        Healthy since the pneumonia

SOCIAL HISTORY: Lives alone on his farm
FAMILY HISTORY: Negative

PHYSICAL EXAMINATION: Significant aspects:
        He is alert and oriented to person, place, and time
        All vital signs are normal
        On mouth exam: He cannot open it completely
        Pupils react normally and extraocular movements are intact
        Neck is stiff
        Abdomen is tense; you note that all of the muscles of his abdominal wall are rigid
        His extremities exam is remarkable for all of the muscles of his extremities being rigid
        During the exam, especially with his reflexes, you note tonic-clonic motor activity

While examining him, a loud, boisterous nurse walks in and startles you both; he develops opisthotonic posturing with flexion of the arms and extension of his legs. He does not lose consciousness but experiences severe pain with this episode.

Of the following, what is the likely etiology for this man's condition?

   A.   *Clostridium botulinum*
   B.   *Clostridium perfringens*
   C.   *Clostridium septicum*
   D.   *Clostridium tetani*
   E.   *Corynebacterium diphtheriae*

218.

A 30-year-old woman is found to be HIV-seropositive. She has no medical complaints. She was diagnosed on routine screening while donating blood. Her physical examination is normal, except she has noticed that she bruises more easily than normal.

LABORATORY:

WBC:	3500/cu mm; 60% polys, 30% lymphocytes
Hemoglobin:	13 mg/dL
Platelet count:	40,000/cu mm
CD4 count:	250 cells/cu mm
HIV viral load:	150,000 copies

Bone marrow examination is requested.

Which of the following should you do now?

A. Begin efavirenz, tenofovir, and emtricitabine.
B. Begin corticosteroid therapy.
C. Begin intravenous gamma globulin therapy (IVIG).
D. Begin trimethoprim/sulfamethoxazole.
E. Infuse platelets.

219.

A 26-year-old African-American woman with transfusion-dependent sickle cell disease presents with a 1-week history of fever, malaise, nausea, diarrhea, and cramping abdominal pain. She has to be monitored closely because of her frequent transfusions. She receives deferoxamine on a daily basis because of severely high ferritin levels.

PAST MEDICAL HISTORY: Recurrent transfusions and use of deferoxamine

SOCIAL HISTORY: Unremarkable

FAMILY HISTORY: Unremarkable

PHYSICAL EXAMINATION:
    BP 95/50 mmHg, P 130, RR 38, Temp 101.5° F

HEENT:	Marked scleral icterus
	PERRLA, EOMI
	TMs clear
	Throat clear
Neck:	Supple
Heart:	RRR with II/VI systolic murmur at apex
Lungs:	Bilateral crackles in both bases with occasional faint wheeze
Abdomen:	Liver is 12 cm in span; no spleen palpated
Extremities:	No cyanosis, clubbing, or edema

Which of the following organisms would you expect to find growing in her blood cultures?

- A. *Escherichia coli*
- B. *Yersinia enterocolitica*
- C. *Klebsiella pneumoniae*
- D. *Haemophilus influenzae*
- E. *Francisella tularensis*

220.

A 50-year-old nurse whom you have been following while on isoniazid (INH) prophylaxis therapy presents today for routine follow-up. She had a PPD conversion about 3 months ago. Active disease was ruled out, and she was started on INH 300 mg daily. Today, she is returning for routine checkup and has no complaints. Her physical examination is completely normal. By mistake, lab is sent, and an AST comes back at 154 U/L (upper limit normal 40) and a serum ALT is 100 U/L (upper limit normal 56). The rest of the laboratory is normal.

Which of the following choices is most appropriate at this time?

- A. Continue INH; add pyridoxine supplementation.
- B. Discontinue INH; repeat liver tests in 2 weeks; if normal restart INH.
- C. Stop INH; start rifampin instead.
- D. Stop INH; start ethambutol, which has little liver toxicity.
- E. Continue INH; repeat serum aminotransferase measurements in one month or sooner if clinically warranted.

221.

Jessica Parker is a 23-year-old woman who is in her second month of pregnancy. She is referred to you by her obstetrician for evaluation of the following laboratory values. She feels well and has never had jaundice that she knows of.

LABORATORY:
    AST 19 U/L
    ALT 25 U/L
    Serum alkaline phosphatase 110 U/L
    Serum total bilirubin 0.5 mg/dL
    Hepatitis B surface antigen (HBsAg): Positive
    Antibody to hepatitis B surface antigen (anti-HBs): Negative
    IgM antibody to hepatitis B core antigen (IgM anti-HBc): Negative
    Hepatitis B e antigen (HBeAg): Negative
    IgG antibody to hepatitis B core antigen (IgG anti-HBc): Positive

The newborn of this woman should receive which of the following?

- A. Hepatitis B vaccine only
- B. Hepatitis B immune globulin at birth; then hepatitis B vaccine at 2 months of age
- C. Both hepatitis B vaccine and hepatitis B immune globulin at birth
- D. Alpha-interferon and ribavirin
- E. No vaccine until 2 months of age

222.

A 50-year-old man fishes regularly on the Chesapeake Bay. While sailing on the bay, he usually listens to Christopher Cross sing "Sailing." However, 3 weeks ago he was listening to Ted Nugent and was distracted. On that day, he caught some crabs, and one of the crabs scratched him on his arm with one of its claws. Over the next 2 weeks, he developed progressive painful swelling of the wound site. He took aspirin and ibuprofen without relief. His wife had some leftover dicloxacillin that he took, which also did not improve his condition.

His physical examination is really unremarkable except for marked swelling and induration of the scar area on the side of his left arm. He does not drink alcohol or smoke.

Which of the following organisms is most likely the cause of his illness?

    A. *Mycobacterium tuberculosis*
    B. *Mycobacterium leprose*
    C. *Mycobacterium marinum*
    D. *Vibrio vulnificus*
    E. *Bartonella crustacea* (crab scratch fever)

223.

A previously healthy 45-year-old man comes to the ER with a history of headache and fever, which he has had for about a day and a half. His wife reports that he has been confused and, at times, she is not able to understand what he is saying. This has progressively gotten worse in the past few hours. They are "outdoorsy" people and camp quite a bit in the Ozark Mountains.

PAST MEDICAL HISTORY: Negative

SOCIAL HISTORY: Airline pilot; no travel outside of U.S.
                               Main route is Little Rock to Dallas

FAMILY HISTORY: Father with Alzheimer's at age 60
                               Mother healthy

PHYSICAL EXAMINATION:
        BP 110/70, P 100, RR 18, Temp 102° F
        Oriented only to person; does not know where he is ("Tiparari") or the current year ("1984")

HEENT:	PERRLA, EOMI
	TMs clear
	Throat clear
Neck:	Stiff with meningismus
Heart:	RRR without murmur, rubs, or gallops
Lungs:	CTA
Abdomen:	Bowel sounds present; no hepatosplenomegaly
Extremities:	No cyanosis, clubbing, or edema
Skin:	No rash
Neuro:	Normal other than mental status testing

CT without contrast preliminary results: no infarct; ventricles normal
EEG shows abnormalities in the right temporal lobe area

Lumbar puncture results:

WBC:	220 WBC/cu mm (30% polys; 70% lymphs)
RBC:	400 RBC in tube 1
RBC:	300 RBC in tube 4
Protein:	65 mg/dL (normal)
Glucose:	80 mg/dL with serum of 120 mg/dL

Gram stain of CSF: No organisms seen
Acid-fast stain: No organisms seen
Cryptococcal antigen assay on CSF: Negative

Which of the following is the most likely cause of his illness?

A. *Borrelia burgdorferi*
B. *Francisella tularensis*
C. *Listeria monocytogenes*
D. *Streptococcus pneumoniae*
E. Herpes simplex virus

224.

A 79-year-old man has a right hip prosthesis. Ten months after his prosthesis is placed, he complains of persistent pain that has not improved since his surgery. He has tried ibuprofen without relief. For the last few weeks the pain has worsened to the point that he will not get out of bed, unless his grandchild helps him. He has not had any fevers during this time.

PAST MEDICAL HISTORY: Lung cancer diagnosed 20 years ago; had resection and cure
Hypothyroidism for 30 years; on replacement therapy
Hypertension for 50 years; on ACE inhibitor for 10 years with good control

SOCIAL HISTORY: Lives with his granddaughter and her 3 kids
Doesn't smoke or drink

PHYSICAL EXAMINATION:
BP 130/70, P 80, RR 18, Temp 99° F

HEENT:	PERRLA, EOMI
	Throat clear
Neck:	Supple
Heart:	RRR without murmurs, rubs, or gallops
Lungs:	CTA
Abdomen:	Benign
Extremities:	Normal muscle strength
	Range of motion in right hip is diminished compared to the left; severe pain produced with movement—"DON'T DO THAT"
	Neurovasculature is intact

Plain films of hip: Lucency of the right hip located where the prosthesis and the femur interact

Which of the following is the next step in workup?

A. Begin oral dicloxacillin
B. Begin oral gatifloxacin
C. Fluoroscope-guided aspiration of the hip
D. Technetium^{99m} bone scan
E. Blood culture

225.

A 40-year-old woman is vacationing in Acapulco, Mexico. She eats salad and tacos at a local café and drinks multiple margaritas during her stay. While on the trip she develops watery, nonbloody diarrhea. Additionally, she has cramping abdominal pain that is relieved with a bowel movement. She has low-grade temperatures to between 99 and 100 degrees F for a day or two. Her symptoms resolve without any treatment after 4 days of illness.

You see her in follow-up after the trip. Her physical examination is normal. She has no symptoms now.

Which of the following organisms was most likely responsible for her illness?

A. Enterotoxigenic *Escherichia coli*
B. *Escherichia coli* O157:H7
C. *Campylobacter jejuni*
D. *Shigella sonnei*
E. Rotavirus

226.

A 20-year-old Mexican-American man is brought into the Emergency Room with a seizure. This is his first known seizure, and he has been in excellent health in the past—he runs marathons for the Mexican Olympic team. He has been training in the United States for 3 years now.

PAST MEDICAL HISTORY: Negative
                         Immunizations up-to-date, including 2nd MMR and hepatitis B

SOCIAL HISTORY: Lives with relatives in San Diego
                         Works as a courier for an express mail company

FAMILY HISTORY: Mother and father both healthy; live in small community outside of Mexico City

REVIEW OF SYSTEMS: Completely negative

PHYSICAL EXAMINATION:
    BP 120/70, RR 16, Temp 98.6, P 50

    HEENT: PERRLA, EOMI
                TMs clear
                Throat clear
    Neck: Supple; no masses
    Heart: RRR without murmurs or rubs; healthy gallop
    Lungs: CTA

Abdomen: Benign
Extremities: Normal, no rashes

LABORATORY:
CT of head: 8 cystic lesions, 1 cm to 3 cm in diameter; two of the lesions enhancing slightly with contrast
HIV ELISA: Negative
CD4: 2000/cu mm

Which of the following is the most likely diagnosis?

A. *Toxoplasma gondii*
B. Cryptococcal meningitis
C. Neurocysticercosis
D. Lymphoma
E. Herpes simplex virus

227.

A 35-year-old man comes to the Emergency Room because of malaise, fever, chills, and a diffuse rash that he has had since awakening this morning. He is a mailman and was bitten by a dog one week ago. Subsequently, he noted some pain, redness, and discharge from the bite wound.

PHYSICAL EXAMINATION:
BP 80/60 mm Hg, P 120, RR 40, Temp 104° F

HEENT:	PERRLA, EOMI
	Conjunctivitis is noted
	Throat: tongue is beefy red and he has large papillae
Neck:	Supple
Heart:	RRR without murmurs, rubs, or gallops
Lungs:	CTA
Abdomen:	Benign
Skin:	Diffuse, pink rash with blotches is noted over his entire body
	A yellowish fluid is draining from his bite wound

LABORATORY:

WBC:	20,000/cu mm; 50% polys, 29% bands
Hemoglobin:	12.5 mg/dL
Platelets:	55,000/cu mm
BUN:	70 mg/dL
Creatinine:	5.0 mg/dL
AST:	500 U/L
Serum albumin:	2.2 g/dL
Urinalysis:	3+ proteinuria

Which of the following is the most likely organism responsible?

A. *Neisseria meningitidis*
B. *Eikenella corrodens*
C. *Pasteurella multocida*
D. *Staphylococcus aureus*
E. *Bartonella henselae*

228.

A 23-year-old woman comes to your office after being told by a local physician that she is HIV-infected. She had been tested as part of a routine physical examination. She has never injected intravenous drugs and has had sexual intercourse in her lifetime with only four men, each of whom reportedly has never used drugs and is healthy.

At the time of physical examination, she is very anxious and tearful. Her complete physical examination is normal except for 2 lymph nodes in her posterior cervical chain that measure 0.3 cm x 0.5 cm.

Her previous test results from her doctor show an HIV ELISA that is positive and a Western blot assay that is "indeterminate." You repeat her Western blot assay 3 months later, and it shows no bands (negative). A repeat Western blot assay at 6 months shows no bands (negative).

Which of the following is the best interpretation of her initial lab result that prompted her to see you?

    A. Early HIV-1 infection
    B. Resolved HIV-1 infection
    C. HIV-2 infection
    D. She has HIV; the Western blots are now false negatives because of her advanced disease
    E. False-positive HIV ELISA for HIV-1

229.

A 30-year-old man will be traveling to rural areas of Africa for a year. His medical history is unremarkable. His physical examination is normal. He will be outside in the sun for many hours daily. His trip begins in 2 weeks.

Based on this limited information, which of the following agents would be best for him to take for antimalarial chemoprophylaxis?

    A. Mefloquine weekly, starting 1 week before his travel and continuing for 4 weeks after returning to the U.S.
    B. Doxycycline daily, starting 2 days before his travel and continuing for 4 weeks after returning to the U.S.
    C. Chloroquine weekly, starting 1 week before his travel and continuing for 4 weeks after returning to the U.S.
    D. Chloroquine weekly, starting 2 weeks before his travel and continuing for 4 weeks after returning to the U.S.
    E. Primaquine daily, starting 1 week before his travel and continuing for 4 weeks after returning to the U.S.

230.

A 16-year-old female is referred to you by her school nurse because of persistent vaginal discharge. She has had several episodes in the past 2 years that have been self-diagnosed as yeast infections. They have always responded to over-the-counter medications such as clotrimazole. She is a sexually active student who has had multiple male sexual partners in the past. Currently, she has been having sex with 2 different male partners—one on Friday nights and one on Saturday nights. These 2 partners and all previous partners she reports as being "healthy." Recently, she completed another course of topical anti-fungal therapy with no improvement in her discharge. She denies history of vaginal lesions or vesicles.

PAST MEDICAL HISTORY: Currently on oral contraceptives

SOCIAL HISTORY: Doesn't drink or smoke
Goes to the movies with her Friday partner regularly
Goes bowling with her Saturday partner regularly

PHYSICAL EXAMINATION: Completely normal except for slight yellow discharge from the cervical os

Management of this young woman should include which of the following:

A. Pap smear, RPR, HIV testing and counseling, and HSV culturing
B. Pap smear, RPR, HIV testing and counseling, and culture for *Gardnerella vaginalis*
C. Pap smear, RPR, HIV testing and counseling, and gonorrhea and *Chlamydia* culturing
D. Pap smear, RPR, HIV testing and counseling, and culture for *Candida*
E. Pap smear, RPR, HIV testing and counseling, no culture needed, and just treat for *Candida*

231.

A 30-year-old man works as a nurse on the wards in your hospital. He spilled a urine specimen from an HIV-infected patient on his hands 30 minutes ago. The patient has end-stage AIDS with a CD4 count of 1/cu mm and a viral load of 1 million copies/cc. The patient has been on zidovudine/lamivudine/efavirenz for the past year with failure noted because of poor adherence to the regimen, although a recent genotype showed resistance patterns developing to zidovudine and indinavir! The patient is hepatitis B-surface-antigen-negative, and the nurse has received a series of 3 doses of hepatitis B vaccine, which was completed last year when he finished nursing school.

The nurse notes that he has a healing laceration from a cat scratch on his left hand, and that the urine splashed onto this lesion. The lesion is well scabbed over. As soon as he spilled the urine on his hands, he scrubbed them meticulously.

Which of the following do you recommend?

A. A regimen of using agents other than zidovudine and indinavir is indicated because of the known resistance patterns.
B. Zidovudine, lamivudine, and indinavir for 4 weeks.
C. Lamivudine alone is sufficient.
D. Test the remaining urine for HIV RNA and start treatment if the viral load is detectable.
E. No prophylaxis is indicated.

232.

A 50-year-old man is brought into the Emergency Room with a dramatic decrease in his visual acuity. He reports he was fine until yesterday, when he thinks a metal sliver went into his eye. He was trying to pry open a lock with a wrench and a metal screwdriver when he had severe pain in his eye after one of his attempts. He does not remember seeing anything come into his eye. He tried washing his eye out, but the pain has persisted.

PAST MEDICAL HISTORY: Hypertension for 20 years; on thiazide diuretic
History of cellulitis of right foot 10 years ago; resolved with oral medications

SOCIAL HISTORY: Drinks 2–3 beers daily

PHYSICAL EXAMINATION:

Vital signs:	Normal
Right eye:	Normal
Left eye:	Severely erythematous with severe chemosis
Slit lamp:	Severe corneal deterioration with a ring abscess
	Both chambers full of debris and cells

Plain x-ray: Shows a foreign body in the left eye

Which of the following is the most likely pathogen?

A. *Acanthamoeba*
B. *Bacillus cereus*
C. *Bartonella henselae*
D. *Staphylococcus epidermidis*
E. *Streptococcus oralis*

233.

A 55-year-old man comes to the night clinic with a history of acute onset of nausea, severe headache, and facial flushing. He says that the symptoms began while he was sitting at home drinking a beer. On further questioning, you discover that he is receiving an outpatient intravenous antibiotic for a wound infection.

Which of the following antibiotics is most likely responsible?

A. Ceftriaxone
B. Cefotetan
C. Imipenem
D. Clindamycin
E. Piperacillin/tazobactam

234.

A 28-year-old man is referred to you because he is found to be seropositive for Epstein-Barr virus. For a year he has had difficulty falling asleep, as well as frequent awakening during the night. He has had increasing problems with daytime fatigue and reports that he can't concentrate as well. He has lost interest in his hobbies; he used to enjoy playing basketball avidly. He has gained 20 lbs in the last year and says that he "just doesn't feel like exercising."

PAST MEDICAL HISTORY:	Negative; started coming to the local physician about 1 year ago with sleep disturbances
SOCIAL HISTORY:	Divorced about 2 years ago
	Has 2 children; wife has custody
	"Recovered alcoholic"; hasn't had a drink in 5 years
	Smokes 1 pack of cigarettes daily
	No illicit drug use
FAMILY HISTORY:	Mother age 60; history of depression
	Father age 60; hypertension

REVIEW OF SYSTEMS: No fever
No chills
No sore throat
No lymph node enlargement noted
No diaphoresis
No cough
No palpitations
No constipation
No diarrhea
No risk factors for HIV

PHYSICAL EXAMINATION:
BP 120/70, P 90, RR 18, T 99° F (pt. says, "See Doc, I got a fever")
Ht. 5'10" Wt. 190 lbs (moderate truncal obesity)

HEENT:	PERRLA, EOMI
	TMs clear
	Throat clear; no erythema; no obvious dental caries noted
Neck:	Supple
Heart:	RRR without murmurs, rubs, or gallops
Lungs:	CTA
Abdomen:	Bowel sounds present; liver span 6 cm; no spleen palpated
Extremities:	No cyanosis, clubbing, or edema

LABORATORY:

CBC:	Normal
Electrolytes:	Normal
Liver enzymes and panel:	Normal

EBV titers: Only positive is EBV viral capsid (VCA) specific IgG antibody titer at 1:160

Based on your findings, which of the following do you think he needs?

A. Measurement of T-lymphocytes
B. Repeat EBV testing
C. CMV testing
D. Referral to an infectious disease specialist for evaluation of chronic EBV syndrome
E. Further evaluation for depression and referral for counseling

235.

A 34-year-old patient with HIV disease presents with cough, dyspnea, and bilateral infiltrates. A presumptive diagnosis of PCP is made, and he is treated with trimethoprim/sulfa and prednisone. In addition, he is noted to have oral candidiasis, and fluconazole is given.

Labs obtained 48 hours after admission: Na 133, K 7.0, Cl 100, HCO_3 23, BUN 20, Cr 1.2

Of the following, what is the most likely cause for the hyperkalemia?

   A. Trimethoprim/sulfamethoxazole
   B. Prednisone
   C. Fluconazole and prednisone
   D. Fluconazole
   E. Adrenal insufficiency

236.

You are called to evaluate a 74-year-old man with Parkinson disease. He has been hospitalized twice in the last year for urosepsis. Because of incontinence, he has required a chronic indwelling urinary catheter. He is currently afebrile and has no abdominal pain. He has had no mental status changes or recent falls. Lab work from 48 hours ago includes: WBC 8,000, HCT 42%, Na 137, K 3.6, BUN 20, Cr 1.2, and urine culture > 100,000 colonies of *Enterococcus*.

Of the following, what therapy do you recommend?

   A. Ceftriaxone + gentamicin
   B. No therapy at this time
   C. Ampicillin + gentamicin
   D. Ciprofloxacin
   E. Amoxicillin

NEPHROLOGY

237.

Which of the following is true about angiotensin-converting enzyme inhibitors?

A. Not likely to lower blood pressure in patients with renal artery stenosis
B. Not associated with angioedema
C. Associated with cough
D. Unable to prevent progressive renal dysfunction in patients with Type 1 diabetes mellitus
E. Frequently stopped for hyperkalemia

238.

A 35-year-old woman presents with altered mental status. No medical history is available. Other than being stuporous, her exam is unremarkable with normal vital signs, no orthostasis, no edema, and without focal findings. Her serum sodium is 104 mEq/L, creatinine 0.6 mg/dL, U_{Na+} 8 mEq/L, and Uosm 90 mOsm/kg H_2O (low!).

Which of the following is true?

A. Treatment should start with hypertonic saline.
B. Her total body sodium is approximately normal.
C. She has an excess of antidiuretic hormone.
D. Diuretic abuse should be suspected.
E. Water intoxication has been ruled out.

239.

A 50-year-old alcoholic was found down in the street and brought to the ER. The patient has had nausea and vomiting. Vitals show mild orthostasis with tachycardia and low-grade fever. Labs show sodium of 134, potassium of 5.8, chloride of 100, and bicarbonate of 16 mEq/L. The creatinine is 6.8 with a BUN of 36 mg/dL. The calcium is 7.2, phosphorus 9.0 mg/dL, and albumin 3.0 g/dL. Urinalysis shows 3+ blood, 1+ protein; microscopic exam of urine sediment shows rare RBCs and rare muddy brown granular casts.

Appropriate therapy includes which of the following:

A. Free water replacement
B. Volume restriction
C. Dialysis to clear toxins
D. Intravenous calcium chloride
E. Alkalinization of the urine

240.

A 24-year-old man presents for evaluation. A kidney stone passed spontaneously 2 weeks ago. The patient feels well. An uncle also has kidney stones. The patient's exam is normal. Labs show sodium of 140 mEq/L, potassium of 3.2 mEq/L, chloride of 116, and bicarbonate of 14 mEq/L. Creatinine is 0.8 and BUN is 14 mg/dL. Urine electrolytes are sodium 40, potassium 36, and chloride 75 mEq/L. The urine pH is 6.5.

Each of the following may be useful <u>except</u>:

    A. Bicarbonate therapy
    B. Low-calcium diet
    C. Diuretic therapy
    D. High water intake
    E. Potassium citrate therapy

241.

Routine lab tests demonstrate the following: sodium 138, potassium 3.5, chloride 100, and bicarbonate 35 mEq/L. Urine studies show sodium of 35, potassium of 20, and chloride of 70 mEq/L, with a urine pH of 4.8.

Which of the following is most likely associated with these abnormalities?

    A. Renal artery stenosis
    B. Remote diuretic use
    C. Vomiting
    D. Contraction
    E. Hypokalemia

242.

A 70-year-old woman presents with low-grade temps, arthralgias, and hypertension. She has lost 20 lbs over the past 3 months. Other than a blood pressure of 170/100 mmHg and mild edema, the exam is benign. Laboratory exam shows sodium 138, potassium 4.5, chloride 108, bicarbonate 20 mEq/L, creatinine 2.7, and BUN 45 mg/dL. Urinalysis shows 3+ blood, 3+ protein with RBC casts. Complement studies are normal: ANA is +, 1:16 in a speckled pattern; ANCA is +, 1:64 in a perinuclear pattern; and anti-GBM is negative. Renal biopsy shows negative immunofluorescence with a necrotizing capillaritis.

Treatment should be started with which of the following:

    A. Plasmapheresis
    B. Bedrest and diuretics
    C. Azathioprine and pulse steroids for lupus flare
    D. High-dose steroids and cytotoxic drugs
    E. Converting enzyme inhibition

243.

Loop diuretics do all the following <u>except</u>:

A. Inhibit sodium-potassium-2 chloride channel transports in the loop of Henle
B. Promote potassium loss
C. Cause hypercalcemia in some users
D. Increase the risk of gout
E. Effectively treat hypertension in patients with renal insufficiency

244.

A severely mentally retarded 46-year-old is brought to the ER by neighbors after being left alone at his group home. He was found in the open garage of his home. He is obtunded and clinically appears intravascularly volume-depleted. His clothing is soiled with stool and urine. He has a significant fall in his blood pressure and increase in his pulse when he is brought to an upright position. Kussmaul's respirations are noted. Neurologic exam is non-focal.

Na   133
K   2.5
UA: pH 5.0, Na 6 mEq/L, K 12 mEq/L, Cl 24 mEq/L
Cl   118
HCO₃ 5
ABG: 7.25 / pCO₂ 14 / calc HCO₃ 5
BUN   52
Cr   3.4

Of the following choices, what is the acid-base abnormality?

A. Anion gap metabolic acidosis
B. Non-anion gap metabolic acidosis
C. Respiratory acidosis with a metabolic acidosis
D. Anion gap metabolic acidosis with respiratory alkalosis

245.

A 50-year-old man presents for evaluation of renal insufficiency and proteinuria. He has a 10-year history of diabetes and hypertension. He has had treatment for diabetic polyneuropathy and retinopathy within the past year. Exam shows eye and nerve abnormalities, blood pressure of 160/102 mmHg, and mild edema, but is otherwise normal. Labs demonstrate a sodium of 138, potassium 4.0, chloride 108, bicarbonate 20, creatinine 2.2, and BUN 48 mg/dL. The blood sugar is 186 mg/dL, and albumin is 3.4 g/dL. Urine shows a creatinine clearance of 40 mL/min and 3.4 g/day of protein.

The best treatment of his renal condition would include which of the following:

A. Magnetic renal angiography
B. Blood pressure reduction with dihydropyridines
C. Weight gain, blood sugar control, and low-salt diet
D. Renal biopsy
E. Enalapril

246.

Which of the following is a feature more typical of Type 1 (distal) renal tubular acidosis than of Type 2 or 4?

    A. Hyperchloremic acidosis
    B. Associated with Fanconi syndrome
    C. Hyperkalemia
    D. Kidney stones
    E. Normal anion gap

247.

A 46-year-old alcoholic male is brought to the Emergency Room with altered mental status by a friend following a week of "heavy" drinking. He is found to have a glucose level of 45 and, with D50 administration, his mental status returns to normal. He has been drinking a quart of vodka a day for the past 12 years, but for the past week has doubled that amount. On examination, his blood pressure is 110/74, pulse 112, respiration 22; his hands are tremulous, and he has hepatomegaly with a liver span of 14 cm. His initial laboratory studies are: sodium 135, potassium 3.9, CO_2 16, chloride 94, BUN 7, serum creatinine 0.8 mg/dL. His serum osmolality is 302. ABGs: pH 7.30, PCO_2 30, HCO_3 14. Hemoglobin is 11.3, HCT 35.1%, and WBC 8.7. He is given IV fluids (D5 ½N/S), vitamins, and lorazepam. Studies for hepatitis B and C are negative, and ultrasound of his liver shows no obstruction. Clinically he seems to be improving, but 3 days later, his serum creatinine is noted to be 5.5. Urinalysis at this time: Sp Gr 1.1010, pH 5.5, 3+ blood, no glucose, trace protein, 0–1 RBCs/HPF, 3–5 hyaline casts, and 2–3 granular casts. His serum osmolality is 302.

Which of the following is the most likely explanation for this rise in his creatinine?

    A. Isopropyl alcohol intoxication
    B. Acute renal failure secondary to ethylene glycol
    C. Methanol intoxication
    D. Acute renal failure secondary to rhabdomyolysis associated with hypophosphatemia
    E. Hepatorenal syndrome

248.

A 52-year-old patient with diabetes mellitus Type 2 for 20 years is seen for follow-up of his renal disease. Five years earlier, he first developed proteinuria, and about 1 year ago he developed edema. His past medical history is significant for laser treatment of both eyes over the past 2 years. His current medications include NPH insulin administered twice per day with sliding scale coverage, lisinopril 40 mg daily, furosemide 20 mg daily, and aspirin one daily. On physical examination, his blood pressure is 126/84, pulse 84 per minute. His funduscopic examination reveals evidence of prior laser therapy, his chest is clear, and there is no S_3. He has 1+ edema of his lower extremities.

His hemoglobin is 8.7 mg/dL with a hematocrit of 27.3%, WBC 11.4, sodium 135, potassium 4.8, CO_2 22, chloride 106, creatinine 3.6, and BUN 42. Serum albumin is 2.6, urinalysis reveals 4+ protein with no other abnormalities, and the 24-hour urine collection reveals 6.5 gm protein per day with 1.2 gm of creatinine.

Ultrasound of the kidneys reveals no evidence of hydronephrosis, and kidney sizes are 11.5–12 cm bilaterally.

Which of the following would be most appropriate in this patient's management at this time?

    A. Discontinue lisinopril.
    B. Refer this patient for dialysis.
    C. Refer patient for renal biopsy to exclude other causes of nephrotic syndrome.
    D. Begin therapy with recombinant human erythropoietin.
    E. Administer a nonsteroidal antiinflammatory drug to reduce proteinuria.

249.

A 65-year-old woman is seen for evaluation of swelling in her legs. She has noted this off and on for the last 3 months, worse when she has been standing for long periods of time. Her past medical history is significant only for hemicolectomy for diverticulosis 10 years previously, during which time she required three units of blood. On physical examination, her blood pressure is 134/84 with a pulse of 82 per minute. She is well dressed and appears younger than her stated age. Her physical examination is remarkable only for 2+ edema of her lower extremities, extending up to her knees. Her CBC and electrolytes are normal; her BUN is 22 with a serum creatinine of 1.1 mg/dL. Serum albumin is 1.6. Urinalysis is remarkable for 4+ protein and oval fat bodies. Serologic studies were significant for hepatitis B surface antigen positivity. Her 24-hour urine reveals 12.6 gm protein per day with a urine creatinine of 1.050 gm/day. She undergoes renal biopsy, and a diagnosis of membranous glomerulopathy is made. A decision is made with her not to initiate therapy at this time and to follow her closely.

Four months later, she notices that her urine looks very dark, so she returns for a follow-up visit. At this time, her serum creatinine is 4.5 mg/dL and her urinalysis reveals 4+ protein, 4+ blood, and, on microscopic examination, has too many red cells to count.

The initial approach to evaluate the change in her renal function should be which of the following:

    A. Initiate therapy with prednisone.
    B. CT scan of the renal veins.
    C. Obtain urgent angiography to exclude bleeding from the renal biopsy.
    D. Refer the patient to a hepatologist for interferon therapy for hepatitis B.
    E. Urology consultation.

250.

A 65-year-old gentleman presents to the Emergency Room complaining of shortness of breath. He has a history of ischemic cardiomyopathy and has been experiencing progressive dyspnea, worsening orthopnea, and more frequent paroxysmal nocturnal dyspnea over the past 2 weeks. He has a history of 2 MIs. Four months ago, he underwent triple vessel coronary artery bypass grafting. A recent echocardiogram showed an ejection fraction of 15%. His medications are captopril 25 mg tid, furosemide 120 mg bid, digoxin 0.25 mg daily, carvedilol 2.5 mg bid, and warfarin 5 mg daily. On physical examination: blood pressure 102/68, pulse 98 per minute and regular, temperature 98.6°F, respiration 16 per minute. In general, he is a thin, elderly gentleman in moderate respiratory distress. His central venous pressure is 16 cm and his chest has bibasilar crackles throughout both lung fields. The PMI is displaced to the anterior axillary line with a regular S_1 and an S_3 gallop. There is a III/VI holosystolic murmur heard at the apex radiating to the axilla. His abdomen is unremarkable; there is 2+ peripheral edema. ECG: no acute ST-T changes, old inferior and anteroseptal myocardial infarction with sinus rhythm. Chest x-ray: pulmonary vascular congestion with cardiomegaly. Electrolytes: sodium 121, potassium 3.2, chloride 96, CO_2 32, BUN 73, creatinine 1.2. CBC: normal. U/A: specific gravity 1.020, pH 5.5, pro-trace, otherwise negative.

This patient's hyponatremia is most likely due to which of the following:

    A. Renal sodium losses secondary to furosemide
    B. Hypothyroidism
    C. Water retention
    D. SIADH
    E. Adrenal insufficiency

251.

A 26-year-old HIV-infected male presents with shortness of breath. His past medical history was negative. On physical examination, he becomes short of breath with any minimal activity; chest exam reveals scarce bilateral crackles, and the rest of his exam is unremarkable. Chest x-ray: bilateral interstitial infiltrates. ABGs on room air: PO_2 52, PCO_2 32, pH 7.48; electrolytes normal; serum creatinine 1.1; urinalysis normal. The patient is started on oxygen, trimethoprim/sulfamethoxazole, and prednisone and begins to show improvement; but one week later, his creatinine has risen to 3.4 mg/dL. Urinalysis demonstrates pH 1.015, trace protein, trace blood with no glucose. Microscopic: 4–6 WBCs, 0–2 RBCs, and occasional hyaline casts.

Which of the following studies would be most helpful in establishing the etiology of his acute renal failure?

    A. Urine electrophoresis
    B. Urine eosinophils
    C. Ultrasound of the kidney
    D. 24-hour urine for protein and creatinine clearance
    E. ANCA

252.

A 42-year-old Caucasian male is evaluated for shortness of breath. He has a 3-week history of progressive dyspnea on exertion; more recently, he began coughing up blood and now is seeking medical attention. His past medical history is unremarkable, except for a long history of chronic allergic rhinitis for which he has used nasal steroids and over-the-counter antihistamines. His past medical history is otherwise unremarkable. On physical examination, his blood pressure is 150/90, pulse 110 per minute, respiration 20 per minute, temperature 98.7° F. In general, he is a thin white male who gets short of breath periodically during the history taking. His HEENT examination is unremarkable. He has no lymphadenopathy. His chest has scattered crackles. The rest of his examination is normal. His electrolytes demonstrate sodium 136, potassium 3.9, chloride 110, HCO_3 26, BUN 62, creatinine 3.1, hemoglobin 10.5, hematocrit 32.5%, WBCs 11,500. ABGs on room air: PO_2 56, PCO_2 29, pH 7.33, bicarbonate 26. Urinalysis: specific gravity 1.015, pH 5, 2+ protein, 3+ blood, no glucose. Microscopic: 15–20 RBCs per high-power field, 0–2 RBC casts, 5–7 WBCs. Chest x-ray: diffuse bilateral patchy infiltrates. Renal biopsy is performed and demonstrates epithelial crescents, with negative immunofluorescence.

Which of the following statements is correct?

A. c-ANCA is likely to be positive.
B. Plasmapheresis should be initiated immediately.
C. p-ANCA is likely to be positive.
D. This patient is likely to have a significant eosinophilia.
E. Complement levels will be low.

253.

A 22-year-old Caucasian college student was seen for evaluation of progressive swelling in his ankles over the last 10 days. The patient's roommate notes that his eyes look swollen in the morning. The patient has no previous medical history and is taking no medications. On physical examination, his blood pressure is 116/78, and the rest of the vital signs are normal. The examination is remarkable only for edema that is 3–4+ pitting, extending all the way up to the thighs with 2+ presacral edema. CBC is normal, sodium is 131, potassium 3.9, chloride 103, HCO_3 26, BUN 22, and creatinine 0.9. Urinalysis: pH 5, specific gravity 1.008, 4+ protein, no blood. On microscopic examination, oval fat bodies are present. Further evaluation reveals serum cholesterol-387, serum albumin 0.9, and a 24-hour urine protein is 14.3 gm per day. A calculated creatinine clearance is 112 mL per minute.

Which of the following statements is true?

A. Treatment should be initiated with cyclosporine.
B. Treatment should be initiated with steroids and cytotoxic therapy to prevent progressive renal disease.
C. The most likely diagnosis is focal and segmental glomerulosclerosis.
D. This patient is not likely to develop progressive renal failure.
E. ACE inhibitor therapy should not be used in patients with heavy proteinuria.

254.

A 19-year-old Caucasian male is seen for evaluation of hematuria. He has always been healthy with no medical problems; but yesterday, he developed an upper respiratory infection. Last night, when he urinated, he noted that his urine was initially very dark and then appeared to be grossly bloody. Quite concerned about this problem, he made an appointment for an office visit the following morning. This is the first time this has ever happened, and he has no family history of anyone having any similar problems. His physical examination is entirely normal. CBC and electrolytes are normal. His BUN is 11 and the serum creatinine is 0.8. Urinalysis demonstrated blood-tinged urine with 4+ blood and trace protein. There are too many red blood cells to count microscopically, and there are occasional red blood cell casts.

Which of the following is the most appropriate next step in the evaluation and management of this patient?

A. Immediate referral for renal biopsy.
B. Referral to urologist.
C. Order complement levels.
D. Begin prednisone 60 mg daily.
E. Hearing evaluation.

255.

A 32-year-old motorcycle enthusiast was brought to the Emergency Room following a collision with a sport utility vehicle. He was trapped under the vehicle and was extracted with the "jaws of life." He suffered severe injuries to his pelvis and legs and was rushed to the ER as soon as he was freed. In the ER, his initial blood pressure was 85/palpable with a heart rate of 136/minute. His blood pressure improved with 3 liters of normal saline and 4 units of blood. Further evaluation revealed multiple fractures of his pelvis and both tibias. His initial hemoglobin was 8.9, hematocrit 28.4%; but his electrolytes, urinalysis, and liver function tests were normal. His BUN was 13 and serum creatinine was 1.0. Following an open reduction and fixation of both tibias, he was brought to the SICU for observation. The next day the patient's urine output began to fall, and his serum creatinine rose to 2.9. His urinalysis revealed specific gravity of 1.010, pH 5.5, 4+ blood, trace protein, 1–2 RBCs per high-power field, and 4–6 granular casts. A CPK was 25,500, K^+ was 7, and urine myoglobin was pending. His heart rate began to slow and an ECG demonstrated a rate of 45 with no P waves, and widening of the QRS.

The immediate next step in the management of this patient is which of the following:

A. Perform fasciotomies.
B. Temporary pacemaker placement.
C. Administer sodium polystyrene sulfonate (Kayexalate®, Kionex®, Marlexate®) enemas.
D. Initiate dialysis therapy.
E. Administer calcium gluconate.

256.

A 17-year-old woman is brought to the Emergency Room by her parents, because she has become lethargic and seems to have trouble breathing. They have noticed that, over the last several weeks, she has been going to the bathroom more frequently and appears to have lost some weight. She has always been a good student, but recently she has felt poorly and has had difficulty completing her homework assignments. For the last two days, she has completely lost her appetite, has had nausea, and she vomited 5–7 times during the day before she was brought in. She has no previous medical history. On physical examination, her blood pressure is 95/60, pulse 114 per minute, respirations 24, temperature afebrile. In general, she is a thin and lethargic but arousable 17-year-old woman who is breathing deeply. Her skin turgor is markedly decreased, and her neck veins are not visible. She has a hyperdynamic precordium, but the examination is otherwise unremarkable. Laboratory studies: sodium 124, potassium 5.9, chloride 80, CO_3 18, BUN 31, creatinine 1.4, hemoglobin 15.1, hematocrit 47%. Urinalysis: specific gravity 1.010, pH 5, 4+ glucose, 2+ ketones. ABGs on room air: PO_2 105, pH 7.25, PCO_2 20, bicarbonate 12. The patient is immediately given 3 liters of .9 NS, and an insulin drip is initiated with improvement in her sensorium.

Which of the following acid-base abnormalities does she have?

A. Metabolic acidosis, respiratory acidosis, metabolic alkalosis
B. Respiratory acidosis, metabolic acidosis, metabolic alkalosis
C. Metabolic acidosis, respiratory alkalosis, metabolic alkalosis
D. Metabolic acidosis, respiratory alkalosis
E. Respiratory acidosis, metabolic alkalosis

257.

A 35-year-old woman comes in for a routine physical examination. Her only complaint is that lately she has been feeling "weak," but is otherwise able to work and perform all of her normal activities. She has no medical problems, denies any special diet, and takes no over-the-counter medications. Her family history is unremarkable. On physical examination, her blood pressure is 116/76, pulse 86, with the rest of the examination being normal. Screening laboratory studies were obtained with everything returning normal except for her electrolytes, which revealed sodium 136, potassium 3.8, chloride 91, CO_3 34, BUN 11, and creatinine 0.9. Urine chloride is 45.

Which of the following is the most likely diagnosis?

A. Renal artery stenosis
B. Liddle syndrome
C. Primary hyperaldosteronism
D. Addison disease
E. Bartter syndrome

258.

A 29-year-old Type 1 diabetic male has maintained excellent control of his blood sugars with a hemoglobin A1C of 6.9%. He is seen routinely for follow-up with no known complications; however, for the last three visits, his blood pressure has been 150–160/85–95. His last year's protein:creatinine ratios were normal. Currently, his only medications are insulin and simvastatin for hyperlipidemia. On physical examination, blood pressure is 162/98 and pulse is 82 per minute. In general, he is a well-appearing 29-year-old man. There is no retinopathy, and the rest of the examination is unremarkable. Electrolytes are normal, BUN 14, creatinine 0.7. Urinalysis: no proteinuria.

Which of the following agents is your initial choice for treatment of his hypertension?

    A. Minoxidil
    B. An ACE inhibitor
    C. Thiazide diuretic
    D. Nifedipine
    E. Beta-blocker

259.

A 24-year-old Caucasian male presents for evaluation of kidney stones. His history began at age 2 with a bladder neck obstruction secondary to stones requiring surgical intervention. At age 9, he was noted to be below the 5th percentile for height and weight, and his long bones showed "ricketic" changes. He had pyelonephritis and stones at age 10; and one year later, he had pyelolithotomy and *Pseudomonas* urinary tract infection, but no further stones. He did well until he was 19, when he presented to a local Emergency Room with severe muscle weakness and arrhythmias and was found to have a potassium of 1.8 mEq/L. He was placed on potassium supplements and now comes in for follow-up. His family history is significant for two maternal uncles with stones, and his father, paternal grandfather, and paternal aunts and uncles with hearing loss.

On physical examination, his blood pressure is 120/80, and in general he is short in stature, has significant hearing loss, and is wearing bilateral hearing aids. His examination is remarkable only for surgical scars on his abdomen.

Labs: Na 139, K 2.8, Cl 117, CO_3 12, BUN 31, Cr 1.8
Urinalysis: Sp Gr 1.010; pH 7; No protein, blood, or glucose; + calcium oxalate crystals
ABGs: pH 7.29, pCO_2 25, HCO_3 12
Urine Lytes: Na 130, K 20, Cl 110

Abdominal flat plate: Calcium deposits in periphery of both kidneys

The most likely diagnosis is which of the following:

    A. Type 2 RTA
    B. Type 1 distal RTA
    C. Type 4 RTA
    D. Chronic diarrhea
    E. Salicylate intoxication

260.

A 75-year-old man with long-standing hypertension and diabetes mellitus presents to the Emergency Room complaining of shortness of breath of 3 to 4 days duration. He ran out of his furosemide and oral hypoglycemic agent 1 month ago. He admits to noncompliance with his diabetic diet and with his dietary salt restriction. He denies cough, fever, orthopnea, or weight gain. He has nocturia 1 to 2 times per night and has noted a decrease in the strength of his urinary stream for the past 2 years.

His physical exam shows a mildly obese African-American man with a blood pressure 150/100 mmHg supine and standing, P 50 bpm, RR 28/min, and he is afebrile. He has no jugular venous distention or carotid bruit. Lungs are clear. Cardiac exam shows regular slow rate without murmur or gallop. He has no peripheral edema.

Laboratory evaluation shows:
Hb 13.9 g/dL, HCT 40%, WBC 8000/mL, platelets 240,000/mL.
Na 133 mEq/L, K 6.8 mEq/L, Cl 100 mEq/L, bicarbonate 23 mEq/L, BUN 31 mg/dL, Cr 1.8 mg/dL, glucose 170 mg/dL.
Urinalysis shows Sp Gr 1.015, pH 5.7, 100 mg% protein, trace glucose.
ECG shows sinus bradycardia with 1st-degree AV block.
Arterial blood gases show pH 7.30, pCO_2 50, pO_2 75 on room air.
Chest radiograph shows clear lung fields and mild left ventricular hypertrophy.

Which of the following is the most likely cause of his hyperkalemia?

    A. Pseudohyperkalemia
    B. Potassium movement into the extracellular fluid due to acidosis
    C. Chronic renal failure due to diabetes mellitus and hypertension
    D. Impaired renal excretion due to Type 4 renal tubular acidosis
    E. Excessive dietary potassium intake

261.

A 37-year-old man with no prior history presents at the urging of his wife for evaluation of nocturia. He states that he has always liked to drink water frequently and urinates several times per day and 3 or 4 times every night. He had no childhood illnesses that he is aware of, except enuresis up until the age of 10.

Physical exam shows a young man with BP 130/70 mmHg, P 68 bpm, RR 10/min; he is afebrile. His general physical exam is completely within normal limits.

Laboratory evaluation shows:
Hb 14.2 g/dL, HCT 43%, WBC 7,000/mL, platelets 367,000/mL
Na 147 mEq/L, K 4.2 mEq/L, Cl 118 mEq/L, bicarbonate 24 mEq/L, BUN 13 mg/dL, creatinine 1.0 mg/dL, glucose 80 mg/dL
Urinalysis: Sp Gr 1.012, pH 5.5, negative dipstick and microscopic analysis
Urine: Na 57 mEq/L, K 42 mEq/L, Cl 110 mEq/L, osmolality 270 mOsm/kg
24-hour urine volume: 6,500 mL

Of the following, which therapy would be most appropriate for this man?

A. Request urgent psychiatric evaluation.
B. Begin vasopressin tannate in oil, nightly injection.
C. Begin nasal installation of des-amino arginine vasopressin (DDAVP®) twice a day.
D. Begin water restriction 2000 mL/day.
E. Begin hydrochlorothiazide 25 mg/day.

262.

A 40-year-old man with lymphoma presents for follow-up. He has a 24-hour urine test done that shows he is excreting 2.1 grams of protein on a daily basis. However, you note that his urine dipstick is negative for protein.

Which of the following best explains this discrepancy?

A. Dipsticks detect only negatively charged proteins like albumin.
B. Tamm-Horsfall proteins block the reaction.
C. The test strip recognized only heavy chain proteins.
D. His urine was too diluted with the dipstick testing.
E. The test strip cannot pick up the smaller proteins.

263.

A 21-year-old man is being evaluated because of increased polyuria and polydipsia.

His laboratory is as follows:
Serum Lytes: Sodium 143 mmol/L, K 4.0 mmol/L, Cl 105 mmol/L, HCO$_3$ 25 mmol/L
BUN: 20 mg/dL
Serum Glucose: 98 mg/dL
Urine electrolytes: Na 27 mmol/L, K 33 mmol/L
Urine osmolality: 197 mosmol/kg water

After 12 hours of fluid deprivation, his body weight has fallen 6 kg! Laboratory testing now shows:
Serum Lytes: Sodium 152 mmol/L, K 4.2 mmol/L, Cl 110 mmol/L, HCO$_3$ 25 mmol/L
BUN: 22 mg/dL
Serum Glucose: 96 mg/dL
Urine electrolytes: Na 24 mmol/L, K 36 mmol/L
Urine osmolality: 202 mosmol/kg water

One hour after the subcutaneous administration of 5 units of vasopressin, urine values are as follows:
Urine electrolytes: Na 30 mmol/L, K 29 mmol/L
Urine osmolality: 198 mosmol/kg water

Which of the following is the most likely diagnosis?

A. Salt-losing nephropathy
B. Osmotic diuresis
C. Nephrogenic diabetes insipidus
D. Psychogenic polydipsia
E. Occult diabetes mellitus

264.

Which of the following lab values are consistent with a young man drinking ethylene glycol?

A. Na 140, K 5.2, Cl 102, HCO_3 20, Serum Creatinine 3.5, Arterial pH 7.36
B. Na 135, K 4.5, Cl 106, HCO_3 22, Serum Creatinine 3.5, Arterial pH 7.37
C. Na 140, K 2.6, Cl 115, HCO_3 13, Serum Creatinine 3.5, Arterial pH 7.31
D. Na 143, K 4.8, Cl 100, HCO_3 10, Serum Creatinine 3.5, Arterial pH 7.25
E. Na 140, K 6.2, Cl 109, HCO_3 20, Serum Creatinine 3.5, Arterial pH 7.36

265.

Which of the following lab values are consistent with a middle-aged woman who has been given amphotericin B for the treatment of disseminated histoplasmosis?

A. Na 143, K 4.8, Cl 100, HCO_3 10, Serum Creatinine 3.5, Arterial pH 7.25, Urine pH 5.0
B. Na 140, K 2.6, Cl 115, HCO_3 13, Serum Creatinine 3.5, Arterial pH 7.31, Urine pH 6.2
C. Na 135, K 4.5, Cl 106, HCO_3 22, Serum Creatinine 3.5, Arterial pH 7.37, Urine pH 5.0
D. Na 140, K 5.2, Cl 102, HCO_3 20, Serum Creatinine 3.5, Arterial pH 7.36, Urine pH 5.0
E. Na 140, K 6.2, Cl 109, HCO_3 20, Serum Creatinine 3.5, Arterial pH 7.36, Urine pH 5.0

266.

A 17-year-old boy has had acute post-streptococcal glomerulonephritis. He is improving and is feeling better.

Which of the following laboratory values are consistent with someone in a recovery period like his?

A. Na 136, K 5.0, Cl 102, HCO_3 20, Serum Creatinine 3.5, Arterial pH 7.36, Urine pH 5.0
B. Na 140, K 2.6, Cl 115, HCO_3 13, Serum Creatinine 3.5, Arterial pH 7.31, Urine pH 6.2
C. Na 143, K 4.8, Cl 100, HCO_3 10, Serum Creatinine 3.5, Arterial pH 7.25, Urine pH 5.0
D. Na 135, K 4.5, Cl 106, HCO_3 5, Serum Creatinine 3.5, Arterial pH 7.22, Urine pH 5.0
E. Na 140, K 6.2, Cl 109, HCO_3 20, Serum Creatinine 3.5, Arterial pH 7.36, Urine pH 5.0

267.

Which of the following laboratory values support the diagnosis of Type 4 renal tubular acidosis?

A. Na 135, K 4.5, Cl 106, HCO_3 22, Serum Creatinine 3.5, Arterial pH 7.37, Urine pH 5.0
B. Na 136, K 5.2, Cl 102, HCO_3 20, Serum Creatinine 3.5, Arterial pH 7.36, Urine pH 5.0
C. Na 140, K 2.6, Cl 115, HCO_3 13, Serum Creatinine 3.5, Arterial pH 7.31, Urine pH 6.2
D. Na 143, K 4.8, Cl 100, HCO_3 10, Serum Creatinine 3.5, Arterial pH 7.25, Urine pH 5.0
E. Na 140, K 6.2, Cl 109, HCO_3 20, Serum Creatinine 3.5, Arterial pH 7.36, Urine pH 5.0

268.

Which of the following laboratory values are consistent with multiple myeloma?

A. Na 140, K 2.6, Cl 115, HCO$_3$ 13, Serum Creatinine 3.5, Arterial pH 7.31, Urine pH 6.2
B. Na 140, K 6.2, Cl 109, HCO$_3$ 20, Serum Creatinine 3.5, Arterial pH 7.36, Urine pH 5.0
C. Na 136, K 5.2, Cl 102, HCO$_3$ 20, Serum Creatinine 3.5, Arterial pH 7.36, Urine pH 5.0
D. Na 135, K 4.5, Cl 106, HCO$_3$ 22, Serum Creatinine 3.5, Arterial pH 7.37, Urine pH 5.0
E. Na 143, K 4.8, Cl 100, HCO$_3$ 10, Serum Creatinine 3.5, Arterial pH 7.25, Urine pH 5.0

269.

The hyperlipidemia of nephrotic syndrome is best characterized by which of the following:

A. Elevation of total cholesterol but no increase in atherogenesis
B. Elevation of all lipids but no increase in atherogenesis
C. Selective elevation of LDL cholesterol with increased atherogenesis
D. Very high (> 30%) risk of myositis in those treated with lipid-lowering agents
E. Doesn't respond well to HMG-CoA reductase inhibitors

ENDOCRINOLOGY

270.

A woman comes to your clinic complaining of galactorrhea. She is 55 years old with no significant past medical history except for an uneventful hysterectomy for fibroids at age 45. She is not on any hormone therapy, not involved in a sexual relationship, wears loose-fitting clothing, and denies nipple stimulation. You notice that she is very tired and moves slowly. She even seems to talk slowly. On physical examination, you can easily express thin, white fluid from both breasts. She has no breast masses or tenderness. Her skin is dry. A recent mammogram was unremarkable. You order a prolactin level and a CT of her pituitary. She returns for follow-up, and you find her unchanged. The prolactin was mildly elevated at 80 ng/mL (normal: 1.4–24.2 ng/mL), and she has a pituitary macroadenoma.

Which of the following is the next best step in patient care?

A. Start bromocriptine.
B. Check TSH.
C. Because of her age, re-check the prolactin in 6–12 months.
D. Refer her to a neurosurgeon.
E. Look for an unknown non-pituitary cancer.

271.

Your favorite patient comes to your clinic. He is 45 years old and has a recently diagnosed 5-mm prolactinoma, which you started treating with low-dose bromocriptine. He complains to you about constant nausea and vomiting since starting bromocriptine. He retches several times in your presence.

Of the following, what is the next best thing to do?

A. Try some prochlorperazine or other anti-nausea drug.
B. Stop the bromocriptine and follow his prolactinoma with serial MRIs.
C. Refer him to a neurosurgeon for resection of the prolactinoma.
D. Switch him to cabergoline.
E. Add cabergoline to bromocriptine.

272.

You are asked to see a patient admitted to the medicine service. He was found to have a large pituitary tumor that is extending toward the optic chiasm, but without any significant changes in his visual fields. The tumor is a prolactinoma. The primary physician is very concerned because of the size of the tumor. He wants to have the patient operated on immediately, even though it's Christmas Eve, and the best neurosurgeon is out of town for the next few days.

Of the following, what would be the best advice to give?

A. Begin a trial of high-dose glucocorticoids.
B. Find any neurosurgeon in the phone book who is willing to operate on Christmas Day.
C. Transfer the patient to a hospital with a competent neurosurgeon who happens to be in town for the holidays.
D. Begin pre-op evaluation in preparation for surgery in three days.
E. Start cabergoline and repeat the CT/MRI in a few days.

273.

A 28-year-old male is involved in a motor vehicle accident while riding a motorcycle and experiences loss of consciousness, despite wearing a helmet. He regains consciousness while en route to the hospital and denies any sequelae. On arrival at the hospital, the Emergency Room staff notes a mildly obese young man with central obesity, blood pressure 160/90, and multiple mild lacerations, but otherwise unremarkable. Routine labs are within normal limits. Other than general soreness, he has no complaints. A CT of the head is normal except for a 3-mm well-visualized pituitary mass. He is discharged from the ER after a period of observation and comes to see you several days later for follow-up. Your exam is similar to the ER staff's except that now his blood pressure is 140/85.

Which of the following would be the most appropriate next step at this time?

A. Check an ACTH stimulation test, TSH, and a total testosterone.
B. Refer him to a neurosurgeon for transsphenoidal resection of the pituitary mass.
C. Discharge him from your clinic on a drug to treat hypertension and encourage him to stop riding motorcycles.
D. Have him return to your clinic in a few weeks to recheck his blood pressure.
E. Check serum IGF-1 and 24-hour urine cortisol.

274.

A 38-year-old woman is referred to you by a neurologist who was seeing her for severe headaches. His final diagnosis was stress headaches, but because a head MRI showed an empty sella, the neurologist wanted you to see her. On questioning, you learn that she has seven children and all are healthy. When the first child was born, she experienced a difficult delivery and considerable bleeding that required a transfusion. All subsequent deliveries were uneventful. The review of systems was otherwise negative. Physical examination shows normally pigmented abdominal striae. The blood pressure is 100/60. You order some blood tests and find that the electrolytes, glucose, and TSH are normal.

Which of the following is the most correct thing for you to do next?

A. Tell her that everything is normal and discharge her from your clinic.
B. Refer her to a neurosurgeon for exploration of her pituitary gland.
C. Diagnose Sheehan syndrome and begin replacement therapy.
D. Evaluate for pituitary hypofunctioning.
E. Evaluate for pituitary hyperfunctioning.

275.

A 60-year-old man comes to your clinic complaining of weight loss and reports losing 25 pounds over the last year. He recently moved to your town hoping that a change of pace might make him feel better. He has been somewhat depressed for the last two years. He doesn't get much exercise and often feels tired. He has smoked about a pack a day since he was in his twenties. He admits to feeling stressed in your office, because he hasn't seen a doctor for over 20 years. His affect is somewhat flat and his pulse is 101. Otherwise, your examination is unremarkable. Because of his smoking history and unexplained weight loss, you suspect lung cancer and order a chest x-ray. He returns for follow-up and is unchanged from the earlier office visit. The radiologist reports the chest x-ray as normal.

Of the following, what should you do next for this patient?

    A. Begin an anti-depressant and have him return to clinic for follow-up.
    B. Refer him to a psychiatrist for evaluation of depression.
    C. Check FT4 and TSH.
    D. Encourage better eating habits and more exercise.
    E. Refer him to an oncologist for workup of an occult cancer.

276.

A 50-year-old man is in your clinic for follow-up 1 year after a subtotal thyroidectomy for cancer. He had a 2-cm thyroid nodule with papillary cancer. The surgeon reported no spread to adjacent tissue and no lymph node involvement. After surgery, he received high-dose radioactive iodine ablation. A total body scan was negative. He is now on suppressive thyroxine. Current labs are TSH 0.25 mU/L (0.5–5.0) and FT4 1.5 ng/dL (0.7–1.5). He asks you about his risk for cancer recurrence.

Of the following, which is the most accurate response?

    A. Increased risk due to his gender
    B. Increased risk due to his age
    C. Increased risk due to the size of the nodule
    D. Increased risk due to the type of cancer
    E. No increased risk

277.

A psychiatrist in your community refers a patient to you who is an 80-year-old woman being treated for depression. She reports generalized weakness, fatigue, dry skin, weight gain, and constipation. Her past medical history includes CHF and stable angina. Your examination reveals periorbital edema, skin that is cool and dry, loss of the lateral third of her eyebrows, mild bradycardia, and slow relaxation phase of her deep tendon reflexes. You strongly suspect hypothyroidism and check TSH and FT4. The TSH is 95 µIU/mL (normal: 0.3–5.0 µIU/mL) and the FT4 is 0.1 ng/dL (normal: 0.7–1.5 ng/dL). She obviously has severe hypothyroidism.

Which of the following should you do next?

   A. Administer thyroxine 500 μg IV every day for 5 doses.
   B. Administer thyroxine 500 μg IV and triiodothyronine 20 μg IV qd x 3.
   C. Begin thyroxine 150 μg PO qd.
   D. Begin thyroxine 25 μg PO qd.
   E. Begin thyroxine 300 μg PO qd.

278.

You are asked to see a patient in the surgical ICU who is doing poorly 7 days after emergency repair of a perforated colon. He is 68 years old and developed mesenteric ischemia, which resulted in his perforation. He is now septic and requires ventilator support. You note numerous laboratory derangements, including abnormal WBC, HCT, HCO_3, creatinine, hepatic enzymes, and arterial pH. He also has a mildly depressed TSH and FT4. He is receiving adequate and appropriate care in the ICU, but the surgeon wants your opinion about his thyroid dysfunction.

Which of the following should be your response?

   A. The patient has mild hypothyroidism that doesn't need treatment.
   B. The patient has mild hyperthyroidism that doesn't need treatment.
   C. The patient probably does not have any thyroid problems.
   D. The patient has mild pituitary dysfunction and should start thyroxine therapy.
   E. The patient has mild hypothyroidism and should start thyroxine therapy.

279.

A 62-year-old man comes to see you because of a lump in his throat that has been there for about 1 year. You palpate a 2-cm firm nodule in the left lower lobe of his thyroid. The mass is nontender and movable. The remainder of his thyroid is non-palpable, and he has no palpable lymph nodes in his neck. You find him to be clinically euthyroid. You order thyroid tests and have him return to your clinic in 1 week. The nodule has not changed, and his TSH and FT4 are both within normal limits.

Of the following, what is the next best step in patient care?

   A. Begin thyroxine therapy in the hope that the nodule may shrink.
   B. Refer him for a thyroid fine-needle biopsy and aspiration (FNA).
   C. Refer him to a surgeon for a near-total thyroidectomy.
   D. Refer him to a surgeon for a hemithyroidectomy.
   E. Follow him for several years, watching for any changes in the nodule.

280.

A 65-year-old man has had benign prostatic hypertrophy for several years. He is still able to urinate effectively, but his symptoms have started to worsen. His urologist has scheduled a TURP for next week and referred him to you for a medical preoperative evaluation. Besides the expected prostate enlargement, your examination shows mild tachycardia and atrial fibrillation. Suspecting hyperthyroidism, you order thyroid function tests. The results are TSH 0.1 µIU/mL (normal: 0.3–5.0 µIU/mL) and FT4 2.5 ng/dL (normal: 0.7–1.5 ng/dL).

Which of the following is the best advice for you to give the urologist?

A. Begin antithyroid medication now and postpone the surgery until he is euthyroid or nearly so.
B. Proceed with the operation and begin antithyroid medication afterward.
C. Give an ablative dose of radioactive iodine immediately before the operation.
D. Recheck his thyroid function postoperatively.
E. Postpone the surgery and ask the urologist to refer the patient to a cardiologist for treatment of his atrial fibrillation.

281.

A patient of yours comes to see you and complains about being tired. She gave birth to a healthy child about 6 months ago, and she tells you that the baby is doing fine. Her obstetrician reported to you that the pregnancy and delivery were uneventful. You ask your patient to tell you more, and she says that at first everything was perfect. She had plenty of energy to take care of the baby and to do all of the housework; she easily lost the weight that she had gained; and she had no problem staying up at night to feed the child. After about one month, she began to get tired. At first she was able to ignore it, but her fatigue steadily worsened until she could barely function. She can no longer keep up with the baby's needs or the housework. She is having difficulty with nursing. She blames herself for everything that's wrong and begins to cry.

Which of the following should you do next?

A. Tell her that the symptoms of her "postpartum blues" will soon pass.
B. Begin anti-depressants.
C. Begin stimulants.
D. Order TSH and FT4, suspecting hypothyroidism due to postpartum thyroiditis.
E. Refer her to a psychiatrist for evaluation.

282.

A mildly overweight 25-year-old man comes to your office because of an elevated glucose. He attended a health fair where his glucose was checked with a glucometer. His random glucose was found to be 220 mg/dL, and he was advised to have his glucose checked again. He reports more frequent urination and greater thirst than usual. The fasting glucose is 126 mg/dL. Metabolic panel otherwise is normal with a creatinine of 0.7 mg/dL.

Which of the following should you tell him?

A. He is not diabetic.

B. He has diabetes and must talk with a diabetes educator and dietitian to begin a diet, exercise program, and metformin.

C. He has impaired glucose tolerance and should be rechecked in one year.

D. He may have diabetes and needs to be rechecked again next year.

E. He has diabetes but doesn't need treatment until his glucose reaches 140 mg/dL.

283.

A 45-year-old man comes to your office for a routine follow-up. He has Type 2 diabetes mellitus and hypertension. In your office today his blood pressure is 128/76. He has his glucometer log book, which shows relatively good glycemic control. Your exam, including his feet, shows no abnormalities. His current medications are metformin 1,000 mg twice daily and aspirin 81 mg daily. You order routine fasting blood work, which comes back with the following values:

Na^+	138 mEq/L	(135–143 mEq/L)
K^+	3.9 mEq/L	(3.5–5.0 mEq/L)
Cl^-	105 mEq/L	(100–109 mEq/L)
HCO_3^-	23 mEq/L	(22–30 mEq/L)
Urea nitrogen	13 mg/dL	(8–18 mg/dL)
Creatinine	1.5 mg/dL	(0.6–1.2 mg/dL)
Glucose	84 mg/dL	(65–110 mg/dL)
HbA1c	7.0 %	(4.9–6.2 %)
TChol	167 mg/dL	
LDL	98 mg/dL	
HDL	45 mg/dL	
Trigylcerides	120 mg/dL	

Random urine microalbuminuria screen 12 µg/mg (< 30 µg/mg).

After reviewing the lab results, you call him.

Which of the following choices is most appropriate?

A. Begin an ACE inhibitor for better blood pressure control.

B. Add a thiazolidinedione.

C. Begin a statin drug.

D. Don't change anything and have him come back to the office in 6 months.

E. Stop taking the metformin and have him come to your office tomorrow.

284.

A woman with Type 1 diabetes comes to your office. She has been followed by another physician but hasn't been feeling right and wants to try a different physician. She heard that you are the best internist in town. She is 50 years old and has had diabetes for 35 years. She has retinopathy (being followed by an ophthalmologist) and mild microalbuminuria. Her medications include NPH insulin 15 units every morning and 60 units at bedtime; a rapid-acting insulin analogue 6–12 units with each meal, which she adjusts depending on the pre-meal capillary glucose level; an ACE inhibitor every evening; and aspirin 81 mg daily. Her glucometer log shows glucose levels generally okay except for the morning fasting glucose, which is elevated. The physical examination is unremarkable except for some retinal microaneurysms. She has her most recent laboratory tests from last week, which are generally okay. The HbA1c is 5.8%. She is very proud of her HbA1c and reports that her other physician had been increasing the evening NPH in an attempt to lower the morning fasting glucose, which has been steadily high despite increasing the evening insulin. She reports to you that she has been experiencing terrible, vivid nightmares during the night and often wakes up in a cold sweat, but attributes this to a scary movie that she saw two months ago.

Which of the following is the most appropriate action to take at this time?

A. Begin an anxiolytic to help her nightmares.
B. Reduce her evening NPH insulin and follow closely.
C. Increase the evening NPH insulin again to reduce the morning fasting glucose levels.
D. Add an insulin sensitizer to reduce her insulin needs.
E. Switch her to 70/30 insulin mix twice daily.

285.

A patient of yours comes to your office for a routine follow-up. He is 50 years old and has had Type 2 diabetes for 8 years. He is mildly overweight with a BMI of 28, has lost a few pounds over the past 4 months, is watching his diet as best he can, and is walking 1–2 miles every evening after work. You have been treating him with a thiazolidinedione, a statin, and a baby aspirin every day for the past 3 years. Three days before coming to your office he went to the lab for the routine tests that you asked him to get. Your physical examination is unremarkable. His blood pressure at the last visit was 132/80 and today is 134/82. His fasting LDL is 98 mg/dL; the liver function tests, including ALT, are well within normal limits; electrolytes are all normal; the creatinine is 0.8 mg/dL; the random urine microalbuminuria screen is 180 μg/mg.

Which of the following is the best next step in care?

A. Increase the statin.
B. Tell him to keep up the good work and continue to lose weight.
C. Add an ACE inhibitor or an angiotensin-receptor blocker (ARB).
D. Add a calcium-channel blocker for his hypertension.
E. Start a low-dose diuretic such as hydrochlorothiazide 12.5 mg every morning.

286.

A patient develops a kidney stone and comes to see you. He is a "health freak" and takes megadoses of vitamins and supplements of calcium. The following labs are all elevated: calcium, ionized calcium, 25OH-Vitamin D, 1,25(OH)$_2$-Vitamin D, and intact PTH. You briefly entertain a long differential diagnosis because of his megadoses of vitamins and minerals, but you quickly discard all of them except one.

Which of the following is the most likely diagnosis?

A. Pseudopseudohypoparathyroidism
B. Vitamin D intoxication
C. Vitamin A intoxication
D. Primary hyperparathyroidism
E. Secondary hyperparathyroidism

287.

You are asked to see a woman recently hospitalized for a hip fracture and found to have hypocalcemia. She is 75 years old and has been in poor health for quite some time. She lives alone and is reluctant to leave her house. Her granddaughter does the shopping and laundry for her, but admits that her grandmother doesn't eat very much. Her only medication is hydrochlorothiazide 50 mg every morning for mild hypertension; she rarely goes to her internist for scheduled appointments. When you examine her, you find a frail-looking elderly woman with moderate dementia. She has a right hip fracture that she attributes to falling down the steps to her front door. The orthopedic surgeon is currently deciding whether to operate. In the meantime, full DVT precautions are in place. Her labs, including the additional tests ordered by you, come back as the following:

Na^+	142 mEq/L	(135–143 mEq/L)
K^+	3.6 mEq/L	(3.5–5.0 mEq/L)
Cl^-	105 mEq/L	(100–109 mEq/L)
HCO_3^-	28 mEq/L	(22–30 mEq/L)
Urea nitrogen	22 mg/dL	(8–18 mg/dL)
Creatinine	1.2 mg/dL	(0.6–1.2 mg/dL)
Glucose	86 mg/dL	(65–110 mg/dL)
Calcium	7.6 mg/dL	(8.9–10.5 mg/dL)
Phosphate	1.8 mg/dL	(2.5–4.5 mg/dL)
Magnesium	2.9 mg/dL	(1.4–2.5 mg/dL)
25OH-Vitamin D	6 µg/L	(10–55 µg/L)
$1,25(OH)_2$-Vitamin D	12 ng/L	(18–62 ng/L)
Intact PTH	81 pg/mL	(10–65 pg/mL)

Bone density at hip z-score is -2.8 SD.

Which of the following is the most likely cause of her hypocalcemia?

    A. Hypermagnesemia
    B. Vitamin D deficiency
    C. Hypophosphatemia
    D. Thiazide diuretic
    E. Primary hyperparathyroidism

288.

A patient of yours comes to the clinic for his routine follow-up. He is 47 years old and has Type 2 diabetes. He is moderately obese, has mild hypertension treated effectively with an ACE inhibitor, and has hypercholesterolemia treated with a statin. Before you started the statin, his LDL-cholesterol was 170 mg/dL. His glycemic control has been difficult, and he is currently taking a thiazolidinedione, metformin, and a rapid-acting secretagogue, all at the maximum dose allowed. Despite three drugs, his glycemic control has worsened during the past 6 months along with his weight. He states that he is tired of watching his diet and admits to gaining 21 pounds in the last 6 months. The blood pressure today is 126/74. The physical examination is unchanged; his feet are fine.

Labs 6 months ago (fasting):

Na^+	140 mEq/L	(135–143 mEq/L)
K^+	4.0 mEq/L	(3.5–5.0 mEq/L)
Cl^-	107 mEq/L	(100–109 mEq/L)
HCO_3^-	24 mEq/L	(22–30 mEq/L)
Urea nitrogen	11 mg/dL	(8–18 mg/dL)
Creatinine	1.0 mg/dL	(0.6–1.2 mg/dL)
Glucose	102 mg/dL	(65–110 mg/dL)
HbA1c	8.5 %	(4.9–6.2 %)
TChol	169 mg/dL	
LDL	92 mg/dL	
HDL	38 mg/dL	
Triglycerides	195 mg/dL	

Random urine microalbuminuria screen is 12 µg/mg (< 30 µg/mg).

Labs today (fasting):

Na^+	139 mEq/L	(135–143 mEq/L)
K^+	4.1 mEq/L	(3.5–5.0 mEq/L)
Cl^-	105 mEq/L	(100–109 mEq/L)
HCO_3^-	24 mEq/L	(22–30 mEq/L)
Urea nitrogen	12 mg/dL	(8–18 mg/dL)
Creatinine	1.0 mg/dL	(0.6–1.2 mg/dL)
Glucose	179 mg/dL	(65–110 mg/dL)
HbA1c	10.2 %	(4.9–6.2 %)
TChol	198 mg/dL	
LDL	98 mg/dL	
HDL	36 mg/dL	
Triglycerides	320 mg/dL	

Random urine microalbuminuria screen is 17 µg/mg (< 30 µg/mg).

Of the following, which is the best choice to address the hypertriglyceridemia?

A. Stop the statin and begin a fibrate.
B. Add a fibrate and another statin to his current statin.
C. Discontinue his oral agents for glycemic control and switch him to insulin.
D. Add an α-glucosidase inhibitor to his diabetic regimen.
E. Continue his statin and add a second statin.

289.

You are asked to see a woman recently admitted to the ICU with hypotension. She is unable to give a history, and no family members or friends are available. Witnesses report that she was sitting at the airport waiting for a connecting flight when she passed out. The person sitting next to her noticed that she became quite agitated when it was announced that the flight would be delayed for 6 hours, just before she passed out. There is no evidence of a pulmonary embolism. During your examination, you note that she is very thin, lacks axillary hair, has sparse pubic hair, and has extra pigmentation on her gums and buccal mucosa. The blood pressure was 40/palp with a heart rate of 130 when she first arrived, but is now 100/64 with a heart rate of 78 with saline running. Her temperature is 98.2 °F; the cardiac rhythm is sinus; the routine chemistry tests show a hyperkalemic metabolic acidosis; and the renal status is compatible with prerenal azotemia.

Which of the following should you do now?

  A. Begin dexamethasone 4 mg IV and order an ACTH stimulation test.
  B. Measure ACTH and TSH before beginning prednisone 60 mg and thyroxine 100 µg every day.
  C. Measure cortisol and FT4 levels before beginning thyroxine and methylprednisolone.
  D. Begin hydrocortisone 100 mg IV every 8 hours and order an ACTH stimulation test.
  E. Begin hydrocortisone 100 mg IV every 8 hours.

290.

A 74-year-old man is admitted with mental status changes.

On physical exam BP was 134/86 without orthostatic changes, P 86

Face:	Unilateral ptosis
Thyroid:	Difficult to feel
Lungs:	Decreased air entry
Abd:	No abnormalities noted
GU:	Enlarged prostate without masses
Extremities:	Normal without edema
Pre-sacrum:	Normal without edema
Mental Status:	Oriented to name and place but does not know time of day or most recent meal

CXR:	Mass in right upper lobe with volume loss
Laboratory:	Na 121, K 3.3, Cl 105, HCO_3 24, BUN 12, Cr 1.2, Ca 9.9
	H/H 13.8/39%, normal LFTs with albumin 3.1 g/dL

Which of the following is the correct treatment for his hyponatremia?

  A. NS with 20 mEq KCL @ 75 cc/hr
  B. Fluid restriction to 800 cc/day
  C. Hypertonic saline
  D. Desmopressin

291.

A 40-year-old man is referred to you after a DEXA scan done at a health fair screening indicated low bone density with a T-score of -1.6. He tries very hard to stay healthy by exercising and taking mega-doses of vitamins. On examination, nothing unremarkable is found. Chem-7, LFTs, and albumin are normal.

	Patient's	Normal
Calcium	10.7 mg/dL	8.5–10.5
Phosphorus	4.7 mg/dL	1.5–4.5
25(OH)-Vit D	60 microgram/L	9–52
1,25(OH)$_2$-Vit D	13 ng/L	16–60
iPTH	5 pg/mL	18–73
Testosterone	550 ng/dL	260–1000

Of the following, which is the most likely cause of his osteopenia and elevated Ca?

A. Primary hypoparathyroidism
B. Excess calcium in his diet
C. Surreptitious use of anabolic steroids
D. Vitamin A intoxication
E. Vitamin D

292.

Pituitary tumors may cause which of the following:

A. Hyperthyroidism
B. Mass effect
C. Hypothyroidism
D. Cushing disease
E. All of the choices are correct

293.

A 79-year-old woman comes to you accompanied by her daughter visiting from out of town. The patient insists she is fine. The daughter confirms the patient's assertion that there's been no difficulty with swallowing or breathing, nor has there been a change in her mother's voice. The family reports weight loss, irritability, and anxiousness. P 104, regular. She has tremor of her outstretched arm and an irregularly textured thyroid. The trachea is not deviated. She cannot resist your pressure against raising her leg from the exam table. T4 is 17 and TSH < 0.1 mIU/mL.

Of the following, the most appropriate evaluation would be:

A. MRI of head
B. CT neck
C. Thyroid ultrasound
D. Thyroid scan
E. Thyroid scan and uptake

294.

A 37-year-old man is referred to you for cholesterol of 256 mg%. He states he has decreased intake of meat, fried foods, and dairy other than low- or no-fat products, and has trouble jogging due to leg cramps. Despite diet change, his weight increased 5 pounds in the past 3 months. Pulse is 66 and BP is 146/88. His thyroid is difficult to feel in his large neck. His hair is not shiny, his skin is dry, and there are no bruits, xanthomas, or xanthelasma.

He returns in two weeks, training for a half triathlon, with his LDL 196 and triglycerides 123; total cholesterol is 252 and HDL 21.

Which of the following pharmacologic treatments is best to begin at this time?

    A. Atorvastatin
    B. Gemfibrozil
    C. Bile acid resins
    D. Nothing; wait longer for diet to take effect
    E. Nitroglycerin

295.

A 28-year-old woman takes paroxetine (Paxil®) for depression, diagnosed when her family suggested she see a therapist because she lacked interest in her usual activities. Six months later, the therapist asked for evaluation because there was no improvement on this antidepressant nor with the 2 other antidepressants tried before. She has lost 12 pounds, which she associates with multiple flu-like episodes she's experienced over the preceding 18 months.

BP 94/54, P 98
She is thin and pale. She has no tremor or diaphoresis and otherwise has no focal findings. She has a family history of thyroid disease and has been having GI symptoms during this time period.

Of the following, which should be the next test you order?

    A. MRI of head
    B. CBC
    C. Basal plasma ACTH and cortisol ACTH stimulation test
    D. T3
    E. Dental evaluation for etched enamel

296.

A 42-year-old woman G2P2 had menarche at age 13 followed by regular q 27-day menses with 4 days flow in the ensuing years, until 9 months ago. She also reports increased pigmented facial hair and some scalp hair thinning.

BP 138/84
Facial and trunk acne is present
Temporalis hair recession
Deep voice
Pigmented hair on chin, chest, shoulders, extremities, and gluteal region

Laboratory is ordered and the results show: DHEA-S extremely high (1183), testosterone high (371ng/dL), LH low (2.7), FSH low (2.2), estradiol low (31).

Of the following, what is the most likely diagnosis?

    A. Menopause
    B. PCOS (polycystic ovary syndrome)
    C. Hypogonadotrophic hypogonadism
    D. Adrenal cancer
    E. Hyperthyroidism

297.

A 32-year-old man comes to see you because his wife cannot conceive. He reports normal development, was taller than his peers, and he's had no change in sexual interest or activity.

BP 112/68, P 88, Wt 220, Ht 71″, Span 72″

He has 2 cm of glandular tissue under the areola, minimally excess abdominal adipose, and testes 2 x 1 cm. His scrotum has rugae and terminal hair.

Of the following, the most likely diagnosis is:

    A. Kallmann syndrome
    B. Klinefelter syndrome
    C. Pituitary adenoma
    D. Prolactinoma
    E. Hereditary small gonad syndrome

298.

A 24-year-old woman comes in tearfully to discuss her Type 1 diabetes. She is on insulin lispro (Humalog®) and NPH. She has increased her NPH from 14 units in the morning and 12 units at bedtime to 16 units in the morning and 16 units at bedtime because she has high morning glucoses. Her log shows FBS 42→325, noon 112→201, supper 68→167, bedtime 189→220. She notes that her sleep is restless, and she has been having increased nightmares and never feels rested in the morning.

Of the following, which is the next appropriate step in patient care?

    A. Make no changes at this time.
    B. Increase both supper Humalog® and bedtime NPH.
    C. Increase a.m. Humalog® and NPH, and increase bedtime NPH.
    D. Decrease noon Humalog® and a.m. NPH, and increase bedtime NPH.
    E. Increase the supper Humalog®, and decrease the bedtime NPH.

299.

A patient with a severe asthma attack was treated with prednisone 50 mg daily for 5 days. The pulmonologist says the patient no longer needs steroids and signs off on the case.

Which of the following steps should you take now?

A. Stop the prednisone abruptly.
B. Switch to 5 mg/day and periodically check for return of adrenal function.
C. CRH stimulation test to assess pituitary function.
D. An insulin tolerance test to assess hypothalamic function.
E. ACTH stimulation test to assess adrenal function.

300.

A 78-year-old woman was last seen for her annual pap smear 1 year ago. At that time she was fatigued and had several yeast infections, which she treated with OTC preparations. She continues to be fatigued, has nocturia twice nightly, and has had several yeast infections. She takes no medications and occasionally takes calcium. Her mother died of an MI, her aunt of a stroke, and her uncle was on dialysis due to diabetes before his death due to myocardial infarction. You find BP 146/94; P 84, regular; Wt 187 lbs.; Ht 65.5″. There is no retinopathy, no bruit; she has decreased sensation to fine touch.

FSBG (fasting serum blood glucose) 238 mg%, cholesterol 287 mg%, triglycerides 681 mg%

After receiving these numbers you start her on diet, exercise, and an ACE inhibitor for her hypertension. She returns in 3 months with the following values:

FSBG is 189 mg%, cholesterol 224 mg%, triglycerides 187 mg%, weight 182 lbs., and BP 122/78, having taken your prescription. Her creatinine is 0.7 mg/dL.

At this point, which of the following is the next appropriate treatment?

A. Metformin
B. Rosiglitazone
C. Glyburide
D. NPH insulin
E. Nothing

301.

You are asked to see a 68-year-old woman who became dizzy and fell last week. She reports becoming shaky, sweaty, and slumping to the floor while shopping about 11:30 a.m. She recovered after lying on the floor for several minutes and eating candy. She takes calcium and multivitamins. Past medical history includes a Billroth II for ulcers in 1962, C-section, and penicillin allergy. She had met a friend for breakfast at a donut shop that morning. Her usual breakfast consists of a boiled egg, brown toast and butter, and fruit. She generally eats a late-morning snack, and a meat-containing salad and hard roll for lunch at 1 p.m. She occasionally has similar, milder episodes, but in the past 10 years has had very few such episodes. She runs 3 miles three times weekly, does yoga daily, and works out with free weights twice weekly. She has no cardiac history, and her parents are still alive in their late 80s, as are their siblings. Physical exam reveals BP 116/78 and P 68. Musculature in upper arms and calves is well developed and delineated. Other than well-healed surgical scars on the abdomen, the exam is physiologic.

The above is a prelude to asking you to identify "Whipple's Triad."

Which of the following comprise Whipple's triad?

    A. Low serum glucose, abdominal pathology, and symptom relief with glucose
    B. Symptoms of hypoglycemia, pancreatic lesion, and low serum glucose
    C. Symptoms of hypoglycemia, low serum glucose, and symptom relief with glucose
    D. High serum glucose, symptom relief with insulin, and symptoms of hyperglycemia
    E. Symptoms of hypoglycemia, pancreatic lesion, and high serum glucose

302.

A 69-year-old man tells you he has leg pain just above the knee, which limits his hobby of gardening and prevents him from dancing. The pain has no aggravating or alleviating features. Physical exam finds Heberden nodes and crepitance without effusion or pain on motion in the knees. Neurologic exam is physiologic. His chemistry panel reveals normal liver enzymes and bilirubin, CBC, and calcium. An alkaline phosphatase is 3 times normal.

Which of the following is the most likely diagnosis?

    A. Stress fracture
    B. Osteoarthritis
    C. Iron deficiency anemia
    D. Chondrocalcinosis
    E. Paget disease

303.

A 35-year-old man presents with a slow onset of fatigue, headache, muscle weakness, and paresthesias.
PHYSICAL EXAMINATION:
BP 150/80, P 100, RR 16, Temp 98.6° F

General:	Coarse facial features
HEENT:	Significant for "a large tongue"
	Wide spacing of his teeth
Heart:	RRR without murmurs, rubs, or gallops
Lungs:	CTA
Abdomen:	+BS, soft abdomen, no HSM
Skin:	"Doughy appearance"

Which of the following laboratory values would <u>not</u> support your diagnosis?

    A. Serum prolactin 35 ng/mL (elevated)
    B. Growth hormone concentration 0.2 micrograms/L 1 hour after oral administration of 100 g glucose (normal = suppression below 1 micrograms/L)
    C. Serum glucose 155 mg/dL (elevated)
    D. Elevated insulin-like growth factor (IGF-I)
    E. Elevated IGF binding protein 3

304.

A 35-year-old transcriptionist is referred to you for evaluation. During the past 4 months, she has noted increasing fatigue, weight loss of 12 pounds despite a good appetite, and increased diaphoresis. Recently, she has noticed a tremor in her right hand that makes typing more difficult. Also, she has had severe mood swings and frequently gets angry with herself for outbursts that she makes to other people.

FAMILY HISTORY: Mother with surgery for "overactive" thyroid

PHYSICAL EXAMINATION: Firm, nontender thyroid enlargement about twice normal size
                                              Fine tremor of outstretched arms
                                              Generalized hyperreflexia

LABORATORY:
   Serum Thyroxine: 15.0 micrograms/dL (high)
   Serum T3:   290 ng/dL (high)
   Resin T3 uptake: 40.1% (high)
   TSH: < 0.1 μIU/mL
   Radioactive iodine uptake (RAIU): 24-hour uptake of 2.7% (normal 5–25%)

All of the following are possible diagnoses for this patient <u>except</u>:

   A. Silent thyroiditis
   B. Subacute thyroiditis
   C. Struma ovarii
   D. Graves disease
   E. Excess iodine ingestion

305.

A 21-year-old man is brought into the Emergency Room after being run over by a motorcycle. On routine lab he is found to have a serum calcium of 11.5 mg/dL and a phosphorus of 3.0 mg/dL (normal is 2.5–4.5 mg/dL). He remembers that his mother told him that his sister or brother might have a "high calcium," but that is all he knows.

His examination is normal except for a tire mark on his chest.

LABORATORY:
         Serum intact PTH of 72 pg/mL (normal 10–65 pg/mL)
         1,25-dihydroxyvitamin D of 40 pg/mL (normal 15–60 pg/mL)
         24-hour urinary calcium of 30 mg (normal 100–300 mg/24 hour)

Of the following, what is the appropriate therapy at this time?

   A. Low calcium diet
   B. Bilateral neck exploratory surgery
   C. Do nothing at this point
   D. Oral phosphates
   E. Steroids

306.

A 60-year-old diabetic woman presents to your clinic as a referral from your favorite orthopedist following a wrist fracture in which he found a serum calcium of 10.9 mg/dL. She reports that she has been having "bone pain" in her hips and knees for several years. Looking over her records, you see that she has been on dialysis for 5 years or so.

Which of the following is most likely true?

    A. Hypercalcemia in this setting is usually acute and life-threatening.
    B. The patient likely has tertiary hyperparathyroidism.
    C. Osteitis fibrosa is unlikely.
    D. Aluminum salts are contraindicated.
    E. Parathyroid hormone half-life is decreased.

307.

A 37-year-old female, three months postpartum, presents with tremor, palpitations, and heat intolerance. She is no longer nursing.

On physical exam, she has a BP of 160/60, P 120, and T 99° F. She has an enlarged thyroid on exam.

Lab: TSH: < 0.03 (low), T_4: 20 (high), T_3RU: 40% (high)

Which of the following tests would be most useful in planning therapy?

    A. Radioactive iodine uptake
    B. Thyroid ultrasound
    C. CT scan
    D. Thyroglobulin

308.

A 70-year-old female presents with complaints of constipation and leg and back pain. She had problems with rectal bleeding six months ago and was found to have a polyp on colonoscopy. This was removed, and the site cauterized. At the time of workup, she had a HCT of 27% with an MCV of 78. She was started on $FeSO_4$.

Two months ago, she returned for her annual exam and was found to be in good shape except for complaints of constipation and pruritus. Her cholesterol was 300, and she was started on simvastatin. Today, she has even more problems with constipation than before. Her pruritus continues.

Meds: simvastatin 20 mg qd, $FeSO_4$ 325 mg tid, levothyroxine sodium 0.1 mg qd, ranitidine, psyllium 1 TBS qd, felodipine 10 mg qd.

On exam, VS: BP 120/70; P 55; Chest clear; Abd soft, tympanitic; Skin—xerosis present; Rectal—heme negative; Ext—tenderness over the muscles on palpation.

Which of the following options would best explain her symptoms?

A. Drug interaction between simvastatin and felodipine
B. Colon cancer
C. Rhabdomyolysis due to HMG CoA reductase inhibitor
D. Interaction between levothyroxine sodium and FeSO$_4$
E. Interaction between ranitidine and simvastatin

HEMATOLOGY

309.

Bleeding disorders are a frequently encountered problem on Board exams.

If you find an increased PT, a normal PTT, and a normal platelet count, that would indicate which one of the following types of deficiency or abnormality?

    A. Anti-platelet antibody
    B. Factor X deficiency
    C. Factor XIII deficiency
    D. Factor I deficiency
    E. Warfarin administration

310.

A 30-year-old woman presents with complaints of her gums bleeding and easy bruisability for the past 7 months. She notes that her menses have been heavier than usual during the past few months.

Which of the following is appropriate in the initial workup?

    A. To be cost effective, start with a coagulation factor deficiency workup initially.
    B. CBC with platelet count, PT, PTT, and bleeding time.
    C. CBC with platelet count, PT, PTT, bleeding time, Factor VIII and IX level.
    D. CBC with platelet count, PT, PTT, antiplatelet antibody, Factor VIII level.

311.

Which of the following is associated with the Philadelphia chromosome, t(9,22)?

    A. Acute myelogenous leukemia (AML)
    B. Chronic lymphocytic leukemia (CLL)
    C. Chronic myelogenous leukemia (CML)
    D. Acute lymphocytic leukemia (ALL)
    E. Chronic myelodysplastic syndrome X

312.

A 20-year-old Caucasian woman is referred to you for evaluation of a hemolytic anemia that was diagnosed recently. Her laboratory values now show that she has mildly decreased hemoglobin and hematocrit levels. Her reticulocyte count is elevated, as well as her mean corpuscular hemoglobin concentration (MCHC). Osmotic fragility of the red cells is increased, and red cell survival is shortened. The physical examination reveals that she has splenomegaly. On further questioning, you determine that her grandmother and father both had gallstones at an early age.

Based on your new history findings and the laboratory results, which of the following is the most likely diagnosis?

    A. Hereditary spherocytosis
    B. Sickle cell disease
    C. Glucose-6-phosphate dehydrogenase deficiency
    D. Aplastic anemia
    E. Thalassemia

313.

A 45-year-old man with a history of recurrent fevers and bleeding gums has recently noted an increased tendency toward bruising and has lost 12 lbs unintentionally. He is admitted to the hospital with urosepsis, with *Klebsiella* identified as the organism. Because of other findings, a bone marrow biopsy is done and demonstrates a leukemic infiltrate, and the leukemic cells show resistance to tartrate inhibition. Cytoplasmic projections are noted.

Based on your findings, which of the following is true?

    A. A splenectomy is curative.
    B. Neutropenia is uncommon.
    C. This disease is associated with defects in antibody production only.
    D. A cutaneous vasculitis may also appear in this condition.
    E. The finding of cytoplasmic projections is uncharacteristic for this disorder.

314.

An 82-year-old woman presents to her local ER with complaints of a mass under her tongue. Evaluation reveals it to be a large hematoma, and she is sent home with instructions to use local measures such as ice for treatment. A week later, the mass resolves, but she develops tender swelling in her left thigh with no known trauma to the area.

CBC : WBC 11,300; normal differential; Hgb 10; HCT 30; MCV 78; Plts 202,000
       PT 11.5 secs; PTT 80 secs; fibrinogen 350

The next appropriate studies for this patient's workup would be which of the following?

    A. Lupus anticoagulant and anticardiolipin studies
    B. 1:1 mix of patient and normal to measure the PTT
    C. Repeat CBC
    D. Platelet aggregation studies

315.

A 40-year-old woman with a deep venous thrombosis is started on coumarin and develops skin necrosis.

Which of the following deficiencies should be considered in her?

A. Antithrombin III deficiency
B. Protein C deficiency
C. Factor VIII deficiency
D. Factor XIII deficiency
E. Plasminogen deficiency

316.

A 19-year-old African-American man is being evaluated for a pre-sport physical. His history and physical examination are normal. Laboratory values are listed below.

CBC: WBC 8,000/mm^3 with normal differential
Hemoglobin 16.0 mg/dL
Hematocrit 55%
MCV 71 fL

You order a hemoglobin electrophoresis and it is normal.

Which of the following explains his laboratory findings?

A. Sickle cell trait
B. β-thalassemia trait
C. α-thalassemia trait
D. Sickle β-thalassemia
E. Sickle C disease

317.

A 28-year-old woman with sickle cell anemia has been fairly well during the last few years. She presents today, however, with severe pain in her chest and abdomen. She notes that about a week ago she had an upper respiratory infection but seemed to recover from it without incident. She has had some mild nausea with the pain.

PHYSICAL EXAMINATION:
BP 110/70, P 110, RR 25, Temp 99.2° F
HEENT: PERRLA, EOMI; sclera icteric
TMs clear
Throat clear
Neck: Supple without masses
Heart: RRR with II/VI systolic flow murmur
Lungs: CTA
Abdomen: No hepatosplenomegaly noted; non-tender examination
Extremities: No cyanosis, clubbing, or edema noted

Laboratory evaluation is consistent with accelerated hemolysis. CXR and abdominal x-rays reveal no abnormalities.

The most appropriate initial intervention/procedure at this point is which of the following?

A. Analgesia only at this point
B. Hydroxyurea
C. Exploratory laparotomy
D. Anti-pneumococcal antibiotics
E. Hydration and analgesia

318.

A 30-year-old woman was diagnosed with hyperthyroidism. She was placed on propylthiouracil (PTU) about 4 weeks ago. She presents to you today with painful mouth ulcers. She has not had any other problems, and she notes that her tremor from her hyperthyroidism has resolved.

PHYSICAL EXAMINATION:
>   Vital signs normal
>   HEENT: Mild exophthalmos (no change)
>   PERRLA, EOMI
>   Throat: small oral aphthous-like ulcers on her buccal mucosa
>   Neck: Supple
>   Heart: RRR without murmurs, rubs, or gallops
>   Lungs: CTA
>   Abdomen: No hepatosplenomegaly
>   Extremities: No cyanosis, clubbing, or edema

LABORATORY:
>   WBC 150/µL (10% neutrophils, 80% lymphocytes, 10% monocytes)
>   Rest of CBC (hemoglobin, hematocrit, and platelets) normal

Which of the following should be done next?

A. Stop PTU and schedule a follow-up appointment.
B. Stop PTU and arrange for HLA typing of any available siblings.
C. Stop PTU and start prednisone.
D. Stop PTU and start piperacillin/tazobactam and ciprofloxacin.
E. Continue PTU and start prednisone.

319.

A 21-year-old woman has been healthy her whole life. She presents to the Emergency Room with confusion and fever. Her boyfriend has noted this morning that she appeared to be yellow.

PAST MEDICAL HISTORY: Negative

SOCIAL HISTORY: Works as a waitress in a local pub, the "Flying Dog"
                                              Doesn't smoke or drink alcohol

FAMILY HISTORY: Negative

REVIEW OF SYSTEMS: Faint rash noted by boyfriend

PHYSICAL EXAMINATION:
    BP 100/70, RR 20, Temp 102° F, P 100
    HEENT: PERRLA, EOMI
                Scleral icterus
                TMs clear
                Throat: palatal petechiae
    Neck: Supple
    Heart: RRR without murmurs or rubs
    Lungs: CTA
    Abdomen: Benign
    Extremities: Scattered petechiae on her lower extremities

LABORATORY:
    Hematocrit   28%
    WBC: 13,000/μL with 85% neutrophils
    Platelet count: 11,000/μL
    Total Bilirubin: 6 mg/dL
    Direct Bilirubin: 0.7 mg/dL
    BUN: 70 mg/dL
    Creatinine: 4.8 mg/dL
    PT: 12 secs (normal)
    PTT: 32 secs (normal)
    Peripheral smear: Fragmented red blood cells and nucleated red blood cells

The best initial therapy for this condition is which of the following?

    A. High-dose glucocorticoids
    B. High-dose aspirin therapy
    C. Low-dose aspirin therapy
    D. Plasmapheresis
    E. Splenectomy

320.

A 30-year-old woman presents with severe anemia that has been refractory for almost 4 months. She has required monthly transfusions of 2 units of packed red blood cells during this time period. One week ago she received a transfusion of 2 units of packed red blood cells for a hematocrit of 21%. Two days after receiving the transfusion, her hematocrit was noted to be 27%. However, today (1 week after the transfusion), her hematocrit is again 21%. She has been ill for 2 days with low-grade fever, and her husband has noted that she is jaundiced in appearance.

Which of the following is <u>not</u> correct?

    A. ABO incompatibility is unlikely.
    B. Intravascular hemolysis has likely occurred.
    C. A potential Rh mismatch may have occurred, and therefore the Rh status of donor and recipient should be rechecked.
    D. If the patient is Rh-negative, you need to look for anti-Kell or anti-Duffy antibodies in the patient's serum.
    E. A positive direct Coombs test is likely.

321.

A 40-year-old woman with sickle cell disease presents with profound fatigue and a hematocrit of 18%. She requires transfusions on a frequent basis. Four units of blood are ordered for type and match, but the blood bank calls back and says that it will take at least a day before they can get the packed cells ready for transfusion.

Which of the following is the most likely reason for this problem in providing appropriate blood for this patient?

    A. She has a rare blood group.
    B. She has developed autoantibodies in her serum.
    C. She has developed alloantibodies in her serum.
    D. Careful screening is required in sickle cell patients to prevent blood-borne infection with organisms like *Yersinia*.
    E. She has developed anti-HLA antibodies in her serum.

322.

A 60-year-old woman presents with the diagnosis of pernicious anemia. She has antiparietal-cell antibodies. She is about to be started on therapy for her anemia.

Which of the following is something to be concerned about as therapy begins?

    A. Severe hypokalemia
    B. Severe hypocalcemia
    C. Severe hyperkalemia
    D. Severe hypercalcemia
    E. No reticulocytosis for 3 weeks

323.

A 40-year-old woman is diagnosed with anemia. You are concerned about the possibility of pernicious anemia in her because she has evidence of a megaloblastic anemia on her peripheral smear.

Which of the following is true concerning pernicious anemia?

A. Antiparietal-cell antibodies are found in fewer than 50% of persons with pernicious anemia.
B. Folate in large doses can correct the megaloblastic anemia, and it does correct the neurologic abnormalities.
C. Folate in large doses cannot correct megaloblastic anemia.
D. Folate in large doses can correct the megaloblastic anemia, but it does not correct the neurologic abnormalities.
E. Gastrin levels are usually decreased in patients with pernicious anemia.

324.

A 40-year-old woman presents with a long history of rheumatoid arthritis. She is being evaluated for anemia and is diagnosed as most likely having "anemia of chronic disease."

Which of the following is a likely mechanism that may cause this type of anemia?

A. Iron deficiency of the bone marrow
B. Defective porphyrin synthesis
C. Hemolysis
D. Lengthening of red cell lifespan, resulting in impaired feedback loop
E. Abnormalities of iron metabolism with trapping of iron in macrophages

325.

An 18-year-old woman with AIDS presents with hemolysis after taking dapsone for her *Pneumocystis* prophylaxis. She is fine now and is on pentamidine mist therapy.

Which of the following is true about glucose-6-phosphate dehydrogenase (G6PD) deficiency?

A. The Mediterranean variant is less severe than that occurring in African-American patients.
B. It is autosomally transmitted.
C. Hemolysis is commonly induced by infection.
D. G6PD levels are usually increased in older red cells.
E. Heinz bodies are seen on Wright staining of peripheral smears.

326.

A 45-year-old woman presents with a pure red blood cell aplasia with normal white cell and platelet production. Various studies are done in her workup.

Which of the following would you expect?

    A. A reticulocyte count greater than 3%
    B. Normochromic, normocytic red blood cells
    C. Decreased serum erythropoietin levels
    D. Ferrokinetic studies to show increased iron turnover
    E. A bone marrow examination to show marked hypocellularity

327.

A 25-year-old woman has had severe menorrhagia and is referred to you by her gynecologist. She reports that she has had difficulty with this as long as she can remember and frequently has to go on iron supplements for treatment of iron deficiency anemia. She is on no medications.

PAST MEDICAL HISTORY: Essentially negative

FAMILY HISTORY: Sister with similar bleeding tendencies; bleeds easily after minor trauma

SOCIAL HISTORY: Doesn't smoke or drink
                            Works as a gas station attendant

Physical examination is unremarkable.

LABORATORY:
        Platelet count 300,000/μL
        PT: 24 seconds (control 12 seconds)
        PTT: 27 seconds (control 29 seconds)

Based on her findings, which of the following laboratory tests should you order now?

    A. Check an α_2-antiplasmin level.
    B. Check Factor VIII level.
    C. Screen for coagulation factor inhibitors.
    D. Check Factor VII level.

328.

Here is another "simple knowledge" question to give you a break from the long tedious questions. (Aren't you sighing in relief at this point?)

Which of the following types of patients is <u>least</u> likely to have thrombocytosis?

A. Iron-deficiency anemia
B. Polycythemia vera
C. Acute bacterial infection
D. Hemolytic uremic syndrome
E. Sickle cell pain crisis

329.

A 20-year-old woman is referred to you by her dentist. Today she underwent dental extraction, and the dentist had difficulty controlling the bleeding. Family history is significant for a few family members with increased tendency for bleeding, including male and female relatives.

LABORATORY:
Platelet count is 358,000/μL
Factor VIII coagulant activity is 56% normal
von Willebrand factor (vWF) antigen is 47% normal
Ristocetin cofactor is 14% normal
A normal spectrum of vWF multimers in the patient's plasma on SDS-agarose electrophoresis is found

Which of the following drugs should she avoid?

A. Prednisone
B. Acetaminophen
C. Aspirin
D. Ranitidine
E. Itraconazole

330.

Which of the following conditions will give you an elevated PTT and a normal PT, but no clinical bleeding disorder?

A. Factor XII deficiency
B. Platelet deficiency
C. von Willebrand disease
D. Factor VII deficiency
E. Glanzmann thrombasthenia

331.

Which of the following is true in Bernard-Soulier Syndrome (Giant Platelet)?

A. Patients have an extremely high platelet count.
B. Patients lack glycoprotein IIB-IIIa complex.
C. Patients have increased platelet adhesion.
D. Patients lack glycoprotein 1b.
E. It is an X-linked congenital disease (only males are affected).

332.

An 18-year-old woman with a severe bleeding disorder has recently been diagnosed with Glanzmann thrombasthenia.

Which of the following is true about her disease?

A. It is due to the inability to bind to von Willebrand factor.
B. It is due to a deficiency of glycoprotein IIb-IIIa complex.
C. It is an autosomal dominant disease.
D. Platelet counts are usually below 20,000/μL.
E. Fibrinogen can cross-connect in this disease.

333.

A 30-year-old African-American woman with a history of menorrhagia and dysmenorrhea presents to you with the chief complaint of fatigue. She says that she "wears out" halfway through the day and needs to take a nap frequently when she gets home from work as a personal trainer.

PHYSICAL EXAMINATION:
    Skin: Pallor
    HEENT: Cheilosis
    Extremities: Spoon nails
    Heart: Tachycardic with any type of activity.

Which of the following is the most likely diagnosis?

A. Myelodysplastic syndrome
B. Occult GI bleed
C. Colon carcinoma
D. Ovarian carcinoma
E. Iron deficiency anemia

334.

A 25-year-old African-American woman with a history of menorrhagia and dysmenorrhea presents to you with the chief complaint of fatigue. She says that she "wears out" halfway through the day and needs to take a nap frequently when she gets home from work as a personal trainer.

LABORATORY:

Hemoglobin:	10.5 mg/dL
MCV:	69
Peripheral smear:	Microcytosis

Which of the following is <u>not</u> a likely diagnosis?

A. Iron deficiency anemia
B. Anemia of chronic disease
C. Myelodysplastic syndrome
D. Thalassemia
E. Sideroblastic anemia

335.

A 65-year-old man presents to your office complaining of fatigue. He has had exertional dyspnea for 3 months, but has not had any chest discomfort during this time period. His wife cooks 3 meals a day for him, and he has "a good steak" on a weekly basis.

PAST MEDICAL HISTORY: HTN x 30 years
Currently on hydrochlorothiazide

SOCIAL HISTORY: Smoking: 1 pack/day for 30 years
Alcohol: 1–2 six-packs of beer daily

PHYSICAL EXAMINATION:

Vitals:	BP 180/70, HR 100, Temp 98.5° F, RR 15
HEENT:	Anicteric sclera
	PERRLA
	Conjunctiva are very pale
	No cheilosis.
Heart:	RRR with II/VI systolic murmur heard in the past without change
Lungs:	Coarse wheezing
Abdomen:	Liver palpable and non-tender
	Spleen tip not palpated
Extremities:	Mild clubbing noted of fingers

LABORATORY:

WBC:	4,000/µL
Hematocrit:	27%
Platelets:	99,000/µL
MCV:	109
Reticulocyte count:	0.8%
Peripheral smear:	Shows targeting of large red cells without a leukoerythroblastic picture

AST:	70
ALT:	50
LDL:	Normal

Which of the following is the most likely etiology for his anemia?

A. Dietary vitamin B_{12} deficiency
B. Myelodysplastic syndrome
C. Hemolysis
D. Iron deficiency anemia
E. Alcoholism

336.

A 65-year-old man presents with fatigue. He is rather stoic and denies any other symptoms. He is "dragged in" by his wife.

PAST MEDICAL HISTORY: Negative

SOCIAL HISTORY: Retired from the Air Force

PHYSICAL EXAMINATION (pertinent findings only):
General: Splenomegaly noted

LABORATORY:
WBC: 2800/μL
Hematocrit: 30%
Platelets: 100,000/μL
Red cell: Morphology normal; 12% monocytes, 14% granulocytes, 74% lymphocytes

A bone marrow aspirate and biopsy are done. "The aspirate is **dry**." The biopsy is pending.

Which of the following is the most likely diagnosis for this man?

A. Chronic myeloid leukemia
B. Chronic lymphocytic leukemia
C. Hairy cell leukemia
D. Multiple myeloma
E. Myelofibrosis

337.

A 45-year-old man, with a history of an enlarged liver and elevated hematocrit without apparent cause, had been well until earlier today, when he developed sudden onset of pain in his right upper quadrant.

PHYSICAL EXAMINATION:
General: Afebrile
Vitals: BP 140/90, P 100, RR 18
HEENT: WNL
Heart: RRR without murmurs, rubs, or gallops

Lungs:	CTA
Abdomen:	Markedly enlarged liver that is very tender on its edge
	Enlarged spleen
	Abdominal fluid wave

LABORATORY:

CBC:	Pending: but he has known hemoglobins in the 17–18 mg/dL range
AST:	80
ALT:	70

Which of the following procedures should you consider next?

A. Hepatic venography or magnetic resonance (MR) venography
B. Paracentesis
C. Ultrasound without Dopplers
D. Radionucleotide liver-spleen scan

338.

A 15-year-old refugee from Iran bleeds significantly after an inguinal hernia repair. The patient has no siblings, and there is no family history of bleeding problems.

LABORATORY:

Platelet count:	Normal
Bleeding time:	Normal
PT:	Normal
PTT:	Normal

Which of the following is the most likely diagnosis?

A. Protein S deficiency
B. Factor XII deficiency
C. Thrombasthenia
D. Factor XIII deficiency
E. Prekallikrein deficiency

339.

You are seeing a patient who has protein C deficiency. She is doing well and asks about future generations and other general questions about Protein C deficiency.

Which of the following is <u>not</u> true about Protein C deficiency?

A. It is autosomal dominant in inheritance.
B. Normal levels of protein C rules out the disease.
C. Spontaneous thrombosis may occur in the absence of thrombotic risk factors.
D. The most common sites of thrombosis include the lower extremity deep veins, iliofemoral veins, and mesenteric veins.
E. It can be acquired as well as inherited.

340.

A 70-year-old woman with a history of primary biliary cirrhosis develops a deep vein thrombosis in her left common femoral vein. She is started on warfarin 10 mg daily. On the 3rd day of treatment she develops a tender purpuric lesion on her right breast. It is quite large, measuring 3 x 4 cm. She is afebrile, and her INR is 2.6.

Which of the following would <u>not</u> be given as a treatment?

    A. Fresh frozen plasma
    B. Vitamin K
    C. IV heparin
    D. Protein C concentrate
    E. Protamine sulfate

341.

A 53-year-old man with Zollinger-Ellison syndrome presents with a 3-month history of anemia. Physical exam is unremarkable. He painted his house 2 years ago. He denies alcohol use except at holidays.

CURRENT MEDICATIONS:
    Hydrochlorothiazide
    Sildenafil
    Sertraline
    Omeprazole
    Diphenhydramine

LABORATORY:
    Hb: 10
    HCT: 30
    MCV: 114
    WBC: 3.6

Which of the following is the most likely cause for his anemia?

    A. Lead toxicity because of paint exposure
    B. Alcohol
    C. Folate deficiency due to sildenafil use
    D. B$_{12}$ deficiency due to omeprazole use
    E. Sideroblastic anemia

ONCOLOGY

342.

A 40-year-old woman is the recipient of an HLA-matched allogenic bone marrow transplant in the treatment of her metastatic breast carcinoma. She has been severely granulocytopenic for over 2 weeks following the transplant. She is on multiple agents, including G-CSF, cyclosporin A and corticosteroids. Currently she is on prophylactic acyclovir and trimethoprim-sulfamethoxazole. In the last few hours, she has developed cough, tachypnea and has fever to 102°. Her central venous catheter site is slightly erythematous.

Which of the following is the correct treatment course?

    A. Remove the central venous catheter and start empiric broad-spectrum antibiotics as well as either liposomal amphotericin B or caspofungin.
    B. Remove the central venous catheter and start either liposomal amphotericin B or caspofungin only.
    C. Do not remove the central venous catheter and await cultures.
    D. Start either liposomal amphotericin B or caspofungin only through the catheter.
    E. Remove the central venous catheter and start IV caspofungin and IV trimethoprim-sulfamethoxazole for presumed *Pneumocystis*.

343.

A 48-year-old man comes in for a routine physical examination. You do a thorough exam and find only a pigmented lesion present on his left calf. He states that the lesion has been present as long as he can remember, probably since he was born. The lesion does not itch or bleed. He has noted, however, that the color has changed a little and is no longer as homogeneous as it has been.

Which of the following statements is true?

    A. One of the first signs of malignancy is bleeding.
    B. Change in the color of the lesion warrants further workup for potential malignancy.
    C. One of the first signs of malignancy is tenderness.
    D. Early diagnosis of this lesion would not affect prognosis.
    E. It is unlikely that the lesion, if it really has been present since birth, would be malignant.

344.

A 60-year-old man with a history of chronic alcoholism and chronic tobacco use (2-3 packs a day for 40 years) presents as a referral from the ER with a new neck mass. He states that the mass is nontender and he just noticed it last week.

PHYSICAL EXAMINATION:
    Vitals: BP 110/70, P 90, RR 18, Temp 99°
    HEENT: PERRLA, EOMI
    TM: Clear
    Throat: Clear without lesions

Neck:	3.4 cm left mid-cervical neck mass
	Mass is firm and nontender to palpation
	No fluctuance is noted
Heart:	RRR without murmurs, rubs, or gallops
Lungs:	Coarse breath sounds with few scattered wheezes
Abdomen:	Liver span 10 cm, slightly tender
Extremities:	No cyanosis, clubbing, or edema noted
Neuro:	Grossly intact

An excisional biopsy is done of the neck mass and shows squamous cell carcinoma.

Which of the following is the most appropriate workup at this time?

A. CT of the neck alone
B. CT of the brain alone
C. Neck dissection followed by radiation therapy
D. Endoscopic visualization of the nasopharynx and larynx, and integrated PET-CT scan
E. Proceed directly to chemotherapy

345.

OK. The Boards sometimes like to ask simple, short, pithy questions. It is rare, but be ready for them. Here is one for you to chew on.

Which of the following hereditary disorders is <u>not</u> associated with the development of malignancies?

A. Cystic fibrosis
B. Fanconi's anemia
C. Familial polyposis coli
D. Ataxia-telangiectasia
E. Neurofibromatosis

346.

A 50-year-old man will be starting chemotherapy for leukemia. He has been researching chemotherapeutic agents on the Internet and comes in today with lots of questions about his findings.

Which of the following statements regarding toxic effects of chemotherapy is <u>not</u> correct?

A. Vincristine can be administered during periods of low blood cell counts.
B. Cisplatin induces nausea and frequent vomiting, but it can usually be controlled with metoclopramide or dexamethasone or both.
C. Anthracycline agents suppress bone marrow stem cells to a greater degree than they do more "committed" hematopoietic cells.
D. Cisplatin may produce hypocalcemia.
E. Use of melphalan has been associated with secondary leukemias.

347.

A 66-year-old man diagnosed with poorly differentiated adenocarcinoma of the prostate 3 years ago presents with complaints of severe pain in his left hip. Staging at that time revealed no evidence of extraprostatic spread. He underwent radiation therapy, without surgery, because he did not want to lose his ability to have sex. Until recently, he has done well. Physical examination shows marked pain with passive and active movement of the hip joint. No other abnormalities are found on physical examination.

LABORATORY:

Prostate specific antigen:	Elevated
Bone scan:	New areas of uptake in the pelvis and ribs

Today he again says he would like to forego an orchiectomy if possible. He is willing to change his mind, he says, if it will significantly improve his quality of life or chance for survival.

Which of the following is the most appropriate therapy?

A. Biopsy one of the bony lesions first before making any decisions.
B. Perform an orchiectomy since it will improve survival.
C. Administer cisplatin.
D. Perform an orchiectomy and administer cisplatin since the combination will improve survival.
E. Administer leuprolide.

348.

A 55-year-old woman presents with fatigue as her chief complaint. She really has not been ill but notes that she can't seem to get through the day without a nap. Additionally, she reports that she cannot walk as far as she used to in her neighborhood mall-walking program. Her physical examination is essentially normal without any focal findings.

LABORATORY:

WBC 3,800/μL with a normal differential
Hematocrit is 28%
Platelet count is 185,000/μL
Reticulocyte count is only 1.2%
Occult blood on her stool is hemoccult negative x 3
Ferritin and iron studies are normal
Peripheral blood smear does not reveal any abnormalities

A bone marrow is done and shows infiltration with plasma cells, which account for nearly 35% of the total nucleated cells.

Which of the following tests is <u>not</u> useful in this disease process?

A. β_2-microglobulin
B. Bone scan to show increased uptake
C. 24-hour urine protein
D. Serum protein electrophoresis
E. Skeletal survey

349.

A 37-year-old woman presents with hirsutism and a deepening voice noted by her husband. Pelvic examination is done and shows clitorimegaly and a right ovarian mass.

Based on this limited information, which of the following is the most likely diagnosis?

    A. Ovarian cancer of epithelial cell lineage
    B. Ovarian cancer of germ cell lineage
    C. Soft tissue sarcoma
    D. Carcinoid tumor
    E. Lymphoma

350.

A 66-year-old man presents with cervical adenopathy. He reports that recently he has had "bed-soaking" night sweats. Further workup using computed tomography shows that he has a large mediastinal mass as well as abdominal periaortic adenopathy. He undergoes bone marrow biopsies that fail to show tumor. Cervical lymph node biopsy indicates infiltration with moderately immature-appearing lymphoid cells. You send off immunophenotypic studies on the node biopsy, and this shows expression of the following antigens: CD19, CD20, and CD5. Immunochemistry shows involvement of cyclin D_1. Cytogenetic studies show a t(11;14) translocation. Interestingly enough, his CBC is normal.

Based on these findings, which of the following is the most likely diagnosis?

    A. Hairy cell leukemia
    B. Acute lymphoblastic leukemia
    C. Acute myeloblastic leukemia
    D. Diffuse large cell lymphoma
    E. Mantle cell lymphoma (a type of mature-B cell non-Hodgkin lymphoma)

351.

A 60-year-old man presents with stable chronic myeloid leukemia and has been managed effectively with α-interferon for 3 years. Today he presents with his laboratory showing an increased left shift in his white blood cell differential. A bone marrow is done today and shows a hypercellular marrow with increased numbers of basophils. Cytogenetic analysis reveals now there are two Philadelphia chromosomes per cell (previously he had only one).

Which of the following is the most likely explanation for the cytogenetic analysis change?

    A. He has entered an accelerated or blastic phase.
    B. This is an interferon effect.
    C. He was misdiagnosed and actually has agnogenic myeloid myelofibrosis.
    D. Laboratory error.
    E. He has been exposed to ionizing radiation.

352.

A 25-year-old male presents with painless swelling of his scrotum for 2 months. The swelling is worsening and has begun to worry him. He is otherwise healthy. His physical exam confirms scrotal swelling with testicular enlargement.

Which of the following should the initial workup include?

A. MRI of the head
B. CT of the abdomen
C. Ultrasound of the testicle
D. Laparoscopic removal of the testicle

353.

An 18-year-old man is diagnosed with Hodgkin disease stage 1B. He receives mantle radiation only without chemotherapy.

Which of the following is a possible complication of his mantle radiation therapy?

A. Upper extremity paresthesia
B. Testicular carcinoma
C. Increased incidence of AML
D. Early onset coronary artery disease
E. Hyperthyroidism

354.

A 26-year-old female is back in your office after the return of her pap screening. It showed a low-grade squamous intraepithelial lesion. No inflammation was present. She was found to be HIV negative; a pap smear 2 years previously was negative.

Which of the following is the most appropriate next step in her treatment?

A. Colposcopy
B. Conization
C. Cryo or laser therapy
D. Return (4 to 6 months) for repeat pap smear
E. Hysterectomy

355.

A 75-year-old woman presents to your clinic complaining that yesterday her urine smelled very unusual. She is found on pelvic exam to have a firm, enlarged right ovary. Subsequent workup reveals she is BRCA1 positive and has an elevated CA-125 level, but the alpha-fetoprotein and HCG are normal. Transvaginal ultrasound finds the right ovary to be about twice its expected volume.

At this point, which of the following is the most likely diagnosis?

A. Choriocarcinoma
B. Serous or mucinous epithelial cancer
C. Germ cell carcinoma
D. Clear cell carcinoma
E. Metastasized clear cell carcinoma

356.

Your next patient is a 30-year-old woman who presents for a pre-employment physical examination. She is ordinarily in good health and takes no medications. Family history reveals that her mother was treated for breast cancer 10 years ago at age 40. The physical exam is negative except for a subtle but suspicious breast density. The laboratory exam was unremarkable. Mammography reveals a small suspicious lesion that corresponds to the palpated mass. Ultrasound is indeterminate. A radiography-guided core needle biopsy finds invasive ductal carcinoma! At surgery a small, approximately 1/2 cm tumor is removed that is estrogen-receptor and progesterone-receptor positive. In addition, a single positive lower axillary node is found.

Which of the following is the most appropriate course of therapy following this lumpectomy?

A. Radiotherapy & chemotherapy
B. Radiotherapy & chemotherapy & tamoxifen
C. Radiotherapy, no other adjuvant therapy
D. Chemotherapy & tamoxifen
E. Tamoxifen only

357.

A 21-year-old college student presents to your office for a physical exam for participation in varsity football. He is a smoker, social drinker, on no medications, and has been in good health. His family history is negative. The review of systems is negative except for a lump in his scrotum that he has noticed for over a month. He thinks it has been getting larger. There is no pain, and there has been no penile discharge or dysuria. Physical exam is unremarkable except for an indurated mass almost a centimeter in diameter on the left testis. Inguinal nodes palpate "normal" bilaterally. Laboratory exam is unremarkable, including LDH, liver enzymes, AFP, and β-hCG.

Which of the following is the most likely diagnosis of this mass?

A. Nonseminoma
B. Seminoma
C. Sertoli cell cancer
D. Testicular torsion
E. Hydrocele

358.

A 45-year-old woman presents with findings of acute leukemia. A complete workup is done as well as physical examination. She has anemia, granulocytopenia, and thrombocytopenia.

If splenomegaly is found, which of these is the <u>least</u> likely diagnosis?

  A. Acute myelogenous leukemia (AML)
  B. Chronic myelogenous leukemia (CML)
  C. Hodgkin disease
  D. Hairy cell leukemia
  E. Myelofibrosis

359.

A 50-year-old woman presents with acute leukemia. A bone marrow is done and shows that she has decreased normal elements but overall hypercellularity due to leukemic blasts. She has pancytopenia on peripheral smear. It is noted that she does not have any significant palpable lymphadenopathy or splenomegaly.

Which of the following is the most likely diagnosis?

  A. Acute lymphoblastic leukemia (ALL)
  B. Acute myelogenous leukemia (AML)
  C. Hodgkin Disease
  D. Hairy cell leukemia
  E. AIDS-induced leukemia

360.

A 30-year-old woman presents with a history of fatigue and pallor noted by her family. She has had low-grade fevers of 99° to 100° for the past several weeks. She has noted easy bruisability and bleeding gums when she brushes her teeth.

PAST MEDICAL HISTORY:	Negative; had 2 normal deliveries 5 and 7 years ago Pap smear done 2 years ago was normal Breast exams done monthly reveal no masses
SOCIAL HISTORY:	Doesn't smoke or drink alcohol Attends physician assistant (PA) school Lives at home with husband (carpenter) and 2 children ages 7, 5
FAMILY HISTORY:	Mother alive and healthy; HTN Father alive and healthy; HTN Maternal aunt with breast cancer at age 45
REVIEW OF SYSTEMS:	Increased fatigue over the past 2 weeks Can't walk up 2 flights of stairs without stopping to catch her breath Nicked herself shaving last week, and it took 20 minutes to stop the bleeding

PHYSICAL EXAMINATION:
>   Bruises noted over her calves and thighs
>   Few petechia on her hard palate as well as her pre-tibial areas and arms where blood pressure cuff was located
>   Bleeding gums noted
>   Severe gingival hyperplasia
>   No splenomegaly

LABORATORY:
>   Peripheral smear: Pancytopenia without blast forms seen

Which of the following is the most likely etiology for her condition?

>   A. Acute lymphocytic leukemia
>   B. Acute myelogenous leukemia
>   C. Acute erythroleukemia
>   D. Endocarditis
>   E. Jean-Luke Picard syndrome

361.

A 16-year-old male with newly diagnosed ALL (acute lymphocytic leukemia) is going to undergo standard chemotherapy with prednisone, vincristine, and daunorubicin/doxorubicin.

With regards to vincristine, which of the following toxicities should you be most concerned about?

>   A. Cardiac toxicity
>   B. Glaucoma
>   C. Interstitial lung fibrosis
>   D. Neurotoxicity
>   E. Spastic colon

362.

You are presented a man with pancytopenia and prominent splenomegaly. You are concerned about the possibility of hairy cell leukemia because you note one lymphocyte with "cytoplasmic projections."

Which of the following is true concerning hairy cell leukemia?

>   A. Bone marrow aspirate will likely be quite useful in showing cells.
>   B. Bone marrow biopsy will likely show many cells.
>   C. On immunophenotyping, CD11c marker is likely to be present.
>   D. 2-chlorodeocyadenosine (2-CdA) is unlikely to produce complete remission in most patients.
>   E. Hairy cell leukemia is a T-cell malignancy.

363.

An 18-year-old male with confirmed Hodgkin lymphoma by lymph node biopsy of a left axillary node presents for evaluation. Staging is initiated and includes a complete history and physical examination, chest X-ray, CT of his chest and abdomen, and a bone marrow aspiration and biopsy.

Complete history and physical reveal just the left sided axillary node and occasional night sweats.

Chest x-ray: Normal; no masses
CT of chest and abdomen: Significant nodes in the retroperitoneal space near the splenic flexure
PET scans confirm CT findings

Based on these findings, which of the following should you do next?

A. Perform laparotomy and do splenectomy; then proceed with combination chemotherapy if nodes positive.
B. Proceed with radiation therapy only.
C. Perform laparotomy with splenectomy; proceed with radiation therapy.
D. Proceed with combination chemotherapy without laparotomy.
E. Do lymphangiogram of lower extremities; if negative then just do radiation therapy.

364.

A 60-year-old man is diagnosed with non-Hodgkin lymphoma. Testing confirms that he has follicular lymphoma.

Non-Hodgkin lymphoma is typically which of the following?

A. > 75% are B-cell lymphomas.
B. > 75% are T-cell lymphomas.
C. About 50% are T-cell and 50% are B-cell lymphomas.
D. Follicular lymphomas are typically very aggressive.
E. Burkitt lymphoma is seen in Africa and associated with human herpes virus 6 infection.

365.

A 50-year-old man presents for workup of worsening renal failure and fatigue. It is noted that he has lytic punched out lesions of his femur and pelvis on plain films. A bone marrow aspirate and biopsy shows plasmacytosis > 10%. Urine and serum monoclonal proteins are ordered. Rouleaux formation is seen on the peripheral blood smear.

Which of the following would a bone scan in this patient be expected to show?

A. The bone scan would be consistent with infection because these patients have increased rates of infection due to abnormal functioning immunoglobulins.
B. The bone scan would show "hot" spots consistent with new bone formation.
C. Bone scan is contraindicated in these patients because of renal failure.
D. A bone scan is contraindicated because of the presence of Rouleaux formation.
E. The lytic lesions on plain films would **not** "light up" on the bone scan.

366.

A 50-year-old woman with breast cancer presents with confusion. You determine that her calcium level is 11 mg/dL with an albumin of 2.5 mg/dL. Besides confusion, no other abnormalities are found, and her ECG is currently unremarkable.

Which of the following should be done initially to manage her hypercalcemia?

A. Water restriction followed by zoledronic acid
B. Vigorous hydration with normal saline with hydrochlorothiazide to maintain urine output at 100–150 cc/hour followed by zoledronic acid
C. Vigorous hydration with normal saline to maintain urine output at 100–150 cc/hour followed by zoledronic acid
D. Zoledronic acid alone
E. Vigorous hydration with 1/4 normal saline with furosemide to maintain urine output at 100–150 cc/hour followed by zoledronic acid

367.

A 21-year-old woman presents for routine physical examination. You discuss safe sex practices and learn that she has been sexually active for 3 years and rarely uses condoms. She notes that she has had "growths" in her genital area for the last year or so. She denies fever, chills, weight loss, or other constitutional symptoms.

PAST MEDICAL HISTORY:	Negative
	Immunizations: due for Tdap booster
FAMILY HISTORY:	Mother with breast cancer at age 50
	Father with HTN and alcoholism
	Sister age 15, healthy
SOCIAL HISTORY:	Works as a bartender while attending college—dream is to be an accountant
REVIEW OF SYSTEMS:	Negative
PHYSICAL EXAMINATION:	Essentially normal except for genital warts

Which of the following increases her risk for cervical carcinoma?

A. If the genital warts are due to human papillomavirus type 19 or 21
B. If the genital warts are due to human papillomavirus type 16 or 18
C. If the genital warts are due to human herpes virus
D. If the genital warts are due to *Treponema pallidum*
E. If the genital warts are due to varicella zoster

368.

A 54-year-old woman with history of rectal bleeding was found to have adenocarcinoma 3 cm below the peritoneal reflection. She had a full metastatic workup that was negative for other disease. She had resection of her tumor with primary reanastomosis. Pathology report showed a well-differentiated adenocarcinoma of the rectum with 3 of 10 adjacent lymph nodes positive for carcinoma. She has had no other medical problems except for mild hypertension.

Which of the following therapies is the most appropriate next step?

A. Pelvic irradiation alone
B. Chemotherapy alone
C. Combination of pelvic irradiation and chemotherapy
D. Observation
E. Pelvic and mantle irradiation

369.

A 60-year-old man is newly diagnosed with prostate carcinoma. He underwent transrectal ultrasonography with a needle biopsy showing adenocarcinoma. He is asymptomatic, and this was only found after an elevated PSA (20 ng/dL) was discovered.

Which of the following would be the first test to order in staging for his prostate cancer?

A. Full body plain film x-rays
B. Bone scan
C. CT of head
D. CEA level
E. Repeat PSA now

370.

A 25-year-old Caucasian male comes in for a routine physical examination for work. He is healthy and reports no medical problems.

SOCIAL HISTORY: Doesn't smoke
                    Drinks 2 beers on the weekends
                    Lives with boyfriend

PHYSICAL EXAMINATION:
        HEENT: PERRLA, EOMI
        TM: Clear
        Throat: Clear
        Heart: RRR without murmurs, rubs, or gallops
        Lungs: CTA
        Abdomen: + Bowel sounds, no hepatosplenomegaly
        Extremities: No cyanosis, clubbing, or edema
        GU: Tanner V male;
                     Solid firm mass in left testicle

He is found to have a seminoma with Stage I. He undergoes orchiectomy and completes radiation therapy without complications.

Which of the following is his expected cure rate?

    A. 95%
    B. 50%
    C. Not enough information to ascertain
    D. 35%
    E. 10%

371.

A 50-year-old post-menopausal woman is diagnosed with breast cancer. She has a 5 cm primary lesion, is node-negative, and is hormone receptor positive (HR+).

Which of the following is/are the best treatment regimens for her?

    A. Lumpectomy and radiation therapy
    B. Modified radical mastectomy and chemotherapy but not tamoxifen
    C. Modified radical mastectomy alone
    D. Modified radical mastectomy and tamoxifen for 5 years
    E. Modified radical mastectomy with chemotherapy and tamoxifen

372.

A 35-year-old woman is diagnosed with breast cancer. She has a 5 cm primary, is node-negative, and is hormone receptor positive (HR+).

Which of the following is/are the best treatment regimens for her?

    A. Modified radical mastectomy and tamoxifen for 5 years
    B. Modified radical mastectomy with chemotherapy and tamoxifen for 5 years
    C. Lumpectomy and radiation therapy
    D. Modified radical mastectomy and chemotherapy but not tamoxifen
    E. Modified radical mastectomy alone

373.

A 28-year-old woman is recently diagnosed with ovarian carcinoma. She is doing well and has finished all of her chemotherapy. She took birth control pills and wonders if they are a risk and also knows that her sisters are on birth control pills.

She asks you what risk factors are associated with her cancer, because she is concerned for her sisters as well as her nieces.

Which of the following is <u>not</u> associated with increased risk of ovarian cancer?

A. Positive family history
B. Nulliparity
C. BRCA1 positivity
D. BRCA2 positivity
E. Oral contraceptive use

374.

A 70-year-old male smoker presents with severe back pain and pain in the pelvic girdle. X-ray shows osteoporosis of the spine.

LABORATORY:
WBC:	6,000/μL
HCT:	26
Calcium:	12
Bone scan:	Negative

Which of the following is the most likely diagnosis?

A. Multiple myeloma
B. Metastatic prostate cancer
C. Prolonged corticosteroid use
D. Metastatic lung cancer
E. Avascular necrosis

375.

A 44-year-old woman had a biopsy of an enlarged left axillary lymph node that revealed a metastatic adenocarcinoma. Physical examination of her breasts was unremarkable, and a mammogram was normal.

Which of the following is the most likely diagnosis?

A. Breast cancer
B. Lung cancer
C. Gastric carcinoma
D. Colon carcinoma

376.

Six months ago a 40-year-old male presented with gynecomastia that had developed during the preceding two months. A chest x-ray revealed a right upper lobe lung mass, and he underwent a biopsy and subsequent lobectomy, which revealed a large cell poorly-differentiated carcinoma. He now presents with recurrent multiple pulmonary masses and complains of an enlarged testis.

Which of the following is his most likely original diagnosis?

A. Large cell carcinoma of the lung
B. Metastatic germ cell tumor of the testis
C. Anaplastic large cell lymphoma
D. Anaplastic colon carcinoma

377.

Which of the following drugs is <u>not</u> associated with peripheral neuropathy?

A. Paclitaxel (Taxol®)
B. Cisplatin
C. Vincristine
D. Vinorelbine (Navelbine®)
E. Doxorubicin (Adriamycin®, Doxil®)

378.

Retinoids reduce the risk of which of the following?

A. Ovarian cancer
B. Colon cancer
C. Head and neck cancer
D. Breast cancer

379.

Which of the following is most commonly associated with SIADH?

A. Squamous cell carcinoma of the lung
B. Ovarian epithelial carcinoma
C. Non-seminoma germ cell tumor of testis
D. Small cell lung cancer

380.

Which of the following shows reduced risk with the use of oral contraceptives?

A. Ovarian cancer
B. Colon cancer
C. Breast cancer
D. Head and neck cancer

NEUROLOGY

381.

A 46-year-old man develops a severe headache this morning while working at his car dealership. He also has nausea and has had one episode of emesis. He has shoulder and neck stiffness that developed today. He denies any history of migraine headaches or any similar headaches.

Which of the following diagnostic tests should be ordered next?

A. CT scan without contrast
B. MRI scan
C. CT scan with contrast
D. Lumbar puncture
E. None of the choices is correct

382.

A 22-year-old woman presents for evaluation of headaches. She has had headaches for the past 6 months, occurring 4–5 times a month. The headaches are of great intensity, involving the right side of her head with the maximum intensity of pain occurring behind her right eye. Symptoms worsen with exertion. Headaches last 3–6 hours, are sometimes associated with nausea, and on 2 occasions have been preceded by a scotoma in the right eye. Neurologic exam is unremarkable.

Which of the following tests would you recommend next?

A. CT scan without contrast
B. CT scan with contrast
C. MRI
D. MRA
E. No imaging

383.

A 31-year-old female presents with numbness in her left arm and some left leg weakness. She had an episode similar to this 9 months ago, which resolved spontaneously. Exam shows subjective difference in light touch and slight motor weakness in the left leg.

Which one of the following tests would you order?

A. CT without contrast
B. Head CT with contrast
C. MRI of spinal cord
D. Head MRI
E. Nerve conduction studies of left arm

384.

A 27-year-old male with history of IDDM and seizure disorder presents with a 3-week history of fatigue, low-grade fevers, and diffuse lymphadenopathy.

Exam is remarkable for diffuse lymphadenopathy (cervical, axilla, inguinal; nodes 2–3 cm in each area), tender liver, and fever of 101°.

Meds: Phenobarbital, phenytoin, cisapride, and nortriptyline.

Labs – WBC 9.9, HCT 38, SGOT 90, SGPT 78, BUN 20, Cr 1.1, Glu 236, RPR negative.

Which of the following diagnoses is most likely?

    A. Hodgkin disease
    B. Syphilis
    C. Hepatitis B
    D. Tularemia
    E. Reaction to phenytoin

385.

An 80-year-old man presents to the ER following a seizure. He has a history of hypertension and chronic neck pain.

Medications include: Amitriptyline, hydrochlorothiazide, tramadol, benazepril, and stool softeners.

His exam is unremarkable except for post-ictal confusion.

Lab: BUN 20, Cr 1.2, Na 140, K 4.2, Ca 9.8.
Head CT with contrast: no abnormalities.

Which of the following would you recommend next?

    A. Obtain lumbar puncture.
    B. Obtain MRI.
    C. Stop tramadol.
    D. Begin phenytoin.
    E. Stop amitriptyline.

386.

A 36-year-old obese woman presents for evaluation of headaches. She has had increasing problems with headaches over the past 6 months. She has had no visual symptoms. She has occasional nausea but no focal neurologic symptoms.

On physical exam: BP 120/70, P 80, Skin – without lesions, Fundi – normal examination, Neurologic exam – without abnormalities

Medications: $CaCO_3$, oral contraceptive pills, fluoxetine

Which of the following is the most likely etiology for her headache?

A. Glioblastoma
B. Pseudotumor cerebri
C. Tuberous sclerosis
D. Prader Willi syndrome
E. Oral contraceptive pills

387.

An 80-year-old man with HTN, BPH, and CAD develops herpes zoster involving the trigeminal nerve. After the lesions heal he still has severe pain involving his right eye and right side of his forehead.

Which of the following treatments would you recommend next?

A. Hydrocodone/oxycodone
B. Phenytoin
C. Amitriptyline
D. Nortriptyline
E. Gabapentin

388.

An 83-year-old woman comes to the clinic with concerns about worsening dizziness. She has had an increase in disequilibrium recently, including a recent fall. She has no history of CAD or seizure disorder. Her symptoms begin when she stands up and starts to walk. They are improved when she stops for a minute and touches the wall. Medications include: Sertraline, nizatidine, $CaCO_3$, and estrogen.

Which of the following is the most likely diagnosis?

A. Benign positional vertigo
B. Vestibular neuronitis
C. Orthostatic hypotension
D. Multiple sensory deficits
E. Panic attacks

389.

A 56-year-old male presents for routine clinic visit with complaints of dizziness. He states the episodes are particularly common at night when he rolls over in bed. They last for 15–30 seconds and then resolve. The sensation is that of the room spinning around him.

Appropriate diagnostic workup would include which of the following?

    A. Nylen-Bárány maneuver
    B. Audiogram
    C. Electronystagmography
    D. Weber test
    E. MRI

390.

A 66-year-old man presents with complaints of decreased hearing in his right ear. He was recently diagnosed with prostate cancer. He had presented with urosepsis because of urinary tract obstruction. He was successfully treated with gentamicin and ceftazidime. On exam he has cerumen in both ear canals. The Weber test lateralizes to his right ear. A Rinne test shows air conduction louder in the left ear, bone conduction louder in the right ear.

Which of the following is the most likely cause of the hearing loss?

    A. Gentamicin toxicity
    B. Cochlear osteosclerosis
    C. Ménière's disease
    D. Cerumen impaction
    E. Acoustic neuroma

391.

A 45-year-old male patient of yours calls you on a Sunday afternoon. He has been having nausea, vomiting, and diarrhea today. He also has had a headache and mild dyspnea. These symptoms actually improved when he was shoveling snow earlier in the day but have now returned. He reports his wife is sick in bed with the same "flu-like" symptoms.

Which of the following do you recommend next?

    A. Have the patient call 911 for emergency evaluation/transport to ER.
    B. Have the patient see you in the clinic tomorrow if the symptoms persist.
    C. You will make a house call today.
    D. Prescribe amantadine 100 mg bid x 7d for both the patient and his wife.

392.

A 26-year-old man is found unconscious and unresponsive in his well-ventilated apartment. No medical history is available. 15 minutes later, when he arrives in the Emergency Room, he has improved.

PHYSICAL EXAMINATION: His general exam is negative. There is no evidence of trauma. His vital signs are normal. He is afebrile. There are no signs of meningeal irritation. He does not answer questions or follow commands well. Cranial nerves are normal. Formal strength testing is difficult, but he moves both arms and legs equally well. He withdraws all four limbs to painful stimuli. There is no decerebrate or decorticate posturing. Reflexes are 2+ and symmetric. Toes are downgoing bilaterally.

LABS: Normal routine tests

Which of the following is the most likely cause for his diminished mental state?

    A. Drug intoxication
    B. Seizure (post-ictal)
    C. Stroke
    D. Encephalitis
    E. Hyperglycemia (diabetes)

393.

A 26-year-old man is found unconscious and unresponsive in his well-ventilated apartment. No medical history is available. 15 minutes later, when he arrives in the Emergency Room, he has improved.

PHYSICAL EXAMINATION: His general exam is negative. There is no evidence of trauma. His vital signs are normal. He is afebrile. There are no signs of meningeal irritation. He does not answer questions or follow commands well. Cranial nerves are normal. Formal strength testing is difficult, but he moves both arms and legs equally well. He withdraws all four limbs to painful stimuli. There is no decerebrate or decorticate posturing. Reflexes are 2+ and symmetric. Toes are downgoing bilaterally.

LABS: Normal routine tests

Which of the following is the best test to perform in the ER to narrow the differential?

    A. Lumbar puncture
    B. CT scan of the brain
    C. Toxicology
    D. Skull x-ray
    E. Arterial blood gas

394.

A 25-year-old man comes to your office complaining of an excruciating unilateral headache for the past week. He says, "It's like an ice-pick behind my eye." You discover that it occurs 8 times per day, and that each headache lasts 30 minutes. The headache is associated with eye watering on the same side. He had a headache like this 1 year ago. It lasted 6 weeks before resolving spontaneously. His dad gets the same kind of headache.

Physical exam: His general and neurologic exams are normal.

Which of the following is the most likely diagnosis?

    A. Migraine headache
    B. Tension headache
    C. Cluster headache
    D. Subarachnoid hemorrhage
    E. Pseudotumor cerebri

395.

A 25-year-old man comes to your office complaining of an excruciating unilateral headache for the past week. He says, "It's like an ice-pick behind my eye." You discover that it occurs 8 times per day, and that each headache lasts 30 minutes. The headache is associated with eye watering on the same side. He had a headache like this 1 year ago. It lasted 6 weeks before resolving spontaneously. His dad gets the same kind of headache.

Physical exam: His general and neurologic exams are normal.

Which of the following treatments might be helpful?

    A. Prednisone
    B. Verapamil
    C. Oxygen
    D. Valproic acid
    E. All of the choices listed are correct

396.

A 43-year-old woman is brought to the ER by her husband. She had a right middle cranial fossa meningioma removed less than 2 weeks ago. She went home on postoperative day number 5. Four days ago, the staples were removed in the neurosurgeon's office. Ever since the surgery, she has had headaches. She was given acetaminophen with codeine, which initially helped. However, the headaches have worsened over the past 3 days. In addition, she has had a low-grade fever to 100.5°F.

Exam: The surgical wound looks clean (no drainage, fluctuance, or excessive redness). Chest is clear to auscultation. The patient appears slightly sleepy. She does not have signs of meningeal irritation. Cranial nerves are normal. Speech and language are normal. There is mild weakness (4/5) in the left arm. There is a left pronator drift. Reflexes are mildly increased in the left arm. Sensation and coordination appear intact.

Which of the following is the most likely diagnosis?

    A. Hemorrhagic infarct
    B. Abscess
    C. Viral encephalitis
    D. Bacterial meningitis
    E. Ischemic infarct

397.

A 33-year-old woman is referred for episodic dizziness. When you see her, she reports a spinning sensation that is accompanied by nausea, and less often, vomiting. The dizziness is episodic, usually lasting 45 minutes. It first started 4 years ago. She reports ringing in the left ear and has more recently noticed hearing loss in the same ear (left) that is unassociated with the attacks of dizziness. There have been no recent illnesses, fever, chills, or focal neurologic deficits.

Exam: The patient's general exam is negative. Neurological exam reveals mild hearing loss to the tuning fork, but is otherwise unremarkable.

Which of the following is the most likely diagnosis?

    A. Vestibular neuronitis
    B. Benign positional vertigo
    C. Labyrinthitis
    D. Ménière disease
    E. Stroke

398.

A 76-year-old man with a history of hypertension and CABG surgery 5 years ago is brought to the ER with a sudden onset of dizziness and clumsiness. He feels mildly nauseated, but has had no vomiting. He has been in relative good health recently. He denies malaise, fever, and chills.

Exam: His general exam is normal. His vital signs show an elevated BP of 170/90. Neurological exam shows direction-changing nystagmus, and ataxia of both the left arm and leg. Otherwise, his exam is normal.

Which of the following is the most likely diagnosis?

    A. Cerebellar infarct
    B. Ménière's
    C. Labyrinthitis
    D. Vestibular neuronitis
    E. Benign positional vertigo

399.

A 50-year-old man is brought to the ER by his wife. About 2 hours ago, he reported a sudden, severe headache. She went to get him Tylenol, and when she returned, he was lying on the couch and was difficult to arouse. He quickly awakened, but was confused. He seemed to drift off to sleep. When she returned a little later to check on him (hmm..she didn't think this was weird the first time??), he was unable to be aroused, at which point she called 911 (Whew! Thank goodness!). There have been no recent illnesses. He is on no medications.

Exam: His general exam is negative. He has a temperature of 100.2° F. He is unable to be aroused, but withdraws extremities to painful stimuli. Brainstem reflexes are intact. He has meningismus. There are no obvious focal neurological deficits, but your exam is limited.

Which of the following is the most likely diagnosis?

A. Subarachnoid hemorrhage
B. Intracranial tumor
C. Large MCA infarct
D. Herpes encephalitis
E. Bacterial abscess

400.

A 34-year-old woman is referred to your office because of weakness. The problem has been gradually worsening for 10 days. She has no pain, denies trauma, and has had no recent illnesses or fever. She has no other medical illnesses. In college, she said that she had transient blurriness in one eye. This lasted "a few days," and she cannot recall which side was involved. She did not see a physician for the visual symptoms because they resolved spontaneously.

Physical exam: She has a pale, mildly atrophied optic disc on the right. She has 4/5 strength in the left upper and lower extremity, brisk reflexes in the left arm and leg, and an upgoing toe on the left. Tone is normal. Strength and reflexes on the right are normal. Testing of sensation is normal. Coordination is remarkable for slowed rapid alternating movements in the left upper extremity. Her gait is slow.

Which of the following is the most likely diagnosis?

A. Guillain-Barré syndrome
B. Multiple sclerosis
C. Transverse myelitis
D. Cauda Equina syndrome
E. Stroke

401.

A 65-year-old man comes to the office with his wife because, as she says, "he is moving so slow. I know we're not getting any younger, but he is really having troubles." Upon interviewing him, you discover that his voice has become softer, and he has had a tremor in the right hand. He has trouble turning over in bed, getting out of chairs without assistance, and has frequently "felt stuck" when trying to ambulate. His memory and thinking are normal. He is on no medications.

Exam: His general exam is normal. Mental status exam is normal. His cranial nerves are remarkable for masked facies and hypophonic speech. He has increased tone (rigidity) on the right arm and leg, cogwheeling, and a resting tremor on the right. His gait is slow and festinating. He has a stooped posture. When walking he turns "en bloc."

Which of the following is the most likely diagnosis?

A. Shy-Drager
B. Parkinson disease
C. Striatonigral degeneration
D. Progressive Supranuclear Palsy (PSP)
E. Alzheimer's

402.

A 33-year-old woman sees her internist because of intermittent diplopia, and a feeling of overall fatigue for the last month. The double vision occurs mainly at night, usually while watching television. She denies associated symptoms such as dysphagia, dysarthria, weakness, or numbness. Prior to this, she was in excellent health. She has no other medical illness. There is a family history of hypertension. Her grandmother had a stroke at age 80. She is on prenatal multivitamins and is trying to become pregnant. She denies tobacco, alcohol, and drug use.

PHYSICAL EXAMINATION:
Vital signs are normal. General exam is negative. Neurologic exam reveals an alert, articulate woman. Her speech is without errors. Cranial nerve exam is remarkable for a mild left-sided ptosis. When asked to sustain upward gaze for two minutes, she complains of double vision. When she complains of the diplopia, a mild left sixth nerve weakness is evident. The remainder of her cranial nerves exam is normal. Motor, sensory, and coordination are normal.

LABS: Normal.

Of the following tests, which one would you perform first to confirm the diagnosis?

    A. EMG
    B. CT of the chest
    C. MRI of the brain and brainstem
    D. Anticholinesterase antibodies
    E. Tensilon test (if available); if not available, then acetylcholine receptor antibodies (AChR-Ab)

RHEUMATOLOGY

403.

A 23-year-old male presents to the ER with a 2-day history of joint pain and swelling. He has had no previous episodes of joint pain. He also has had a fever, chills, and thinks he has developed a rash on his body that is not itchy. He denies any penile discharge, diarrhea, or mouth ulcers.

On examination: Temp = 102.3°F.
Neck = normal. Abdomen = soft.
Joint exam reveals synovitis of MCPs bilaterally, right elbow synovitis and effusion of the right knee. He was also noted to have a salmon-colored rash over his trunk and abdomen.
WBC = 16.7   Hb = 11.3   ESR = 123.
Urinalysis = neg.   ANA = 1/80, diffuse.
Rheumatoid factor = neg.

Which of the following is the most likely diagnosis?

  A. Whipple disease
  B. Systemic lupus erythematosus
  C. Reiter syndrome
  D. Adult-onset Still disease
  E. Gonococcal arthritis

404.

A 64-year-old woman presents to her internist with swelling of her neck. She has had 5 years of dryness in her eyes and mouth. She has had pain in her knuckles. She is presently on celecoxib and hydroxychloroquine. Her hypertension is controlled with a thiazide.

PHYSICAL EXAMINATION:
Heberden nodes in both hands.
Mild MCP synovitis is noted bilaterally.
Significant caries are noted.
Crackles are noted at both bases.
Several rubbery 2 x 2 cm lymph nodes are noted in her left cervical chain.

White cell count = 2.9   ESR = 83
ANA = 1/1280   RF = neg.   Uric acid = 4.9
Anti-SSA antibody = 1/32

Which of the following is the most likely diagnosis?

  A. Sjögren syndrome with non-Hodgkin lymphoma
  B. Pulmonary fibrosis
  C. Myelodysplastic syndrome
  D. AIDS with tuberculosis
  E. SLE with reactive lymphoid hyperplasia

405.

A 47-year-old woman presents with an acute painful ulcer on her left index finger. She has had classic triphasic color changes in her fingers for the past 18 months, precipitated by cold weather. She has noticed a 10-pound weight loss recently and is struggling to swallow solids. She has a 20-pack/year smoking history and has diet-controlled Type 2 diabetes mellitus.

Physical examination: BP = 137/87
Positive vital capillaroscopy with infarct at tip of index finger. Sclerodactyly noted. Multiple telangiectasia. All pulses intact. No bruits. Lung fields clear.

Which of the following is <u>not</u> likely to be found?

    A. ANA
    B. Anti-SCL70 antibody
    C. Anti-histone antibody
    D. Anti-centromere antibody
    E. Rheumatoid factor

406.

An 84-year-old female presents to her internist with a 6-week history of bony pain, weight loss, and night sweats. She is very concerned by a red swelling over her right index finger. She has a history of NIDDM and a previous history of cholecystectomy.

Examination reveals an emaciated but alert elderly female. Neck is supple. No lymphadenopathy but one finger splenomegaly detected. Asymmetric Heberden and Bouchard nodes noted with erythema and profound tenderness over right second index DIP.

ESR = 123, Hb = 9.3, creatinine = 2.6.
Serum protein electrophoresis reveals a monoclonal spike.
Urine is positive for Bence-Jones protein.

Which of the following is the most likely cause of her joint problem?

    A. Amyloid
    B. Gout
    C. Osteoarthritis
    D. Pseudogout
    E. Ochronosis

407.

A 75-year-old woman presents to her geriatrician with pain in her shoulders and on the sides of her hips. She is being treated for a peripheral neuropathy with vitamin B_{12}. She had a mastectomy 12 years ago, followed by chemotherapy, and has been told recently by her oncologist that she is disease-free.

Examination reveals no evidence of synovitis, with excellent range of joint motion. No clear-cut proximal weakness. No tender points. No heliotrope and no rash. Normal funduscopic examination.

.
Hb = 9.7   WBC = 4.9   ESR = 88
Calcium = 9.9
Chest x-ray normal
Urinalysis negative

Which of the following should she be treated with?

    A. Folic acid 1 mg
    B. Gabapentin
    C. Tricyclic antidepressant
    D. Prednisone 60 mg/day
    E. Prednisone 15 mg/day

408.

A 50-year-old female diabetic presents with left shoulder pain and stiffness, which has been progressive over the past several weeks. The pain wakes her up at night. She had a pacemaker placed 3 months ago, having suffered an anterior myocardial infarction 6 months ago.

Examination: BP = 137/87   Pulse = 76
Left shoulder abduction to 90 degrees, right shoulder abduction to 140 degrees. Mild lower-extremity sensory deficit. Mild sclerodactyly of upper extremity digits.

Which of the following would be an appropriate treatment?

    A. Prednisone 15 mg
    B. Physical therapy
    C. Left subacromial corticosteroid injection
    D. Non-steroidals

409.

A 29-year-old psoriatic patient has noticed an increased stiffness of his lower back. He has a history of iritis. His psoriasis is controlled with local creams alone. His left knee was swollen 6 months ago but resolved spontaneously.

Which of the following is the next most appropriate investigation?

    A. Chest x-ray
    B. HLA B-27
    C. CT scan of joints
    D. Slit-Lamp investigation
    E. Lumbar MRI

410.

A 47-year-old laborer is complaining of numbness and tingling of his right hand, which wakes him up at night. He is on glyburide for his diabetes. He has a history of apparent gout and has taken colchicine intermittently. He injured his left knee in a motor vehicle accident several years ago and has mild pain.

Examination reveals no wasting of the right thenar eminence. Sensory deficit is noted of the thumb and index finger. Crepitus of the right knee is present. Nerve conduction velocities reveal slowing across the carpal tunnel of the median nerve.

Which of the following would <u>not</u> be appropriate?

    A. Vitamin B_6
    B. Right wrist splint
    C. Right carpal tunnel corticosteroid injection
    D. Carpal tunnel release

411.

A 50-year-old male has a lengthy history of sinusitis. He has developed hemoptysis over the last week and feels a little short of breath. His energy levels have declined, and he has noticed increased night sweats. He has had increased hand, elbow, and knee pain over the last week.

Physical examination reveals a cachectic male, blood pressure = 132/94. Crackles at both bases are noted. No synovitis. Erythematous papules in lower extremities are present. Foot drop is present on left.

Hb = 10.1. White cell count = 7.6.
Creatinine = 1.7.
Urine reveals trace protein with red cells and red-cell casts. C-ANCA = positive.
Later that same day, creatinine = 2.6.

Renal biopsy is likely to show which of the following?

A. Minimal change nephritis
B. Rapidly progressive glomerulonephritis with crescents
C. Membranous nephropathy
D. Focal sclerosis
E. Interstitial nephritis

412.

A 47-year-old woman has had severe erosive, nodular, seropositive rheumatoid arthritis for 7 years. She has responded well to a combination of infliximab, methotrexate, and low-dose prednisone.

She presents to the Emergency Room with a 2-day history of hemoptysis. Physical examination reveals mild synovitis of MCP's bilaterally and left knee effusion. Nodules are noted but no vasculitis. She has diminished breath sounds at the right apex. Abdomen is soft and without masses.

LABORATORY:
    ESR: 66
    Hb: 9.7
    Chest x-ray: Cavity at the right apex revealed

Which one of the following investigations would be the most appropriate?

A. ACE levels
B. Rheumatoid factor
C. Bronchoscopy
D. High-resolution CT scan of the chest
E. Sputum for AFB

413.

A 31-year-old physician's assistant is seen for worsening Raynaud's. She has had classic triphasic color changes in her fingers for the past 10 years. She has never had ulcers on her fingers. She has also had a history of gastroesophageal reflux. The only other medical history of note is that she was diagnosed with anorexia nervosa 10 years ago but feels that she is now currently "healed." No joint pain and no rashes of note. No problems swallowing food.

Examination reveals a healthy 5' 2" female whose weight is 104 lbs. She is well-nourished and well-hydrated. Skin is normal without sclerodactyly, telangiectasia, or pulp atrophy. However, 2 of the digits on her right hand reveal an abnormal vital capillaroscopy with dilated capillaries. The remainder of her exam is benign.

Which of the following serologies is <u>not</u> compatible with a diagnosis of primary Raynaud's?

A. Positive anti-centromere antibodies
B. Anti-nuclear antibody
C. Rheumatoid factor
D. Normal ESR

414.

A 47-year-old woman with a 5-year history of reflux and an 18-month history of Raynaud's is seen by her primary care physician with a history of worsening of her reflux and of solids occasionally getting "stuck in her throat." She particularly has problems swallowing pills and more recently has had to cut her food up into much finer pieces in order to get it down, and is using more liquids to do so. She has no joint pain but is concerned that she is losing grip in her fingers. She is unable to crochet the way that she would like to because of loss of dexterity. She is not short of breath. She has had no other major problems. She denies any joint pain. She is taking a proton-pump inhibitor twice daily.

She is well-nourished. Her blood pressure is 137/73 and pulse is 76. Cardiac exam is benign. Respiratory tract is without crackles. Her joints are normal. Cutaneous exam reveals mild sclerodactyly with positive vital capillaroscopy. She has some telangiectasia on her chest.

Lab workup reveals hemoglobin of 11.7, WBC of 4.9, and normal platelet count. Creatinine is 0.9. ANA is positive, and anti-centromere antibodies were strongly positive. UA is clear.

Which of the following investigations would be appropriate as part of her long-term follow-up?

A. Small bowel follow-through
B. Constant monitoring of ANA's
C. Occasional ECHO to estimate pulmonary pressure
D. Serum protein electrophoresis

415.

A 53-year-old African-American gentleman presents with profound weakness and minimal muscle pain. These symptoms began 2–3 weeks ago. Initially, he could no longer weight-train in the way he was accustomed. He is not short of breath or coughing. He denies any rashes or joint pain. His energy levels have been dramatically reduced. He is having no problems with swallowing.

On examination, he is quite weak proximally. He is barely able to rise from a seated position. Proximal muscles in the upper extremities are similarly weakened, but distal muscle strength is normal, and there are no sensory deficits detected. Vital signs are normal. The joints have a good range of motion and are without active synovitis. Cutaneous exam is positive both for heliotrope and Gottron plaques. The remainder of his examination is normal.

Lab findings reveal hemoglobin of 11.3, WBC of 12.1, and normal platelet count. Creatinine is normal. Creatinine kinase is 19,512. A muscle biopsy reveals fairly non-specific lymphocytic and neutrophil infiltrates of some of the muscle fibers, with occasional areas of necrosis.

Which of the following therapies would <u>not</u> be appropriate?

A. IV immunoglobulin
B. 60 mg of prednisone
C. Alendronate 70 mg q week
D. 1,000 mg of elemental calcium per day in divided doses

416.

A 59-year-old female presents to her primary care physician with a history of "finger problems." More specifically, her right index and left ring fingers have been "locking" and "triggering" for the past several months. She is beginning to lose function and is finding this most irritating. She is otherwise in excellent health. She has no joint pain particularly. About 18 months ago, she had a painful shoulder. She was seen by her local orthopedist and sent for a course of physical therapy, with fairly dramatic improvement of her shoulder pain and stiffness. Her diabetes is controlled on diet alone. A recent glycosylated hemoglobin (HbA1c) was normal. Past surgical history is positive for a hysterectomy and right carpal tunnel release 6 months ago. She has no other major symptoms of note at this time.

Her physical examination reveals her to be a well-appearing, slightly obese female in no distress. Her blood pressure is 143/76 and pulse is 78. Cardiac and respiratory exam is benign. Musculoskeletal exam reveals evidence of asymmetric Heberden nodes. She has no active synovitis of the PIPs or MCPs. The wrists and elbows have a good range of motion. Shoulder abduction is full and normal. Lower extremity joints are normal. Her hands reveal evidence of sclerodactyly and slightly diminished grip strength. There is a positive prayer's sign. There is evidence of early Dupuytren contractures and slight thickening of some of her flexor tendons, including the two relevant fingers, which were not clearly demonstrated to trigger.

Which of the following is the most likely diagnosis?

A. Rheumatoid arthritis
B. Progressive systemic sclerosis
C. Diabetic-limited joint mobility syndrome
D. Diabetic autonomic neuropathy

417.

A 51-year-old female presents in an outpatient clinic with a new onset of a rash on her back and chest. This rash began about 2–3 months ago. Initially, she thought it was some form of fungal infection or allergic reaction and applied a 1% hydrocortisone cream without much benefit. The rash was not particularly itchy. At the same time, she had begun to develop some pain in her shoulders and hips but no early morning stiffness and certainly no swelling of the joints of her fingers or toes. In general, her history is fairly benign. At age 16, she had presented with unexplained painful nodules on her lower extremities, but the cause of this was never fully understood and she has never had any recurrence. During her second normal pregnancy, she developed a weakness of one side of her face and was told that she had a Bell palsy. Her facial expression returned to normal fairly soon after the birth of her child. Her internist had been concerned because he had found mild elevations of her calcium levels 3 years ago and again 6 months ago, but these have normalized on their own. There was no particular explanation found for this at that time.

On examination, she was well appearing. Height was 5' 7", weight was 136, BP was 127/76, and pulse was 72. Cardiac and respiratory exams were benign. The abdomen was without visceromegaly. Musculoskeletal exam revealed no joint synovitis. Neurological exam was normal without any proximal myopathy. Cutaneous exam revealed several circumscribed, somewhat elevated, 2 x 2 coin-sized lesions on her chest and back. Her dermatologist suggested a biopsy.

Which of the following is the most likely pathological finding that could be obtained from the biopsy of her skin?

A. Eosinophilic fasciitis
B. Non-caseating granulomatous inflammatory changes
C. Panniculitis
D. Interface dermatitis

418.

A 20-year-old student is referred to your office from campus health care. There is a concern that she has a possible connective tissue disease process. She lives at home in Florida during the summer months but attends school in the Northeast during the winter months. Over the last month or two of severe winter weather, she has noticed that her fingers seem to be quite painful and go through some color changes that are brand new to her. Most specifically, they are initially white and then seemingly go a little blue and then remain red for prolonged periods of time. She struggles to complete her projects because she finds it very difficult to type. She thinks her finger joints are a little painful. She readily admits to some alcohol intake and has recently begun to smoke 5–10 cigarettes per day, particularly more so over the weekends. She denies any rashes, swallowing problems, shortness of breath, or cough. She has no problem swallowing food. As part of her workup on campus, she was found to have a strongly positive anti-nuclear antibody. She had been reading about lupus and was very concerned about this condition, particularly from the information that she had gleaned from the Internet.

On examination, she is alert and oriented. BP is 112/57, pulse is 76. All pulses are present and equal. She has no bruits. There is a negative Allen's test. Cardiorespiratory exam is benign. Musculoskeletal exam is benign. Cutaneous exam reveals no rashes, vasculitis, or pulp atrophy. There is a negative vital capillaroscopy.

Lab findings include a positive ANA in a titer of 1:320 (normal is less than 1:40.) Hemoglobin is 11.9, and WBC is 4.9. UA is negative.

Which of the following would be appropriate for further workup?

A. Esophageal manometry
B. ECHO to estimate pulmonary pressure
C. Bronchoscopy
D. Repeat ANA, anti-ds-DNA titers, anti-centromere, and anti-SCL70
E. Upper extremity arteriography

419.

A 29-year-old female is seen in the outpatient setting for painful and swollen knees and feet. These symptoms began about 10 days ago. She describes the pain as incapacitating; she can barely ambulate and is brought in today in a wheelchair. She has never had any joint pain prior to this. She denies any rashes. She thinks that she had a fever about 2 weeks ago, which developed 2–3 days into a week-long trip to Mexico. Toward the end of that trip, she developed fairly significant diarrhea for about 48 hours, which was quickly self-limiting. No rectal bleeding was noted at that time. She has had no urinary symptoms since then.

On examination, her temperature was 97.3° F. She was not pale or jaundiced. BP was 112/72 and pulse was 100. Cardiac and respiratory exams were benign. Cutaneous exam was benign. Musculoskeletal exam revealed no upper extremity joint synovitis. However, she had very significant knee effusions, was very tender over the insertion of the right Achilles and had significant sausaging asymmetrically of a few of the lower extremity digits.

Which of the following is the proper course of action at this time?

A. Inject both knees with corticosteroids.
B. Admit the patient and place her on broad-spectrum IV antibiotics.
C. Check baseline labs to include CBC, sed rate, RF, and aspirate one of the knees.
D. X-ray both knees and ankles.
E. Give systemic corticosteroids.

420.

A 76-year-old frustrated man is seen as an outpatient. He has a 20-year history of joint pain. Initially, he began with some stiffness and swelling of the left knee, which rapidly spread to his right knee. He was told that he had OA and had several unsuccessful corticosteroid injections into both knees. His orthopedist was not inclined to replace the knee joints at that time, given his age. Over the years, the knees slowly began to bother him less but certainly made ambulation uncomfortable. About 5 years ago, he began to develop right groin pain and was told that he had severe "arthritis" in the right hip area. Hip replacement was suggested and, because of ongoing limitation of mobility, this was successfully completed 2½ years ago. More recently, he has begun to experience some pain in the base of his right thumb. He has tried acetaminophen and numerous OTC NSAIDs and had been placed on nabumetone, sulindac, and diclofenac. He developed significant abdominal pain while on the nabumetone and subsequently had an endoscopy and was told that he had a small gastric ulcer. He was told not to take antiinflammatories any longer. More recently, his knees have been bothering him significantly. The rest of the history is fairly benign. He has moderate HTN and is on an ACE inhibitor.

On examination, he is alert, oriented, and well-nourished. BP is 137/91 and pulse is 76. Cardiorespiratory exam is benign. Complete musculoskeletal exam reveals bilateral asymmetric Heberden nodes with some squaring of both thumbs. The elbows and shoulders have a good range of motion. Both hips have reasonable internal and external rotation, but he has fairly significant crepitus of both knees. He has fairly obvious varus deformities with some laxity of the lateral collateral ligaments on both sides. He has marked hallux valgus of the right toe. Cutaneous exam is benign.

Which of the following is <u>not</u> a reasonable therapeutic option?

A. Intraarticular glucocorticoid
B. Celecoxib
C. NSAID + proton pump inhibitor
D. Prednisone 10 mg qd

421.

A 19-year-old Caucasian male is seen for low back pain and stiffness. He has been very used to running and playing basketball and is now finding it increasingly difficult to compete in these activities. For the past 18 months or so, he has developed low back pain, which he wakes up with in the morning. Somewhat surprisingly, he notices that this limbers up on his early morning run. His previous medical history has been benign, except for occasional episodes of diarrhea. He has discussed this with his primary care physician and was told that this possibly was irritable bowel syndrome, because it seemed to be made worse by stress related to exams, which he was taking during his freshman year. On one occasion, he had fairly bloody stools, which lasted about 36 hours, but he failed to report this to his primary care physician. Family history is benign—no family members with arthritis or back problems.

On examination, he is well-nourished and well-hydrated. The general exam is benign. His joints appear quite normal. His neck and lumbosacral movement is full and normal, and he has a negative straight leg-raising sign. Schober's test reveals 6 cm of movement. There is no evidence of psoriasis. Lab investigations revealed a sed rate of 63, hemoglobin of 10.9, WBC of 7.6, and creatinine of 0.8. UA is negative.

Which of the following is <u>not</u> an appropriate investigation?

    A. MRI of the LS-spine
    B. CT scan of the SI joints
    C. Colonoscopy
    D. Referral to ophthalmology for slit-lamp examination

422.

A 58-year-old Caucasian female presents with aching of her shoulders and the sides of her hips. This has been present for the past 3–4 weeks. She has not wanted to go to the YMCA, where she participates in exercise and water aerobics 3–4 times weekly. Her fingers, toes, knees, and elbows have not been painful. She has a history of HTN, which has been treated with a beta-blocker. There is no family history of joint problems.

On examination, she is well-nourished and well-hydrated with normal BP and pulse of 76. Exam is completely without any specific findings. Her musculoskeletal exam is entirely negative without any loss of joint range or mobility. She has no synovitis in any joints and no fibromyalgia tender points. Lab investigations reveal a mild anemia with hemoglobin of 10.2, MCV of 88, and ESR of 99. She is placed on prednisone 15 mg qd.

Which of the following is appropriate adjunctive therapy?

    A. Calcitonin
    B. Alendronate 70 mg q week or risedronate 35 mg q week.
    C. A selective estrogen receptor modulator (SERM)
    D. Estrogen therapy

423.

A 42-year-old gentleman presents with diffuse joint pain and swelling, which has been ongoing for the past 18 months. He initially began with some knee pain and swelling and was unable to continue with his usual habit of cycling. However, the episodes of joint pain were seemingly unrelated to his cycling, and he continued to have episodes of swelling that occurred very spontaneously that would last for 10–12 days and then subside. These paroxysmal episodes then began to involve his wrists and then the 2nd and 3rd MCP joints on both sides. He was seen by his primary care physician, who found him to have a sed rate of 53 and a negative RF and ANA. X-rays of the relevant joints were thought to be negative in the early stages. He never had an episode of podagra. He has no history of renal calculi. The rest of the systemic inquiry was benign. He has no family history of joint problems. There are no problems with his eyes. He tried several NSAIDs; these were generally unsuccessful. He was even prescribed a prednisone dose-pack equivalent.

On examination, he was obese with a BP of 112/76. General exam was benign. Musculoskeletal exam revealed some tenderness over the 2nd and 3rd MCP joints on both sides with no effusions or synovitis. His right wrist had somewhat limited flexion and extension. The knees were without effusions. Repeat lab investigations again found him to be RF negative, and he had a normal sed rate. X-ray of the hands revealed significant osteophytes over the 2nd and 3rd MCP joints bilaterally with right wrist triangular fibrocartilage calcification on the right.

Given the fact that there were no active joints to tap, which of the following investigations would be appropriate at this stage?

A. CT scan of the SI joints
B. Ferritin and calcium levels
C. Bone scan
D. Anti-Jo 1 antibody

424.

A 40-year-old man is evaluated because of a 2-week history of fatigue. However, on further questioning, you learn that he has had dysphagia with severe generalized weakness. He notes dyspnea on exertion at 20 feet and has developed significant joint and muscle pains. Finally, with all of this, he says he developed an itchy widespread rash.

PAST MEDICAL HISTORY: Negative

SOCIAL HISTORY: Works as a used car salesman
                                             Married for 18 years with 2 children, ages 10 and 5

PHYSICAL EXAMINATION:
    VS: BP 120/70, P 100, RR 20, Temp 100.6° F
    HEENT: PERRLA, EOMI
                        Throat: Slight redness noted, no exudates
    Neck: Supple
    Heart: RRR without murmurs, rubs, or gallops
    Lungs: CTA
    Abdomen: Bowel sounds are present
                        No hepatosplenomegaly
    Extremities: No cyanosis or clubbing
                        Swelling and tenderness of the metacarpophalangeal and knee joints bilaterally
                        Flat-surfaced, reddish-to-violet, scaling papules noted on the knuckles
    Motor exam: Weakness of the proximal arm and leg muscles
    Skin: Red papular eruption is noted on his face, chest, and back
                        Scaling noted with cracking on the skin of the palmar surface of his fingers

LABORATORY RESULTS:
    WBC: 15,000/μL; 50% polys, 40% lymphs
    ESR: 50 mm/hr
    AST: 170 U/L
    ALT: 190 U/L
    Serum aldolase: 40I U/mL (NL: 0.8-3.0)
    Rheumatoid Factor: 1:40 (Normal is less than 1:80)
    ANA: 1:1280 in speckled pattern

Which of the following is the most likely diagnosis?

A. Scleroderma
B. Rheumatoid arthritis
C. Systemic lupus erythematosus
D. Dermatomyositis
E. Chronic fatigue syndrome

425.

A 40-year-old medical publishing company executive presents with a 2-month history of episodic left shoulder pain after his weekly bowling match. This resolves after 1–3 days but returns following each time he bowls. He has been taking acetaminophen and ibuprofen to relieve the pain. Otherwise, he is without complaints.

PAST MEDICAL HISTORY: Negative

SOCIAL HISTORY:
    Very boring
    No sexually transmitted disease history
    No alcohol or smoking
    No drug use
    Married with 3 kids

PHYSICAL EXAMINATION:
    Left shoulder: Excellent muscle bulk with no point tenderness
    Passive abduction to 90 degrees causing pain in the deltoid region
    With the upper arm held at 45 degrees of abduction, resisted active abduction, and adduction reveals normal strength without pain
    Internal and external rotation is normal without pain

Which of the following best describes his condition?

    A. Bursitis of the subacromial bursa
    B. Rotator cuff tear
    C. Impingement syndrome
    D. Osteoarthritis of the shoulder
    E. Thoracic outlet syndrome

426.

A 50-year-old man swims daily in an indoor YMCA pool. Approximately 2 years ago (yes, 2 years ago) he injured his left foot while in the pool. Pain and swelling developed at the site of injury, which was just proximal to the 3rd digit on his left foot. Traumatic synovitis was diagnosed, and he was started on oral ibuprofen and local corticosteroid injections. During the next 2 years, the pain and swelling have persisted, and now have spread to the plantar surface of his foot and to his ankle. He has not had any fever or chills. Three synovectomies have been performed, and each showed non-caseating granulomas. Special stains revealed no mycobacteria or fungi. Cultures have not grown anything at 2 months since the last synovectomy. He comes to you today because it is worsening again.

Which of the following organisms is most likely causing his infection?

    A. *Mycobacterium marinum*
    B. *Nocardia brasiliensis*
    C. *Mycobacterium tuberculosis*
    D. *Blastomyces dermatitidis*
    E. *Sporothrix schenckii*

427.

A 60-year-old Hispanic man comes in with recurrent episodes of palpable purpura with joint aches.

PHYSICAL EXAMINATION:
> Significant for scattered purpuric papules on his lower extremities bilaterally
> Mild tenderness of the proximal interphalangeal joints of both hands and feet
> No synovial thickening is noted

LABORATORY:

Hemoglobin:	10.5 g/dL
WBC:	7,000/μL
MCV:	88
ESR:	40 mm/hr
AST:	50 U/L
Alkaline phosphatase:	90 U/L
ANA:	Negative
Rheumatoid factor:	1:2080 (< 1:40 normal)
Serum cryoglobulins:	Markedly elevated
Biopsy of skin:	Leukocytoclastic vasculitis

Which one of the following tests will help you confirm your diagnosis?

A. Serum and urine immunoelectrophoresis
B. Anti-DNA
C. CT of chest
D. Antineutrophil cytoplasmic antibodies
E. Hepatitis C serology

428.

A 50-year-old woman with systemic lupus erythematosus (SLE) for 20 years comes to the clinic with a complaint of sudden onset of left hip pain. The pain is much worse when she tries to walk or move the hip. She has been on chronic steroids for most of those 20 years. Her SLE has been under fairly good control for the past 5 years.

PAST MEDICAL HISTORY:
> Last hospitalization was 5 years ago for lupus nephritis exacerbation
> Hospitalized before that for lupus cerebritis 10 years ago

SOCIAL HISTORY:
> Lives with her boyfriend, a 20-year-old computer operator
> Doesn't smoke or drink

FAMILY HISTORY:
> Mother with SLE died at age 45
> Father aged 70 and healthy
> Sister aged 55 with SLE

PHYSICAL EXAMINATION:
VS:	BP 120/70, P 100, RR 19, Temp 98.7° F
HEENT:	PERRLA, EOMI
	TMs Clear
Throat:	Clear

Neck:	Supple
Heart:	RRR with II/VI systolic murmur (no change; heard in the past)
Lungs:	CTA
Abdomen:	Benign
Skin:	No rash
Extremities:	Left hip is painful with any type of movement
	Internal rotation is limited
	X-ray of left hip shows osteopenia

Which of the following is the most likely diagnosis?

A. Chronic osteomyelitis
B. Avascular necrosis of the hip
C. Acute osteomyelitis
D. Slipped epiphyseal head of the femur
E. Fracture of the hip

429.

A 65-year-old woman is coming in for a routine physical examination. She is concerned about postmenopausal osteoporosis. She currently performs in the circus and is worried about bone density problems when she jumps off of the trapeze.

Which of the following tests would be the best to detect and monitor osteoporosis?

A. Dual-photon absorptiometry
B. Dual-energy x-ray absorptiometry
C. Radiography
D. Quantitative CT scan
E. Single-photon absorptiometry

430.

A 50-year-old woman comes in with complaints of dysphagia. She has a 4-month history of proximal muscle pain, Raynaud phenomenon, and a new rash on her hands.
PHYSICAL EXAMINATION:
    Skin: Periungual telangiectasia and scaling, hyperpigmented rash over the dorsum of the
    metacarpophalangeal joints
    Muscle strength testing: Proximal muscle weakness in upper and lower extremities
    Neurologic exam besides above is normal
Barium swallow is done
You determine she has systemic sclerosis.

Which of the following is the barium swallow most commonly going to show?

A. Zenker diverticulum
B. No abnormalities on barium swallow; requires endoscopy
C. A mass constricting flow of barium
D. Loss of lower esophageal sphincter function
E. Poor initiation of swallowing

431.

A 30-year-old man has had recurrent episodes of asymmetric inflammatory oligoarticular arthritis involving his knees, ankles, and elbows. The arthritis usually lasts anywhere from 2 to 4 weeks. Since age 20 or so, he has had recurrent painful "sores" in his mouth. Today he presents to you with fever, arthritis, and mild abdominal pain. Additionally, he reports a "severe" headache.

Physical examination shows significant arthritis of his bilateral knees with warmth to touch and gross fluid accumulation. Additionally, you find a superficial thrombophlebitis in his left leg.

Which of the following is the most likely diagnosis?

   A. SLE
   B. Regional enteritis
   C. Behçet syndrome
   D. Whipple disease
   E. Ulcerative colitis

432.

A 60-year-old man presents with complaints of a swollen left big toe for 3 days. This has never happened before. He has a negative past medical history. Examination shows a large swollen left big toe. This is likely to be acute gouty arthritis.

Of the following agents, which one would <u>not</u> be useful in the treatment of acute gouty arthritis?

   A. Oral colchicine
   B. Indomethacin
   C. Allopurinol
   D. Oral steroid
   E. Intraarticular steroids

433.

A 50-year-old man presents with swelling in his left knee for 3 days. The knee is painful and he cannot ambulate well. He denies history of trauma to the knee. An aspirate of the knee is done and shows crystals with weakly positive birefringence on compensated polarized light microscopy.

Based on the findings, which of the following is the most likely etiology?

   A. Rheumatoid arthritis
   B. Gout
   C. Infection with a crystal-producing organism
   D. Osteoarthritis
   E. Pseudogout

434.

A 28-year-old man develops swelling, pain, and tenderness in his left ankle and right knee. He had severe diarrhea after a picnic 1 month prior to the onset of his arthritis. In between his episodes of diarrhea and arthritis, he had also developed "pink eye," which was mild and lasted only 3 days. He was treated for "gonorrhea" 2 weeks ago but continues to have some clear penile discharge. He wonders if he needs more antibiotics because "the gonorrhea has never lasted this long before."

Which of the following is the most likely diagnosis?

    A. Reactive arthritis (Reiter syndrome)
    B. Resistant gonococcal arthritis
    C. Gout
    D. Pseudogout
    E. Ankylosing spondylitis

435.

A 45-year-old woman presents with arthritis, malar rash, Raynaud phenomenon, leukopenia, and photosensitivity. She is worried that she may have lupus.

According to current guidelines, which of the following is <u>not</u> a clinical manifestation used to diagnose systemic lupus erythematosus?

    A. Leukopenia
    B. Malar rash
    C. Arthritis
    D. Raynaud phenomenon
    E. Photosensitivity

436.

An 80-year-old woman with rheumatoid arthritis for 30 years presents for follow-up. She has had an extensive history and has developed many complications from her disease.

Which of the following is <u>not</u> a characteristic deformity associated with rheumatoid arthritis?

    A. Swan-neck deformity
    B. Heberden node
    C. Hammer toe
    D. Boutonniere deformity
    E. Ulnar deviation

437.

A 19-year-old woman presents to your clinic with leukopenia, a positive ANA, arthritis, and a rash. You review her laboratory work and notice that her urinalysis shows significant proteinuria, red cells, and red cell casts. Her creatinine is 2.0 (normal < 1.3).

Based on these findings, which antibody listed below should you test for at this time?

    A. ds-DNA antibody
    B. cANCA
    C. RNP antibody
    D. SS-A (Ro) antibody
    E. Anti-histone

438.

A 33-year-old man with low back pain for the past 6 months presents for evaluation. The pain is most intense in the morning and seems to improve with exercise. On physical examination, he is tender on palpation of the sacroiliac joints. He has reduced lumbar lordosis. There is no evidence of peripheral arthritis.

Which of the following is true?

    A. A urine sample should be sent for culture and sensitivity.
    B. He needs treatment with prednisone.
    C. X-rays of the hands should be performed.
    D. You should order a 24-hour urine for protein and creatinine.
    E. X-rays of the sacroiliac joints are indicated.

439.

A 55-year-old man presents for routine physical examination. He gives a 10-year history of intermittent episodes of severe pain and swelling of the joints, occurring about every 3 to 5 months and lasting for about 1 week. He says these episodes "are just like my pappy has." Between the attacks, he has virtually no joint pain. His last attack was about 2 months ago, and he is without symptoms when he sees you today.

PAST MEDICAL HISTORY: Essentially negative

FAMILY HISTORY: His father is 70 years old with similar joint complaints

SOCIAL HISTORY: Lives alone with his 2 cats, Melba and Onion
                            Doesn't smoke
                            Drinks a 6-pack of beer daily

PHYSICAL EXAMINATION:
    Extremities: Hallux valgus (bunion) deformity of both 1st metatarsophalangeal joints
                  Firm, enlargement of the right 2nd and 4th proximal interphalangeal joints and the left 1st and 5th proximal interphalangeal joints
                  Several hard nodules are palpated in the left olecranon bursa, which is swollen but not tender, not warm, and not erythematous

An x-ray of the right foot shows soft tissue density around the 1st metatarsophalangeal joint and an oval bone erosion with an overhanging edge in the 1st metatarsal bone at the metatarsophalangeal joint.

Which of the following is the most likely cause of his complaints?

    A. Tendinosis universalis
    B. Osteoarthritis
    C. Gout
    D. Pseudogout
    E. Rheumatoid arthritis

440.

A 42-year-old Caucasian woman presents to your office with the chief complaint "I may have osteoporosis. Can you test me?" You work for an HMO. On further questioning, you learn that she is a very active woman and works out at a gym 3 times a week doing strength training as well as aerobic exercise. She has never smoked and rarely drinks alcohol. She is still having menses.

Physical Examination is unremarkable. She is 5'10" and weighs 140 lbs.

Based on your findings, which of the following is the best thing to do concerning her "osteoporosis"?

    A. Tell her that her case requires referral to a specialist.
    B. Tell her that her risk of osteoporosis is very low, and no testing is required at this time.
    C. Tell her that she is at risk for osteoporosis, and you will send her to get a DEXA scan to assess bone mineral density.
    D. Tell her you are worried that she may have a systemic disease, and you order lumbar spine films, CBC, thyroid function tests, and urinalysis.
    E. Start her on estrogen/progesterone.

441.

A 45-year-old African-American man works as a construction worker. He has a long history of tobacco use and presents to you with a complaint of low back pain that started about 3 weeks ago. He was referred to you by a pulmonologist in your practice. He has a history of asthma. He cannot remember what medications he is taking. You suspect he may have osteoporosis even though he is a male.

Which of the following medications could he be taking that would put him at risk for osteoporosis?

    A. Chronic oral steroid use
    B. ACE inhibitors
    C. Ranitidine
    D. Warfarin
    E. Ibuprofen

442.

A 30-year-old woman with carpal tunnel syndrome comes to you after having been treated by another physician in town with non-steroidal antiinflammatories for the past few months without much improvement. She has also been using "splints" without much improvement. She has no loss of motor function.

Before sending her to surgery, which one of the following should you try?

A. Treatment with a tricyclic antidepressant at bedtime.
B. Corticosteroid injection into the carpal tunnel, or oral steroids.
C. Repeat the EMG and nerve conduction studies.
D. Give 2 weeks of broad-spectrum antibiotics.

443.

An 80-year-old woman presents to your clinic with chronic back pain. She says that she is frequently short of breath. Also, when she walks to the grocery store, she frequently feels a pain in her chest. She describes the pain as a mild pressure. When she rests, the pain goes away. On physical examination, she has dorsal kyphosis with a protuberant lower abdomen. You are concerned that she may have osteoporosis.

Which of the following is <u>not</u> a clinical feature of osteoporosis?

A. Pulmonary dysfunction
B. Exertional chest pain relieved with rest
C. Dorsal kyphosis
D. Back pain
E. Protuberant lower abdomen

444.

A 43-year-old heart transplant recipient comes to the hospital for evaluation of severe foot pain. This pain has been present for 12 hours and hurts even with the slightest pressure to the foot. He received his transplant three months ago and has had no problems with function or rejection. He has no prior musculoskeletal problems, no fever, or other new symptoms. PMH: Hx of duodenal ulcer disease and transplant. Meds: nizatidine, prednisone, cyclosporine, amlodipine, and aspirin. Labs: WBC – 13,000, HCT – 40, SGOT – 30, SGPT – 22.

Of the following, what is the most likely cause of this patient's problem?

A. Aspirin
B. Alcohol use
C. Group A Streptococcus
D. Cyclosporine
E. Nizatidine

445.

A 47-year-old man with benign prostatic hypertrophy develops prostatitis. He is placed on terazosin and ciprofloxacin. His other medications include omeprazole (reflux), erythromycin (acne rosacea), and lisinopril (hypertension). He returns 3 weeks later following a ski vacation, with a severely painful left Achilles tendon.

Of the following, what is the most likely explanation?

    A. Adverse effect due to omeprazole
    B. Overuse due to recent ski trip
    C. Drug interaction due to erythromycin/terazosin
    D. Drug interaction due to lisinopril/ciprofloxacin
    E. Adverse effect due to ciprofloxacin

ALLERGY / IMMUNOLOGY

446.

A 23-year-old graduate student with a negative past medical history, except for gonorrhea at the age of 18, presents for evaluation. He says that he began having problems when he started working in the basic science research laboratory of his school. He says that since working there he has had episodes of shortness of breath, stuffy nose, cough, fever, and chills. He feels bad most of the day. He feels better by Sunday evening, but on Monday his symptoms return. He works with mice in a laboratory at the school on Monday through Friday. He says that he has been well the past few days (today is Monday). He doesn't smoke and occasionally drinks a beer on the weekend. On physical examination, you find nothing—everything is normal. However, a chest radiograph is done and shows ill-defined patchy infiltrates. His laboratory studies, including CBC, lytes, BUN, and creatinine, are all normal. His ESR is slightly elevated at 28. Pulmonary function studies are done and show reduced lung volumes.

Which of the following is the most likely diagnosis?

A. Asthma
B. Acute hypersensitivity pneumonitis
C. Wegener granulomatosis
D. Acute bronchitis
E. Leptospirosis

447.

A 25-year-old woman with a history of intermittent wheezing in response to exercise presents for follow-up. She has never had an attack without it being exercise-induced. She presents to you today with shortness of breath. Her attack began earlier today during an aerobics class (her aerobics class is at a center where a short Caucasian man with an afro runs around in little short gym shorts and says **yea baby, yea baby**). Anyway, at this point in your office she is obviously having difficulty breathing and has diffuse wheezes on her lung examination. A quick pulse oximetry shows that her oxygen saturation is 95%. You begin treatment for her acute attack.

Which of the following treatments would most likely prevent her next attack?

A. Inhaled beclomethasone before she exercises
B. Prednisone 30 minutes before she exercises
C. Theophylline therapy
D. Metered dose albuterol inhaler before she exercises

448.

Okay, some of these immunology questions you just have to deal with. The Boards like to ask these, and there are really no patient scenarios to embellish them with. I could make it cute and sweet, but that wouldn't really ease your pain. You know that you hate these questions. So for the immunology sections, just know that you will get a lot of short torture questions that you are expected to know. Here is one of those now.

During B-cell development, which of the following is expressed the earliest?

  A. Surface immunoglobulin G
  B. Surface immunoglobulin M
  C. Cytoplasmic μ chains
  D. Surface immunoglobulin E
  E. Surface immunoglobulin A

449.

A 35-year-old man presents with episodes of abdominal pain and stress-induced edema of the lips and tongue. Occasionally with severe stress, he will have laryngeal edema also. His examination in between these episodes is completely normal.

With which of the following proteins is he likely to have a low functional or absolute level?

  A. C1 esterase inhibitor
  B. C5A
  C. IgE
  D. Surface immunoglobulin A
  E. Cyclooxygenase

450.

A 40-year-old man presents to you with a history of recurrent rash. He describes an urticarial rash that sometimes leaves a discoloration after the lesions have resolved. He reports intermittent arthralgias with the rash. Otherwise, his physical examination is normal. He currently has some of the lesions. His laboratory is significant for an ESR of 76 mm/hour.

Which of the following should you do next to evaluate his findings?

  A. IgE
  B. Patch test
  C. C1 esterase inhibitor activity level
  D. Skin biopsy
  E. Wheal-and-flare allergy skin test battery

451.

A 40-year-old physician presents for his routine tuberculosis screening. 48 hours after placing his tuberculous purified-protein derivative (PPD), he develops a skin wheal of 11 mm.

Which of the following events at the cellular level is responsible for this finding?

  A. Complement-mediated endothelial cell damage
  B. IL-7-induced B-cell activation and secretion of antibodies
  C. IL-8-induced B-cell activation
  D. CD44-mediated monocyte adhesion to endothelial cells
  E. Monocyte-derived IL-6 activation of T cells

452.

A 20-year-old woman presents with a history of recurrent fevers and associated sputum production. The sputum evidently is fairly foul in its appearance and its smell. She has a past medical history of recurrent upper respiratory infections. Additionally, she has had a *Giardia* diarrheal infection twice in the last 8 years.

Pertinent findings on her physical examination:
Coarse crackles in the left chest with decreased air movement; positive for foul-smelling sputum.
She has an enlarged spleen with a span of 10 cm.

Laboratory:
CBC is normal.
Serum IgG is 80 mg/dL (normal 800–1500 mg/dL).
Serum IgA is 20 mg/dL (normal 90–325 mg/dL).

Which of the following is the most appropriate treatment?

    A. Corticosteroids
    B. Monthly intravenous immunoglobulin
    C. Splenectomy
    D. Bone marrow transplantation
    E. IgA transfusion

453.

Which of the following pertain to the major histocompatibility gene complex (MHC)?

    A. Located on the short arm of chromosome 6
    B. Contains genes involved in the recognition of self
    C. Contains genes involved in antigen presentation to T and B cells
    D. Contains genes involved in the rejection of tissue allografts
    E. All of the answers are correct

454.

A 20-year-old woman presents with recurrent sinopulmonary infections and has developed severe respiratory insufficiency. She has bronchiectasis on a chronic basis. Recently, she has developed progressive cerebellar ataxia and oculocutaneous telangiectasia. She has depressed levels of IgA and IgE on laboratory testing. Additionally, she is noted to have anergy to cutaneous testing. She does not have adenosine deaminase deficiency.

Which of the following is her likely diagnosis?

    A. Ataxia-telangiectasia syndrome
    B. Common variable immunodeficiency
    C. An abnormality on chromosome 12
    D. Severe combined immunodeficiency
    E. Cystic fibrosis

455.

A 40-year-old man with aplastic anemia is administered a treatment. Ten days after beginning therapy with this agent, he develops clinical disease that presents with fever, malaise, arthralgias, and nausea. Soon after, he develops an urticarial rash. He worsens and develops melena and lymphadenopathy. Laboratory is significant for a markedly diminished C3, C4, and CH50. He has high levels of circulating immune complexes.

This is likely due to which of the following therapeutic agents?

A. Gold therapy
B. IVIG
C. Equine antithymocyte globulin
D. Corticosteroids
E. Alkylating agent and corticosteroid

456.

A 45-year-old woman with an abdominal mass palpable in her right upper quadrant is seen for evaluation. You order an abdominal computed tomography exam. While at the radiology suite (which by the way is large and beautiful and without radiologists—because they are at home reading the CT scans), she receives her intravenous contrast. Within minutes of the injection she develops widespread urticaria, facial flushing, and her tongue starts to swell. She also becomes hoarse and says that her "throat is swelling up." She develops stridor and requires emergency intubation with mechanical ventilation.

Which of the following has caused her acute event?

A. An IgE-mediated event against native proteins
B. Direct activation of mediator release from mast cells, basophils, or both
C. A deficiency of C1 esterase inhibitor
D. Contrast dye transformation into formaldehyde
E. An IgE-mediated event against haptens

457.

A 43-year-old woman presents with severe urticaria, facial flushing, and tongue swelling after a bee sting. Her sister had a similar reaction to contrast dye.

Which of the following describes how a bee sting causes anaphylaxis?

A. By causing an IgA-mediated reaction against protein-hapten conjugants
B. By causing an IgE-mediated event against protein-hapten conjugants
C. By causing a direct activation of mediator release from mast cells, basophils, or both
D. It's due to a deficiency of C1 esterase inhibitor
E. By causing an IgE-mediated reaction against the proteins in the sting media

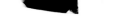

458.

A 42-year-old woman with no prior medical history presents as a new patient. Her eldest sister has a history of anaphylaxis to contrast dye, and her other older sister has a history of anaphylaxis to bee stings. She comes in today with a sore throat. You are able to confirm *Streptococcus pyogenes*, and you start her on the appropriate oral antibiotic for this infection. She returns that afternoon to the ER with a complaint of urticaria, facial flushing, and her tongue starts to swell. She responds to therapy and is observed in the ER.

Which of the following is the mechanism for her anaphylaxis?

A. She has a deficiency of C1 esterase inhibitor.
B. She had IgE recognition of native proteins.
C. She had direct activation of mediator release from mast cells, basophils, or both.
D. She had IgE recognition of protein-hapten conjugants.
E. She somehow got exposed to contrast material while in your office.

459.

A 26-year-old woman has had a 2-year history of recurrent rash. She describes the rash as "small bumps that itch." She describes them as reddish-brown in color. Additionally with these "bumps," she has had flushing of her face, dizziness, and some abdominal pain. If she "pushes" on the skin lesions, they actually itch more and become redder. She has noted that her attacks can occur after she drinks beer or wine or if she takes an ibuprofen. She had an upper GI series done last week that showed an ulcer in her duodenum.

Which of the following is her most likely diagnosis?

A. Common variable immunodeficiency
B. Systemic mastocytosis
C. Anaphylaxis to several agents
D. Familial angioedema syndrome
E. Leukemia

460.

A 17-year-old teen presents with abdominal pain, nausea, and vomiting. With this episode, he has noted a rash and complains of severe arthralgias. He has never had this before.

His physical examination is significant for palpable purpura on his buttocks and lower extremities. None of the lesions are above his waist. Additionally, he has guaiac-positive stool.
Laboratory is sent and is remarkable for a urinalysis that shows mild proteinuria and red blood cell casts. Other studies are normal, including his CBC.

Which of the following is the most likely diagnosis?

A. Henoch-Schönlein purpura
B. Leukemia
C. Anaphylaxis to a hapten
D. Anaphylaxis to a protein
E. Job syndrome

461.

Which of the following is true about T-cells?

A. They lack readily detectable immunoglobulin except for IgE on their membranes.
B. They lack readily detectable immunoglobulin except for IgM on their membranes.
C. They lack readily detectable immunoglobulin except for IgA on their membranes.
D. They lack readily detectable immunoglobulin of **any** class on their membranes.
E. They lack readily detectable immunoglobulin except for IgD on their membranes.

462.

Which of the following is/are true about immunoglobulin A (IgA)?

A. IgA provides defense against local infections in the respiratory, gastrointestinal, and the genitourinary system.
B. IgA is the predominant immunoglobulin in body secretions.
C. IgA exists as 2 subclasses.
D. IgA can prevent virus binding to epithelial cells.
E. All of the statements are true.

463.

A 40-year-old man with a history of recurrent sinopulmonary infections presents for evaluation. He recovers from them fairly quickly, but he has between 4 and 6 episodes a year. Recently, he received an infusion of packed red blood cells after a major motor vehicle accident. During the infusion, he developed anaphylaxis. The blood bank and hospital checked for mismatch and found no evidence of incompatibility.

Which of the following is his likely underlying condition?

A. Isolated IgA deficiency
B. Terminal complement deficiency
C. Systemic mastocytosis
D. IgG deficiency
E. IgD deficiency

464.

Which of the following statements is/are true regarding immune-complex disease?

A. Immune complexes do not have to persist in the circulation for the development of renal manifestations.
B. Signs and symptoms of immune-complex disease develop from the deposition of immune complexes in the reticuloendothelial system.
C. Most immune complexes are removed by the reticuloendothelial system.
D. The rash of cutaneous necrotizing vasculitis is not an example of immune-complex disease.
E. All of the statements are correct.

465.

Class I HLA antigens are expressed on all cells <u>except</u> which of the following?

    A. Mature red blood cells
    B. Reticulocytes
    C. Reticulocytes and mature red blood cells
    D. White blood cells
    E. Purkinje cells

466.

A 33-year-old woman presents with facial pain and nasal congestion. She reports onset of a sore throat and rhinorrhea 5 days ago. Over the past 48 hours, she has had facial pressure over the maxillary sinus and yellow nasal discharge. On exam: T 99.2° F, BP 110/70 mmHg. Nose: swollen turbinates. Neck: no adenopathy. Chest: clear.

Of the following, what would you most likely recommend?

    A. Decongestants/nasal irrigation + amoxicillin
    B. Decongestants/nasal irrigation
    C. Decongestants/nasal irrigation + TMP/Sulfa
    D. Decongestants/nasal irrigation + amoxicillin/clavulanate
    E. Decongestants/nasal irrigation + metronidazole

467.

A 45-year-old woman presents with complaints of episodic abdominal pain. On a few occasions, she reports that she gets swelling of her lips, tongue, and occasionally her "throat." The most recent incident occurred while she was having a dental extraction. All of her "swelling" episodes seem to occur after she has experienced some type of similar stress-induced event.

She is likely to have abnormal functioning levels of which of the following proteins?

    A. T-cell receptor, alpha chain
    B. C5A
    C. IgE
    D. C1 esterase inhibitor
    E. Cyclooxygenase

468.

Each of the following statements concerning <u>anaphylactoid</u> reactions is true <u>except:</u>

    A. They are not immunoglobulin E-dependent (IgE).
    B. Examples include reaction to radiocontrast agents.
    C. They are usually immune responses.
    D. They are systemic reactions.
    E. They have the same symptoms as anaphylaxis.

469.

You are seeing a man with Wiskott-Aldrich syndrome. He has recurrent eczema and bloody diarrhea.

Which of the following is true about his disease?

    A. It cannot be treated successfully with bone marrow transplantation.
    B. It is associated with low IgA.
    C. It is associated with low IgE.
    D. He does not have increased susceptibility to infection.
    E. It is associated with low IgM.

470.

A woman presents to the ER immediately after receiving a bee sting. She has a past history of anaphylaxis and lost her EpiPen®.

She has urticaria but is not having hypotension.

Which of the following should you do next?

    A. Give epinephrine 0.3 mg to 0.5 mg IM
    B. Give epinephrine 1/1000 0.5cc SQ
    C. Give methylprednisolone 2 mg/kg IV
    D. Start beta-blocker
    E. Give epinephrine 1/10,000 0.5 cc SQ

471.

A 36-year-old man works as a school principal. He complains of increasingly frequent episodes of viral illnesses and sinusitis. He has 6–7 colds a year, as well as flu-like episodes that leave him feeling exhausted for several days to weeks at a time. He denies use of drugs or alcohol and states that he has had only one heterosexual partner for the last 5 years. He remembers that as a child he had numerous bouts of tonsillitis, strep throat, and upper respiratory infections.

Which of the following laboratory tests is most likely to help reveal his underlying problem?

    A. HIV test
    B. Serum immunoglobulins
    C. Serum protein electrophoresis
    D. Cold agglutinins
    E. CH50

472.

A 14-year-old student presents to the Emergency Room with a fever of 103° F for 5 days and severe sore throat. She appears toxic and complains of a generalized headache, myalgias, lethargy, and severe malaise. Her physical examination is remarkable for swollen, erythematous lips and tongue. She has cervical lymphadenopathy with one node measuring 2 x 3 cm. She has bilateral conjunctivitis and her palms and soles are thickened, red, and swollen in appearance.

CBC shows a WBC of 15,000 with a mild left shift; platelets are elevated at 550,000; she is not anemic. A rapid streptococcal antigen test is negative, and a Monospot is also negative.

Of the following, what is the most likely diagnosis?

    A. Kawasaki disease
    B. Cryoglobulinemia
    C. Bacterial endocarditis
    D. Toxic epidermal necrolysis
    E. Takayasu arteritis

473.

A patient is scheduled for eye surgery in several weeks. He is currently on a non-steroidal antiinflammatory agent.

Which of the following nonsteroidal antiinflammatory drugs irreversibly inhibits cyclooxygenase?

    A. Acetaminophen
    B. Ibuprofen
    C. Ketoprofen
    D. Aspirin
    E. Diclofenac

DERMATOLOGY

474.

A 16-year-old girl presents with a 3-year history of predominately open and closed comedones of the face, chest, and back. Close inspection reveals an occasional pustule and postinflammatory macules.

Which of the following is the most helpful medication for the acne vulgaris?

   A. Topical sulfacetamide lotion
   B. Topical antibiotic
   C. Topical tretinoin
   D. Systemic tetracycline

475.

A 20-year-old man consults you because of itchy lesions that he has been told are "eczema." He has a lifelong history of asthma and seasonal rhinitis. Your examination reveals popliteal and antecubital lichenification and hyperpigmentation.

Which of the following would you <u>not</u> use for treatment of facial lesions for more than 3–4 weeks?

   A. Lubrication
   B. Topical steroids
   C. Pimecrolimus cream
   D. Tacrolimus ointment

476.

A 70-year-old man comes to the Emergency Room with a 6-week history of progressive weight loss and generalized fatigue. He has difficulty getting up from a sitting position, and complains of room-to-room dyspnea in his home. Your examination reveals erythema and telangiectasia of his cuticles, red papules over the joints of his hands, and proximal muscle weakness.

He most likely has which of the following?

   A. Sarcoidosis and muscle atrophy
   B. Multiple sclerosis and idiopathic myalgia
   C. Dermatitis medicamentosa and myositis
   D. Dermatomyositis and cancer

477.

A 35-year-old African-American woman has a 4-month history of tender nodules on pre-tibial surfaces associated with arthralgias. The remainder of the examination is normal. Biopsy of one of the nodules shows a septal panniculitis. Her chest x-ray shows bilateral hilar adenopathy. Transbronchial lung biopsy reveals non-caseating granuloma.

You diagnose sarcoidosis, and advise her that the lesions on her legs represent which of the following?

A. Cutaneous sarcoidosis
B. Unrecalled trauma
C. Erythema nodosum
D. A viral exanthem

478.

A 17-year-old girl was well until 2 weeks ago when she sustained multiple mosquito bites, which she has been scratching. Today, the lesions are erythematous and covered with honey-colored crusts.

The most likely diagnosis is which of the following?

A. Impetigo vulgaris
B. Erythema nodosum
C. Acne vulgaris
D. A drug eruption

479.

A 65-year-old man has had itchy bullae that come and go on his legs for several years. In the past 2 months, he has developed new bullae in the creases of his arms, medial thighs, and lower abdomen. Some of the bullae are on an erythematous base, and others are on normal skin. Although there are bullae in his mouth, they do not interfere with his eating.

Which of the following is the most likely diagnosis?

A. Erythema multiforme
B. Dermatitis herpetiformis
C. Pemphigus vulgaris
D. Bullous pemphigoid

480.

A 45-year-old man comes to see you because of vesicles on sun-exposed areas, which have been present episodically for 7 years. He has used alcohol to excess for many years. He takes no medications and has not seen a physician for many years. Your evaluation confirms a diagnosis of porphyria cutanea tarda (PCT).

What other diagnosis listed below should you consider?

    A. Paraneoplastic pemphigus
    B. Hepatitis C
    C. Urinary tract infection
    D. Acanthosis nigricans
    E. Hepatitis D

481.

A 69-year-old man consults you because of a diffuse, scaling eruption that almost completely covers his entire body. He reports that the symptoms began shortly after he began to take phenytoin for a seizure disorder. Your examination shows confluent erythematous patches with contiguous scale, generalized lymphadenopathy, and hepatomegaly. Laboratory testing reveals peripheral eosinophilia.

His exfoliative dermatitis is <u>not</u> likely to be associated with which of the following?

    A. Herpetic infections
    B. Drugs
    C. Carcinoma
    D. Lymphoma

482.

This 60-year-old woman comes to you complaining of glossitis, weight loss, diabetes, and a skin rash that has developed over the past 4 months. She has had no other significant illness. Her only medication is a multivitamin with calcium and zinc. Your examination shows erosions of the legs, intertriginous areas, and mucosal surfaces.

Of the following, what is the most likely diagnosis?

    A. Carcinoid syndrome
    B. Primary amyloidosis
    C. Glucagonoma syndrome
    D. Sweet syndrome

483.

A 27-year-old woman comes to your office because of a lesion on her leg, which she believes has slowly changed color over the past 6 months. She has fair skin, blonde hair, and blue eyes. She denies local trauma, and there is no family history of skin disease. Your examination shows an erythematous plaque with variations of brown and black coloration and an irregular border. The lesion is 1 cm in diameter.

Which of the following is the most appropriate treatment?

    A. Remove the lesion with liquid nitrogen.
    B. Perform a 3-mm biopsy of the brown area.
    C. Refer her for excisional biopsy of the lesion.
    D. Advise the patient that no intervention is needed at this time.

484.

A 50-year-old woman is seen for evaluation of rash. She was in her usual excellent state of health until 1 week ago while on vacation in Hawaii, when she developed frequency and dysuria. She was treated with an antibiotic for 3 days, finishing the antibiotic 2 days ago. Physical exam shows severe sunburn.

Which of the following antibiotics did she receive?

    A. Cefixime
    B. Amoxicillin/clavulanate
    C. Nitrofurantoin
    D. Doxycycline

485.

A 35-year-old nurse works in a neonatal intensive care unit. She has to wash her hands multiple times in a day—exceeding 30–40 episodes daily. She has noted a small skin lesion in the 4th interdigital web of her left hand. It is erosive in character.

Of the following, what is the most likely etiology?

    A. Acanthosis nigricans
    B. Cutaneous bacterial infection
    C. Human papillomavirus infection
    D. Psoriasis
    E. Cutaneous candidal infection

486.

A 30-year-old dishwasher presents with scaling of her hands. Recently, she has noted vesicle formation also. She has always had dry scaly lesions on her hands, and they remit and worsen over time. Sometimes, the lesions are quite painful. She has never had asthma or skin problems as a child. Recently, she noted that the small vesicles on the sides of her fingers itch quite a bit.

Of the following, what is the most likely diagnosis?

    A. Herpes simplex I
    B. Dyshidrotic eczema
    C. Atopic dermatitis
    D. Lichen planus
    E. Varicella zoster

487.

A woman with a history of having multiple telangiectasias on her lips, face, feet, and in her nail beds presents for evaluation. The telangiectases are "spider-like"—when you pull the overlying skin over an individual lesion, a central area with radiating vessels is noted. Many members of her family have similar findings, she says.

Which of the following is the most likely diagnosis?

    A. Osler-Rendu-Weber disease
    B. CREST
    C. Actinically damaged skin
    D. SLE
    E. Scleroderma

488.

A 30-year-old homosexual man presents with a diffuse maculopapular rash over his trunk, head, neck, palms, and even his soles! He has had generalized lymphadenopathy for a few days. He has a history of a painless lesion on his anus about 2 months ago.

Which of the following is the most likely diagnosis?

    A. HIV
    B. SLE
    C. Bacterial endocarditis
    D. Syphilis
    E. Dermatomyositis

489.

A 35-year-old pop singer visits his doctor for his yearly checkup. Physical examination is unremarkable except for white patches involving his face, hands, trunk, anus, and genitalia. The white spots have been present for several years.

This condition has <u>not</u> been associated with which of the following?

    A. Vitamin B_{12} deficiency
    B. Diabetes mellitus
    C. Folate deficiency
    D. Hyperthyroidism
    E. Hypothyroidism

OB / GYN

490.

A 29-year-old G1P0 woman with Type I diabetes mellitus presents at 16 weeks with increasing pedal edema. Her BP is 170/110 mmHg. A urinalysis shows 3+ proteinuria. She has no headache and no neurologic symptoms.

Which of the following treatments would you most likely recommend?

    A. Minoxidil
    B. Nitroprusside drip
    C. Lisinopril
    D. Hydrochlorothiazide
    E. Methyldopa

491.

A 27-year-old pregnant woman in her late first trimester presents with dyspnea and pleuritic chest pain. She reports that she has had progressive leg swelling for the last week. ABG shows pH 7.48/PCO_2 22/PaO_2 80 on room air. She is found to have a DVT with probable pulmonary embolus.

The best treatment plan for her includes which of the following?

    A. IV heparin and begin warfarin as soon as PTT is therapeutic.
    B. Subcutaneous low-molecular-weight heparin injections.
    C. IV heparin and begin warfarin on day 3.
    D. Thrombolytics followed by heparin.
    E. Begin warfarin at low dose.

492.

A 23-year-old woman presents for primary care. She reports that she has not had menses in 3 months. A urine pregnancy test is positive.

Of the following choices, what testing would you recommend next?

    A. Urine culture
    B. Serology for HSV II, urine culture, and RPR
    C. RPR
    D. Urine culture, HIV ELISA, and RPR
    E. Serology for HSV II

493.

A 26-year-old woman presents with a 4-month history of vaginal bleeding. During this 4-month time frame, she has had menstrual periods every 10–16 days lasting 3–5 days at a time. She has had no pain and otherwise has felt fine. She states that she is not currently sexually active. Physical examination is normal with a normal pelvic examination and normal uterine size. Pregnancy test is negative.

Which of the following would you recommend for her at this time?

A. Transvaginal ultrasound
B. Dilatation and curettage
C. Begin a trial of an oral contraceptive agent
D. Endometrial biopsy
E. Pelvic CT scan

494.

A 29-year-old woman presents for evaluation of postcoital bleeding. She has had a small amount of bleeding after intercourse 4 times over the past 2 weeks. She has had no pain and no other symptoms. She has had 2 normal pap smears in the past three years.

Which of the following is the most likely finding upon speculum examination?

A. Cervical cancer
B. Cervical HSV
C. Endocervical polyp
D. Nabothian cyst
E. Foreign body

495.

A 32-year-old woman has been having difficulty getting pregnant. She has normal external and internal genitalia and has a history of dysmenorrhea.

Which of the following is most likely the cause of infertility in a menstruating woman over the age of 30 in the absence of a PID history?

A. Leiomyoma
B. Cervical carcinoma
C. Uterine carcinoma
D. Adenomyosis
E. Endometriosis

496.

A 16-year-old female presents for initial evaluation. She has not started menses yet. She denies sexual activity. She has normal sexual characteristics and is at Tanner Stage IV–V for all of her sexual characteristics.

Of the following choices, what is/are the first tests you should order in your evaluation of her primary amenorrhea?

A. Pregnancy test
B. Serum TSH
C. Serum FSH, LH
D. Testosterone level
E. Chromosomal analysis

497.

A couple presents because of infertility. They both have a normal history and physical examination.

Of the options listed below, what is one of the first tests to do for the initial evaluation?

A. Hysterosalpingogram
B. Semen analysis
C. Laparoscopy of the woman
D. Laparoscopy of the man
E. Endometrial biopsy

498.

A 28-year-old woman with HIV disease presents for prenatal care. She was diagnosed 4 years ago with HIV disease. At that time, she had oral and vaginal candidiasis, a CD4 count of 200, and a viral load of 30,000. She was treated with lopinavir/ritonavir + tenofovir/emtricitabine. She now has a CD4 count of 370 and an undetectable viral load. She asks for your advice on what medications she can take during pregnancy.

Which of the following should you advise?

A. Stop antiretrovirals, restart zidovudine at 34 weeks.
B. Stop current regimen and switch to zidovudine now.
C. Switch to ddI/d4T/amprenavir.
D. Continue with current regimen.
E. Stop all antiretrovirals.

499.

A 24-year-old woman with Type I diabetes wishes to become pregnant. She has been using 70/30 insulin twice a day with supplemental regular insulin at meals. Her last three glycated hemoglobins were 7.0, 7.2, and 7.3. She is currently on an oral contraceptive pill.

Which of the following should you advise for her?

    A. Stop the OCP, keep glycated Hb no more than 7.5.
    B. Stop the OCP, keep glycated Hb no greater than 7.
    C. Continue on the OCP, intensify insulin regimen for target glycated Hb 6.
    D. Continue on OCP, keep glycated Hb no greater than 7.

500.

A 76-year-old woman is evaluated for urinary incontinence. She reports a 6-year history of incontinence occurring when she laughs, coughs, or sneezes. Recently, she has had incontinence while standing. UA is normal, BUN 14, Cr 1.1, Glu 111.

Which of the following would you most likely recommend?

    A. Oxybutynin 2.5 mg PO bid
    B. Kegel exercises
    C. Doxazosin 2 mg PO bid
    D. Imipramine 25 mg PO q hs

OPHTHALMOLOGY

501.

A 50-year-old contact lens wearer comes to the Emergency Room with a dramatic decrease in his visual acuity of his left eye. He reports that he was fine until this morning. Earlier in the week while on a business trip, he forgot to bring his contact lens solution. Unable to obtain lens solution, he instead used tap water to store his contact lenses overnight. He does not remember having any foreign bodies get into his eye. He has tried washing his eye out, but the pain and blurry vision have persisted.

PAST MEDICAL HISTORY: Hypertension for 20 years; on thiazide diuretic
    History of cellulitis of right foot 10 years ago; resolved with oral medications

SOCIAL HISTORY: Drinks 2–3 beers daily; no smoking in 30 years

PHYSICAL EXAMINATION:
    Vital signs are normal
    Right eye: Normal
    Left eye: Severely erythematous with severe chemosis
    Slit lamp: Severe corneal deterioration
    Annular infiltration is noted

Which of the following is the most likely pathogen?

A. *Bartonella henselae*
B. *Acanthamoeba*
C. *Bacillus cereus*
D. *Staphylococcus epidermidis*
E. *Streptococcus oralis*

502.

A 70-year-old man with Type 2 diabetes presents with sudden right eye visual loss. He has no other symptoms (no headache, weakness, or history of head injury). He has no history of diabetic retinopathy. Eye exam shows a "cherry red spot."

Which of the following is the most appropriate workup?

A. Cerebral angiography
B. Head CT scan
C. Head MRI
D. Carotid duplex
E. Measure intraocular pressure

503.

A 28-year-old woman presents with the chief complaint of "can't see at my periphery." On visual field testing, she is unable to distinguish objects brought laterally toward the midline, encompassing nearly ½ of the visual field of each eye.

Which of the following lesions is most likely to account for her findings?

 A. Open-angle glaucoma
 B. Pituitary tumor
 C. Closed-angle glaucoma
 D. Multiple sclerosis
 E. Occipital tumor

504.

A 30-year-old woman is being evaluated for anisocoria. Her left pupil is small and round compared to the right pupil in room light. When you place her in a darkened room, this difference is increased. The left pupil responds briskly to light, constricts with pilocarpine administration, and dilates with atropine. Minimal dilatation is produced by 4% cocaine.

Which of the following describes the location of her lesion?

 A. Right occipital lobe
 B. Left iris
 C. Left third nerve
 D. Left optic nerve
 E. Left sympathetic chain

505.

A 65-year-old man presents with severe right-sided eye and facial pain. He has nausea and vomiting. He has noticed "colorful" halos around lights and can no longer see very well. His left eye is quite erythematous, and the pupil is dilated and fixed.

Which of the following is the next test to do to confirm your diagnosis?

 A. Emergent referral to an ophthalmologist for gonioscopy
 B. CT of the head
 C. MRI of the orbits
 D. Cerebral angiography

506.

A 47-year-old man presents with worsening vision over the last few months since taking a new job. He has to read small type and spends hours leaning over a computer with poor lighting.

Of the following, what is the most likely etiology of his vision change?

A. Retinal hemorrhage
B. Acute-angle glaucoma
C. Optic neuritis
D. Presbyopia
E. Gonorrheal ophthalmitis

507.

A 58-year-old woman comes in for follow-up of HTN. She notes that her vision has gradually become more blurred, R > L. She failed the screening eye exam to renew her driver's license last week.

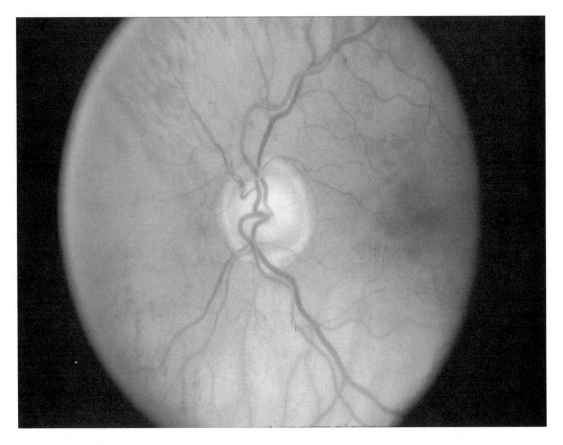

Her eye exam (see figure) is most consistent with which of the following?

A. Macular degeneration
B. Cataracts
C. Hypertensive retinopathy
D. Glaucoma

508.

A 41-year-old male with HIV (CD4 count 410) comes into the clinic for a routine evaluation. Funduscopic exam is done and shows cotton wool spots without hemorrhage. He complains of no visual symptoms.

The most likely etiology for the eye finding is which of the following?

    A. Toxoplasmosis
    B. HIV retinopathy
    C. Cytomegalovirus retinitis
    D. *Cryptococcus*
    E. *Cryptosporidia*

509.

A 36-year-old HIV patient with a CD4 count of 26 presents with the complaint of "floaters" in his vision field. He is on therapy for pulmonary tuberculosis. Funduscopic exam shows scattered fluffy infiltrates peripherally.

The etiology of his visual symptoms is most likely which of the following?

    A. Retinal tuberculosis
    B. Toxoplasmosis
    C. Cytomegalovirus retinitis
    D. HIV retinopathy
    E. *Cryptococcus*

PSYCHIATRY

510.

Which of the following is a true statement about lithium?

A. It is the drug of choice for major depressive syndromes.
B. It can be a very effective treatment for bipolar affective disorder.
C. It has very few drug-drug interactions.
D. Lithium intoxication manifests as increased manic behavior.
E. Hyperthyroidism is a side effect of lithium administration.

511.

A 25-year-old man presents with the new diagnosis of schizophrenia. He works as a writer for a small town paper and is married. His family has a history of mood disorders and schizophrenia.

Which of the following is the best predictor of a good prognosis in the treatment of schizophrenia?

A. Good premorbid functioning
B. Early onset
C. Family history of schizophrenia
D. Poor support system
E. No precipitating factors

512.

The best treatment of schizophrenia is which of the following?

A. Psychosocial treatment alone
B. Antipsychotic medications alone
C. Antipsychotic medications and psychosocial treatment
D. Antipsychotic medications and the use of mind-control elements from radios
E. Electric shock therapy

513.

You are following a 25-year-old man with newly diagnosed schizophrenia. He was started on haloperidol 2 days ago. This morning you receive a call from his wife saying that he has muscle spasms, tongue protrusion and twisting, and can't keep from deviating his head and eyes to the left.

The best treatment for his condition is which of the following?

A. Acetaminophen
B. Dopamine agonist
C. Prolactin
D. Diphenhydramine or benztropine immediately
E. Take a warm shower and it will resolve

514.

Which of the following is true with regard to suicide in the United States?

A. The best predictor of future suicide is a past attempt.
B. Men commit suicide more often than women.
C. Women attempt suicide more often than men.
D. People older than 45 are at greater risk than are younger people.
E. All of the statements are true

515.

A 30-year-old man has a history of suicide attempts. Today when you see him in your office, he seems more depressed than usual. He recently lost his job and has been having marital problems. You ask him if he has suicidal thoughts, and he says that he has on occasion in the last few days. He says that he is "okay" right now, but yesterday he had made a plan to shoot himself.

Based on his history, which of the following should you do at this point?

A. Voluntary hospitalization unless he refuses, then institute involuntary commitment.
B. Voluntary hospitalization; if he refuses, then arrange appropriate follow-up tomorrow.
C. Since he is not acutely suicidal in your office, arrange for visiting nurse to check on him.
D. Since he is not acutely suicidal in your office, arrange for outpatient follow-up tomorrow.
E. Keep him at your office for 3–4 hours and observe; if he is okay then send him home with close follow-up.

516.

Which of the following is/are helpful clue(s) on Board exams (as well as in patients) to diagnose depression?

A. Anxiety
B. Insomnia
C. Anhedonia
D. Poor concentration
E. All items listed are helpful clues

517.

A 50-year-old man presents to you with a complaint of feeling "bummed out" for the last 3 months. He went through a divorce 4 months ago. He leaves work early because of this "feeling." He does not have a change in sleep habits, anxiety, or a change in appetite or psychomotor retardation. His physical examination is normal.

Which of the following is the most likely diagnosis?

    A. Manic-depressive disorder
    B. Major depressive episode
    C. Adjustment disorder with depressed mood
    D. Schizophrenia
    E. Anxiety disorder

518.

A 28-year-old woman is brought in by her husband. He says that she has become a worrywart. She is always worried about her job. She worries about her parents who live 50 miles away. She worries sometimes about her marriage and that her husband doesn't love her. She worries that they don't have enough money to make it through the month. She has never had feelings like she was going to die or major physical complaints from her worrying. She has not had episodes of hyperventilation. She does not relate any sleep disturbances or appetite changes. She says she has been worried "all her life." You diagnose her with generalized anxiety disorder.

In addition to behavioral therapy, which of the following is the best treatment for this disorder?

    A. MAO inhibitor
    B. Buspirone or similar agent
    C. Haloperidol
    D. Clonazepam
    E. Lithium

519.

A 70-year-old woman presents with a 2-year history of recent progressive memory loss and the inability to "pay attention." Now she has progressed to the point that she cannot speak clearly and her judgment appears to be impaired. On occasion, she will exhibit paranoid behavior—says "they are trying to get me."

The plaques that cause Alzheimer's are made up of which of the following?

    A. Fibrillar actin particles
    B. IgD
    C. Cholesterol
    D. Low-density lipoprotein
    E. Beta-amyloid protein

520.

A 30-year-old woman presents with an attack of severe shortness of breath, palpitations, shaking, diffuse numbness, and an intense fear of dying. These attacks are not precipitated by any known factor or event. She is not on any medications and does not drink alcohol. Additionally, she is particularly scared to leave her house unless she can go with someone. Her physical examination is completely normal. A whole "battery" of tests, including thyroid functions, electrolytes, ECG, and Holter monitoring has been normal in the recent past.

Besides cognitive behavioral therapy, which of the following is the best initial therapy for this woman?

    A. Diazepam
    B. Paroxetine
    C. Lithium
    D. Fluphenazine
    E. Flurazepam

521.

A 50-year-old man with long-standing schizophrenia is admitted to your general medicine service for atypical pneumonia. He has been on chlorpromazine for over 15 years. In addition to the findings of pneumonia and schizophrenia, you note that he repetitively smacks his lips and thrusts his tongue (not unlike Mick Jagger). Also you note that he has a stooped posture.

Which of the following is the best way to reverse his neurologic symptoms?

    A. Reduce the dose of chlorpromazine
    B. Give oxazepam
    C. Give propranolol
    D. Give levodopa-carbidopa
    E. Give levodopa only

522.

Which of the following statements is true regarding Wernicke encephalopathy?

    A. In the absence of a response to glucose, thiamine should be administered.
    B. The frontal cortex is most commonly affected.
    C. After the patient responds to emergent therapy, she may develop profound amnesic psychosis.
    D. Alcohol consumption is required to produce the syndrome.
    E. Most patients present with the triad of ophthalmoplegia, ataxia, and encephalopathy.

523.

You are presenting a 45-year-old man with Wernicke aphasia on rounds to a group of 3rd year medical students.

Which of the following is not likely to be elicited on rounds with the students?

   A. Poor language comprehension
   B. Fluent speech output
   C. Paraphasic errors
   D. Left inferior quadrantanopia
   E. Poor repetition

524.

Which of the following is <u>not</u> a routine laboratory test used in the workup of dementia?

   A. TSH
   B. Vitamin B_{12}
   C. RPR
   D. ESR
   E. Serum lytes

525.

A 16-year-old teenager with a history of being "stubborn" all her life, according to her parents, has lately been noted to wash her hands up to 20 times a day. She also has to check and make sure the front door is locked multiple times during the day and night. In the last week, she has had to check her alarm clock to be sure it is set correctly—this has resulted in sleep disturbance, because she can't get to sleep due to worrying that the alarm isn't set correctly.

Which of the following is her most likely diagnosis?

   A. Antisocial personality disorder
   B. Borderline personality disorder
   C. Obsessive-compulsive disorder
   D. Manic-depressive disorder
   E. Narcissistic personality disorder

526.

A 29-year-old male with history of bipolar disorder presents with complaints of nausea, vomiting, and diarrhea. He has no abdominal pain but has been weaker in the past 3 days and has been falling frequently. He was noted to be hypertensive at his last clinic visit 2 weeks ago (200/110 mmHg) and was started on benazepril. He denies any drug use, hepatitis risk, new food experiences, or previous episodes of GI distress. Meds: benazepril, carbamazepine, lithium, melatonin, diphenhydramine, and cimetidine.

On exam, his VS are T 100.4° F, P 120, BP 160/100; skin: perioral acne; chest: clear; abd: soft, nontender; neuro: fasciculations in muscles, reflexes 3–4+ bilaterally, cogwheel rigidity present; gait: marked ataxia.

Which of the following is the most likely cause of this patient's problem?

A. Benazepril/lithium interaction
B. Carbamazepine/lithium interaction
C. Carbamazepine overdose
D. Cimetidine/lithium interaction
E. Benazepril/carbamazepine interaction

527.

The "antidote" of choice for treatment of poisoning with a tricyclic antidepressant is which of the following?

A. Naloxone
B. Flumazenil
C. Sodium bicarbonate
D. Physostigmine
E. Phenytoin

528.

A 20-year-old woman presents to the ER tearful and agitated. She reports that she took a bottle of extra-strength acetaminophen 4 hours ago in a suicide attempt. Her physical exam is normal.
Lab: Hb 13, HCT 39, WBC 9,000. Acetaminophen level 280 mg/mL (elevated above toxic threshold for therapy).

Which of the following is the most appropriate management?

A. Deferoxamine
B. Gastric lavage
C. Activated charcoal
D. N-acetylcysteine
E. N-acetylcysteine + activated charcoal

529.

A 73-year-old woman is admitted with a hip fracture. She has surgery (ORIF) and is doing well. On the 6th hospital day she becomes confused, agitated, and develops a fever of 103° F. She complains of a headache. Physical exam is remarkable for some decreased range of motion of the neck, no skin lesions, and a clear chest. She has a nonfocal neuro exam, but is oriented only to person.

LABORATORY: WBC 17,000, HCT 33, Na 137, K 3.2, HCO_3 26; UA: 20–50 WBCs/ HPF, no RBCs
Chest x-ray is clear. Blood cultures are sent.

Which of the following would you most likely do next?

A. No further testing; begin antibiotics
B. Noncontrast CT scan followed by lumbar puncture
C. Noncontrast/contrast CT scan followed by lumbar puncture
D. Lumbar puncture

MISCELLANEOUS

530.

A 43-year-old heart transplant recipient comes to the hospital for evaluation of severe foot pain. The pain has been present for 12 hours and hurts even with the slightest pressure to the foot. He received his transplant 3 months ago, and has had no problems with function or rejection. He has no prior musculoskeletal problems. He denies having fever or other new symptoms.

MEDS: nizatidine, prednisone, cyclosporine, amlodipine, and aspirin

LABORATORY: WBC 13,000/μL; HCT 40%, SGOT 30 U/L; SGPT 22 U/L

Which of the following is the most likely cause of his problem?

    A. Aspirin
    B. Alcohol use
    C. Group A Streptococcus
    D. Cyclosporine
    E. Nizatidine

531.

A 39-year-old woman is seen for evaluation of rash. She was in her usual state of good health until 1 week ago while on vacation in Hawaii. While there she developed bronchitis and was placed on an antibiotic by a physician —who didn't know **you don't treat viral bronchitis with antibiotics!** Anyway, she was on the antibiotic and developed severe sunburn.

Which of the following antibiotics did she receive?

    A. Amoxicillin/clavulanate
    B. Ciprofloxacin
    C. Nitrofurantoin
    D. Trimethoprim
    E. Cefuroxime axetil

532.

You evaluate an independent 84-year-old woman who has had 3 falls in the past year. She has not sustained serious injury, but her family is worried about her ability to live alone. The patient states she simply slipped, and denies dizziness, chest pain, shortness of breath, palpitations, or other symptoms. Her only medical problems are osteoarthritis and a remote history of peptic ulcer disease. She takes acetaminophen 2 to 3 times a week. Her vision is good.

She does not drink alcohol and is a lifelong non-smoker. The remainder of the history is negative.

Which of the following would be most helpful in evaluating this patient's risk of future falls?

A. Head CT to evaluate for small vessel disease
B. Holter monitoring
C. "Get up and go" test
D. Romberg test
E. Lower extremity electromyelography

533.

Which of the following potential toxins is associated with an osmolar gap and an anion gap acidosis?

A. Aspirin
B. Methanol
C. Isopropyl alcohol
D. Ethanol
E. Paraldehyde

534.

A serum level is useful in the management of poisoning except with which of the following agents?

A. Amitriptyline
B. Acetaminophen
C. Carboxyhemoglobin
D. Aspirin
E. Methanol

535.

In a study of 2,271 patients with a history of colon cancer, fecal occult blood testing (FOBT) is done to screen for recurrent colon cancer. 146 patients have positive FOBT and 2,125 patients have negative FOBT. Colonoscopy is done on all the patients, finding 36 cancers. 12 patients with positive FOBT have colon cancer, and 24 with negative tests have colon cancer.

Of the following choices, what is the correct sensitivity for FOBT?

A. 8.2%
B. 33.3%
C. 94%
D. 98.4%
E. 50%

536.

A study is done to evaluate mammography as a screening tool for women between the ages of 40 and 45. 11,000 mammograms are obtained. 25 women have a positive mammogram and turn out to have breast cancer. 175 women have positive mammograms and do not have cancer. 890 women have negative mammograms and do not have cancer. 10 women with negative mammograms end up having breast cancer.

Of the following choices, what is the correct positive predictive value of the test?

A. 83.5%
B. 98.9%
C. 71.4%
D. 12.5%
E. 31.4%

537.

A study is done to evaluate mammography as a screening tool for women between the ages of 40 and 45. 11,000 mammograms are obtained. 25 women have a positive mammogram and turn out to have breast cancer. 175 women have positive mammograms and do not have cancer. 890 women have negative mammograms and do not have cancer. 10 women with negative mammograms end up having breast cancer.

Of the following choices, what is the correct negative predictive value of the test?

A. 98.9%
B. 96%
C. 93%
D. 12.5%
E. 90%

538.

A prospective randomized study shows that a new treatment will improve survival for squamous cell lung cancer over current standard treatment guidelines. The survival rate increased from 30% survival to 60% in the study. The 95% confidence interval for the study was –2.5 to 80.6. No confounding data were reported, and the patient population was very diverse in character, indicating proper randomization. The prospective aspect of this study was preserved with a very low dropout rate.

Based on this study, which of the following correctly state whether this new therapy provides significant benefit over the standard therapy?

A. Yes, because the survival rate is so poor with this type of cancer that anything is better than nothing.
B. Yes, because the percentage of increase is significant.
C. No.
D. More information is needed to answer this question.
E. Yes, because the study was a prospective, randomized study.

539.

A study is done to test a new treatment for heart failure. Patients received the usual CHF treatment plus new drug X, or usual treatment plus placebo. In this study, 10/50 patients who received the new drug died, and 20/50 patients who received the placebo died.

Of the choices below, which is the correct number needed to treat (NNT) to prevent one bad outcome for this new drug?

    A. 5
    B. 10
    C. 15
    D. 20
    E. 50

540.

A study is done to evaluate mammography as a screening tool for women between the ages of 40 and 45. 11,000 mammograms are obtained. 25 women have a positive mammogram and turn out to have breast cancer. 175 women have positive mammograms and do not have cancer. 890 women have negative mammograms and do not have cancer. 10 women with negative mammograms end up having breast cancer.

Which of the choices below correctly states the sensitivity of mammography?

    A. 12.5%
    B. 98.9%
    C. 71.4%
    D. 83.5%
    E. 31.4%

541.

A study is done to evaluate mammography as a screening tool for women between the ages of 40 and 45. 11,000 mammograms are obtained. 25 women have a positive mammogram and turn out to have breast cancer. 175 women have positive mammograms and do not have cancer. 890 women have negative mammograms and do not have cancer. 10 women with negative mammograms end up having breast cancer.

Which of the choices below correctly states the specificity of the mammography?

    A. 71.4%
    B. 83.6%
    C. 98.9%
    D. 12.5%
    E. 31.4%

542.

An 86-year-old woman who lives in a nursing home is admitted with severe aspiration pneumonia. She is unconscious with a fever of 104° F. ABG 7.22/52/66. She has been started on IV antibiotics and fluids. Her nephew is the durable power of attorney for her health care. The patient has never completed a living will or advance directives. The nephew meets with you, stating that his aunt has become demented over the past few years, and the nephew would like IV fluids and antibiotics discontinued, with comfort care only.

Which of the following statements about the nephew is true?

A. The nephew's instructions can be carried out only if it is determined that he had discussed this issue with his aunt and is carrying out substituted judgment.
B. The patient has a son who is next of kin; and therefore, the nephew can't make medical decisions for her.
C. Since the patient has not left specific advance directives, instructions to discontinue IVF and antibiotics should not be carried out.
D. The nephew's request to discontinue IVF and antibiotics is within his capacity to act as the patient's durable power of attorney for health care.
E. Get an ethics committee consult to determine if the nephew can make these decisions.

543.

A 29-year-old woman presents with hematemesis. She is found to have an HCT of 20. She receives IVF and is typed and crossed for transfusion. A repeat HCT 2 hours later is 14. The patient refuses the blood transfusion when it is brought in because of religious convictions. Her husband, who is in the room with her, supports her stance. She has another episode of hematemesis while you await arrival of the surgeons.

Of the following options, what should you do?

A. Give blood because of the principle of beneficence.
B. Obtain a court-appointed representative.
C. Schedule a hospital ethics consult.
D. Give blood because this is a life-threatening emergency.
E. Do not give blood products.

544.

A 21-year-old college student is brought to the ER by her roommate for symptoms of headache and fever with a stiff neck over the past 18 hours. On exam, she is somnolent but able to be aroused, with a temp of 102.2° F, BP 100/52, P 112. Nuchal rigidity is present. The remainder of her exam is unremarkable. WBC is 24,000. The patient gives consent for a lumbar puncture. You order a stat dose of IV antibiotics, which the patient overhears. She becomes agitated, and refuses the antibiotics.

You carefully explain the high risk of death from untreated meningitis. The patient continues to refuse antibiotics and becomes more agitated.

Of the following options, what should you do?

A. Treat with IV fluids only, because antibiotics carry a risk and shouldn't be given without patient consent.
B. Treat with antibiotics because the patient has a life-threatening condition.
C. Obtain a court order urgently for treatment.
D. Obtain consent from the patient's roommate and give antibiotics.

545.

A 76-year-old man with end-stage COPD (FEV_1 .30) presents unconscious. He is found to have a pCO_2 of 110. He has stated in several clinic visits his desire not to be intubated. His children who brought him in request everything be done, including intubation.

Which of the following is the most appropriate next step?

A. Do not intubate patient; keep him comfortable.
B. Intubate patient.
C. Obtain a court-appointed representative.
D. Obtain an ethics committee consult.

546.

A 79-year-old woman reports problems with urinary incontinence on a daily basis. She has to void many times during the day, yet leaks urine frequently before she can get to the restroom. She has not had hematuria or dysuria. Meds: omeprazole, sertraline, and enalapril. UA is normal.

Of the following, what is the most likely cause of the incontinence?

A. Detrusor underactivity
B. Sphincter dysfunction
C. Detrusor overactivity
D. Side effect of sertraline
E. Side effect of enalapril

547.

A 76-year-old man presents for evaluation of urinary frequency and decreased urinary stream. The symptoms have been present for the past 3 years but have worsened in the past 6 months. He is now getting up 4 times a night to urinate. On exam, his prostate is 3+ enlarged without nodularity. PSA is 3.0.

Which of the following do you recommend as the best initial therapy that will provide symptomatic relief most quickly?

A. Prostate scan
B. Finasteride
C. TURP
D. Terazosin
E. Prostate biopsy

548.

A 74-year-old man reports increasing problems with sexual functioning. He reports normal sexual desire but inability to sustain an erection sufficient for intercourse. He has had these problems intermittently for the past 3 years; now the problem is present whenever he attempts sexual activity. Medications: sertraline, atorvastatin, ranitidine, and gingko biloba.

Which of the following is the most likely cause for his erectile dysfunction?

A. Ranitidine
B. Sertraline
C. Vascular disease
D. Gingko Biloba
E. Low testosterone

549.

A 67-year-old man presents for treatment of erectile dysfunction. He has had problems sustaining erections for the past year. He has a normal libido. Meds: simvastatin, omeprazole, isosorbide mononitrate, lisinopril, and aspirin.

Which of the following would you recommend for therapy?

A. Sildenafil (Viagra®)
B. Intraurethral alprostadil (MUSE®)
C. Testosterone patch (Androderm®)
D. Referral for penile implant

550.

A woman makes an appointment for a physical exam when she turns 65. She has not seen a physician for 12 years. Her last visit was for a skin rash. She has not had a regular doctor because she lacked insurance.

Appropriate preventive care should include which of the following?

A. Breast exam, mammogram, pap smear, and colonoscopy
B. Breast exam, mammogram, and pap smear
C. Breast exam, mammogram, and CBC
D. Mammogram, CBC, and colonoscopy
E. Breast exam, mammogram, and colonoscopy

551.

A 76-year-old man with CAD and Parkinson disease presents for primary care. His exam is remarkable for seborrheic dermatitis, some mild cogwheel rigidity, and a slightly enlarged prostate.

Which of the following tests would you recommend now?

A. Cholesterol, PSA, CBC
B. Cholesterol, PSA
C. PSA
D. Cholesterol
E. No testing

552.

A 36-year-old man with HIV disease (CD4 count 470) and a history of hepatitis C presents for primary care. He reports he has not had any immunizations in the past 10 years. He has a past history of intravenous drug abuse, but none for 5 years.

Labs: Hep C quant 3 million, Hep A IgG antibody negative, Hep B surface antibody+, AST 33, ALT 24, HCT 40, WBC 3.9.

Which of the following immunizations would you recommend?

A. Annual influenza, Tdap
B. Pneumococcal, annual influenza, hep A series, Tdap
C. Pneumococcal, MMR
D. Annual influenza, pneumococcal, hep B booster, Tdap
E. Pneumococcal, hep B booster, annual influenza

Notes

Notes

Notes

Notes

Notes

Notes

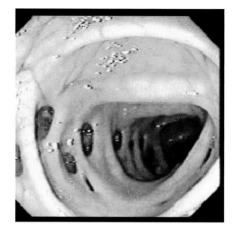

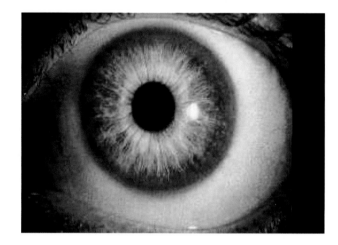

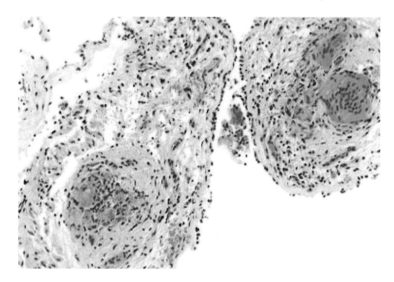

Question 66

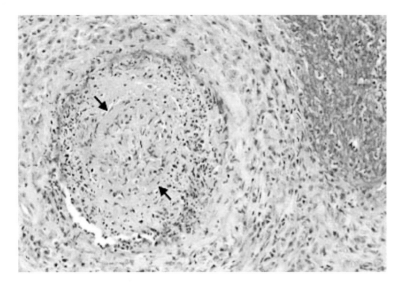

Question 81

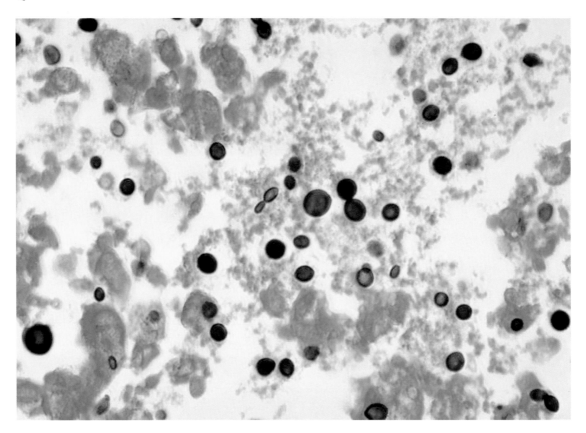

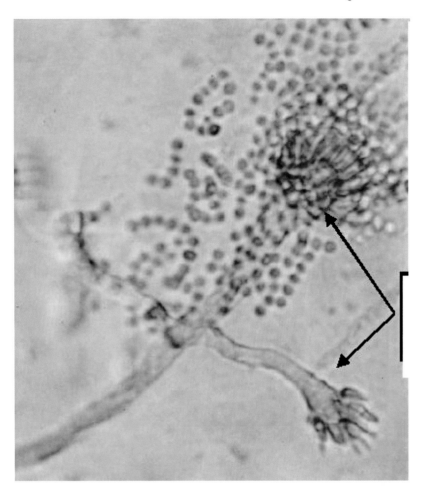

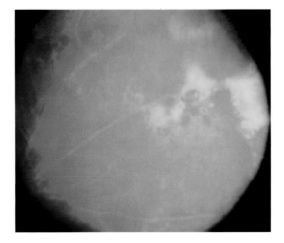

Question 507

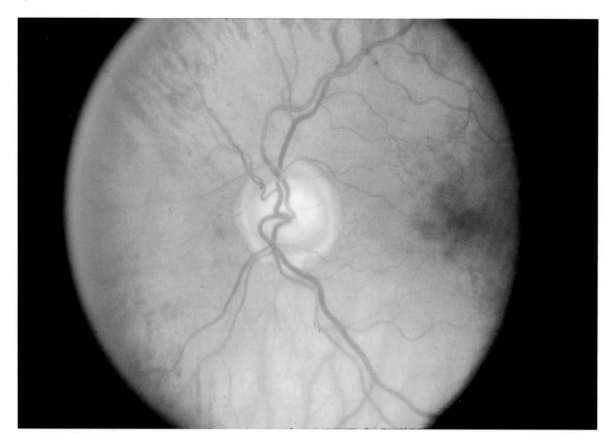